Dermatology and Venereology

U0133034

Chief Editor

Shi Lian

Associate Chief Editor

Wei Zhu

Reviewer

Jianzhong Zhang

Contributors

Xiaoling Chu	Yanqing Gao	Yanling He	Shi Lian
Wenhui Lun	Lin Ma	Zigang Xu	Gaoyun Yang
Xiumin Yang	Guangzhong Zhang	Haiping Zhang	Junying Zhao
Wei Zhu			

高等教育出版社·北京
HIGHER EDUCATION PRESS BEIJING

图书在版编目（CIP）数据

皮肤性病学 = Dermatology and Venereology : 英
文 / 连石主编 . -- 北京 : 高等教育出版社，2012.5
ISBN 978-7-04-034334-2

Ⅰ . ①皮… Ⅱ . ①连… Ⅲ . ①皮肤病学－医学院校－
教材－英文②性病学－医学院校－教材－英文 Ⅳ .
① R75

中国版本图书馆 CIP 数据核字（2012）第 034125 号

总 策 划　林金安　吴雪梅　席　雁

策划编辑　瞿德竑　　责任编辑　瞿德竑　　封面设计　张　楠　　责任印制　毛斯璐

出版发行	高等教育出版社	咨询电话	400 - 810 - 0598
社　　址	北京市西城区德外大街 4 号	网　　址	http：//www. hep. edu. cn
邮政编码	100120		http：//www. hep. com. cn
印　　刷	北京中科印刷有限公司	网上订购	http：//www. landraco. com
开　　本	889mm×1194mm　1/16		http：//www. landraco. com. cn
印　　张	13.25		
字　　数	430 千字	版　　次	2012 年 5 月第 1 版
插　　页	9	印　　次	2012 年 5 月第 1 次印刷
购书热线	010 - 58581118	定　　价	36.00 元

本书如有缺页、倒页、脱页等质量问题，请到所购图书销售部门联系调换
版权所有　侵权必究
物 料 号　34334 - 00

医学教育改革系列教材编委会

《皮肤性病学》编委会

主　编　连　石

副主编　朱　威

主　审　张建中

编　委（以姓氏拼音为序）

褚晓玲　高艳青　何焱玲　连　石

伦文辉　马　琳　徐子刚　杨高云

杨秀敏　张广中　张海萍　赵俊英

朱　威

Foreword

Global developments in medicine and health shape trends in medical education. And in China education reform has become an important focus as the country strives to meet the basic requirements for developing a medical education system that meets international standards. Significant medical developments abroad are now being incorporated into the education of both domestic and international medical students in China, which includes students from Hong Kong, Macao and Taiwan that are taught through mandarin Chinese as well as students from a variety of other regions that are taught through the English language. This latter group creates higher demands for both schools and teachers.

Unfortunately there is no consensus as to how to improve the level and quality of education for these students or even as to which English language materials should be used. Some teachers prefer to directly use original English language materials, while others make use of Chinese medical textbooks with the help of English language medical notes. The lack of consensus has emerged from the lack of English language medical textbooks based on the characteristics of modern medical education in China.

In fact, most Chinese teachers involved in medical education have already attained an adequate level of English language usage. However, English language medical textbooks that reflect the culture of the teachers would in fact make it easier for these teachers to complete the task at hand and would improve the level and quality of medical education for international students. In addition, these texts could be used to improve the English language level of the medical students taught in Chinese. This is the purpose behind the compilation and publishing of this set of English language medical education textbooks.

The editors in chief are mainly experts in medicine from Capital Medical University (CCMU). The editorial board members are mainly teachers of a variety of subjects from CCMU. In addition, teachers with rich teaching experience in other medical schools are also called upon to help create this set of textbooks. And finally some excellent scholars are invited to participate as final arbiters for some of the materials.

The total package of English medical education textbooks includes 63 books. Each textbook conforms to five standards according to their grounding in science; adherence to a system; basic theory, concepts and skills elucidated; simplicity and practicality. This has enabled the creation of a series of English language textbooks that adheres to the characteristics and customs of Chinese medical education. The complete set of textbooks conforms to an overall design and uniform style in regards to covers, colors, and graphics. Each chapter contains learning objectives, core concepts, an introduction, a body, a summary, questions and references that together serve as a scaffold for both teachers and students.

The complete set of English language medical education textbooks is designed for teaching overseas undergraduate clinical medicine students (six years), and can also serve as reference textbooks for bilingual teaching and learning for 5-year, 7-year and 8-year programs in clinical medicine.

We would like to thank the chief arbiters, chief editors and general editors for their arduous labor in the writing of each chapter. We would also like to acknowledge all the contributors. Finally, we would like to acknowledge Higher Education Press. They have all provided valuable support during the many weekends and evening hours of work that were necessary for completing this endeavor.

President of Capital Medical University
Director of English Textbook Compiling Commission
Zhaofeng Lu
August 1st, 2011

Preface

The objective of this book is to meet the requirements of clinical teaching in Capital Medical University (CMU),and better present the achievements CMU has made in clinical teaching mode,teaching contents and other related disciplines.

With the research improvements in all aspects of life science,dermatology and venereology has made rapid progress in recent years.Besides in traditional skin and venereal diseases and cosmetology,growing interaction and multidisciplinary network have been witnessed in dermatology and venereology,immunology,molecular biology and genetics.The development of all these disciplines deepens the knowledge on etiology and pathogenesis of dermatology and venereology,and provides new avenues for disease diagnosis and treatment.Dermatology and venereology has been becoming a clinical and professional subject with plentiful content,extended research fields,fast-changing technology in diagnosis and therapy,and very promising prospects.

All the members in the editorial board and the writers of the present book are academic leaders and core of the middle-aged and the young from various clinical hospitals.They have years' experience in clinical medicine,clinical teaching and research in dermatology and venereology. Their rich teaching experience,carefulness and studied attitude have ensured the scientificness and discipline of the present book,what they know is the key carrier of teaching ideology and the guarantee of teaching quality.

The present book is composed of 27 chapters,which cover kinds of diseases and typical clinical pictures.The general introduction summarizes the achievements in dermatology in recent years and current situations in our country.The following chapters introduce etiology,pathogenesis,differential diagnosis and treatment of various diseases.The brief summary and questions in each chapter can help students grasp the gist of the respective chapters.

I must acknowledge the contributions of the followings,on behalf of the editorial board: Professor Jianzhong Zhang from Peking University People's Hospital, director of Chinese Society of Dermatology Chinese Medical Association, who carefully examined the manuscripts and made many helpful suggestions; Higher Education Press, who gave full support for the publication of the book; Professor Zhihua Wu from the First Affiliated Hospital of Guangzhou Medical University and Professor Tianwen Gao from Xijing Hospital of the Fourth Military Medical University, who provided us with their precious clinic and Pathology pictures(among them 19 pictures by Professor Zhihua Wu,and 8 pictures by Professor Tianwen Gao), and helped us collect and edit the illustrations; doctors and graduates from Dermatology and Venereology Department of Xuan Wu Hospital,who had made great effort in proofreading the book and rearranging the pictures and illustrations.

While every effort has been made to avoid any errors,with the rapid development of new theory,technology and knowledge in dermatology,this may be impossible.We will be able to rectify any errors,if pointed out,at the earliest opportunity.

Shi Lian
July 8,2011

Contributors

Xiaoling Chu 褚晓玲
Beijing An Zhen Hospital
Capital Medical University,Beijing,China

Yanqing Gao 高艳青
Beijing You An Hospital
Capital Medical University,Beijing,China

Yanling He 何焱玲
Beijing Chao-Yang Hospital
Capital Medical University,Beijing,China

Shi Lian 连石
Xuan Wu Hospital
Capital Medical University,Beijing,China

Wenhui Lun 伦文辉
Beijing Di Tan Hospital
Capital Medical University,Beijing,China

Lin Ma 马琳
Beijing Children's Hospital
Capital Medical University,Beijing,China

Zigang Xu 徐子刚
Beijing Children's Hospital
Capital Medical University,Beijing,China

Gaoyun Yang 杨高云
Beijing Friendship Hospital
Capital Medical University,Beijing,China

Xiumin Yang 杨秀敏
Beijing Tong Ren Hospital
Capital Medical University,Beijing,China

Guangzhong Zhang 张广中
Beijing Traditional Chinese Medicine Hospital
Capital Medical University,Beijing,China

Haiping Zhang 张海萍
Xuan Wu Hospital
Capital Medical University,Beijing,China

Junying Zhao 赵俊英
Beijing Friendship Hospital
Capital Medical University,Beijing,China

Wei Zhu 朱威
Xuan Wu Hospital
Capital Medical University,Beijing,China

CONTENTS

Chapter 1

Dermatological Introduction

Dermatology is a branch of medicine dealing with the skin and its diseases. Venereology is a branch of medicine dealing with the study and treatment of sexually transmitted diseases.

It's important to know that the dermis and its underlying structures constitute skin, the largest organ of the human body. The skin can reflect the changes of the human body and response to environment most directly. There are more than 2000 different kinds of skin diseases which affect everyone from neonates to elder people. And, there are numerous subspecialties in dermatology, which including immunodermatology, dermatopathology, phototherapy, laser medicine, cosmetic surgery or Mohs micrographic surgery. With the growing acceptance of plastic surgery, the field of surgical dermatology has been rapid growth.

Compare to other specialties, dermatology is a very interesting specialty. For you can see the problem you are dealing with directly and you can touch it, feel it, sometimes even you can smell it! An experienced dermatologist can recognize the common skin diseases at once without further tests. But if you want to be a good dermatologist, you need extensive knowledge of medicine because a large amount of general medical diseases may present first to the dermatologist.

Nowadays, people take much more care of their skin. Dermatologist must possess good interpersonal skills in dealing with patients. The reason is he/she just handling something extremely important to the patients: their appearance. Even the most minor skin conditions, such as the mild acne, can be scarring in more ways than one.

Finally, being a dermatologist means the stable hours, career flexibility, significant compensation and lower stress. We do a lot of practice in clinical in order to achieve significant gains. Nowadays, in the West, dermatology residencies have been the most competitive in terms of admission. We must try our best to be a good dermatologist!

(**Haiping Zhang** 张海萍)

Chapter

2

The Skin:Basic Structure

▪ Objectives

To master the knowledge of the skin anatomy.

▪ Key concepts

The skin is composed of 3 layers: epidermis, dermis, and subcutaneous tissue. The epidermis mainly contains 4 layers, from bottom to top the layers are: stratum basale, stratum spinosum, stratum granulosum and stratum corneum. There are three types of specialized cells in the epidermis. The melanocyte produces pigment. The Langerhans cell is the frontline defense of the immune system in the skin. The Merkel cell's function is not clearly known.

The dermis is composed of collagen, elastic tissue and reticular fibers. The two layers of the dermis are the papillary and reticular layers. The hair follicles are situated here with the erector pili muscle that attaches to each follicle. Sebaceous glands and apocrine glands are associated with the follicle. This layer also contains eccrine glands, but they are not associated with hair follicles. Blood vessels and nerves course through this layer. The nerves transmit sensations of pain, itch, and temperature.

The subcutaneous tissue is a layer of fat and connective tissue that houses larger blood vessels and nerves.

▪ Introduction

The skin is the body's largest organ, covering the entire surface of the body, while it's an organ that contains many specialized cells and structures, made up of several layers. The total surface area of the skin is about 3000 sq inches (roughly around $1.5m^2$). It's primarily composed of three layers as following (Figure 2 − 1).

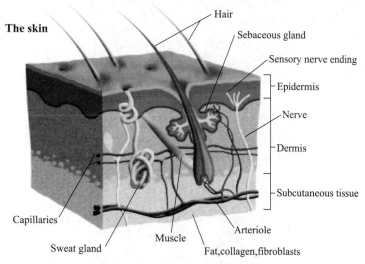

The skin

Hair
Sebaceous gland
Sensory nerve ending
Epidermis
Nerve
Dermis
Subcutaneous tissue
Arteriole
Fat,collagen,fibroblasts
Muscle
Sweat gland
Capillaries

Figure 2 – 1   Anatomy of the skin

2.1   Epidermis

The epidermis is the outer layer of the skin, a stratified squamous epithelium largely composed of keratinocytes that are formed by division of cells in the basal layer, and give rise to several distinguishable layers while they move outwards and progressively differentiate. The epidermis, contains several other cell populations, such as melanocytes, which donate pigment to the keratinocytes, Langerhans cells, which have immunological functions and Merkel cells(Figure 2 – 2). The thickness of the epidermis varies in different types of skin. It's thinnest on the eyelid which is about 0.1 mm and the thickness on the palms and soles which is about 1.5 mm in human.

2.1.1   Keratinocyte

Keratinocytes are the major constituent, constituting up to 95% of the epidermis. Its'primary function is to protect the skin from heat, UV radiation and water loss by forming the keratin layer. The keratinocyte, which moves progressively from attachment to the epidermal basement membrane towards the skin surface, forming several well-defined layers during its transit. The epidermis can be divided into four distinct layers according to its differentiation and characteristics. From bottom to top the layers are named stratum basale, stratum spinosum, stratum granulosum and stratum corneum. The time required for a keratinocyte to move from its origin in the actively dividing cells of the stratum basale to the surface of the epidermis where it is shed is called the turnover

time, which is approximately 28 days in normal skin.

2.1.1.1   Stratum basale

The stratum basal is the bottom layer of keratinocytes in the epidermis, composed of only one row of columnar or cubic cells. This layer is responsible for constantly renewing epidermis cells. Basal cells have large, dark-staining nuclei, dense cytoplasm containing many ribosomes and dense tono filament bundles. The basal cells have desmosomes, gap junctions which act for cell communication, and hemidesmosomes which connect the extracellular matrix with underlying basal membrane.

2.1.1.2   Stratum spinosum

The stratum spinosum is also called prickle cell layer, it is multi-layers composed of cuboidal cells which are found between the stratum granulosum and stratum basale of the epidermis. Cells of the stratum spinosum actively synthesize intermediate filaments called cytokeratins anchoring to the desmosomes, joining adjacent cells to provide structural support, and helping the skin to resist abrasion.

2.1.1.3   Stratum granulosum

The stratum granulosum lies below the stratum spinosum and above the stratum corneum, it formed stratified squamous keratinized thick skin of palms and soles. The layer is composed of two or three layers of flattened cells containing basophilic keratohyalin granules. The cells in the stratum granulosum have lost their nuclei and are characterized by dark clumps of cytoplasmic material.

2.1.1.4   Stratum corneum

The stratum corneum is the outermost layer of the epidermis, composed of about ten sub-layers. The

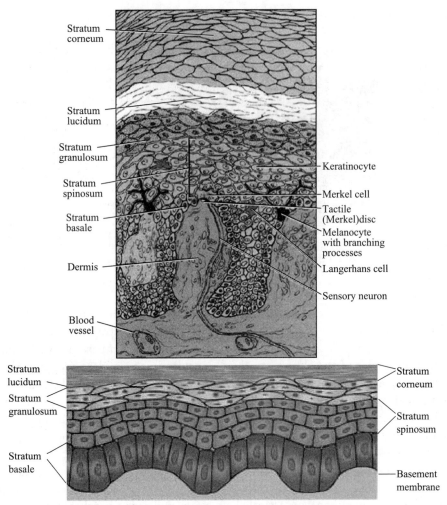

Stratum corneum

Stratum lucidum

Stratum granulosum

Stratum spinosum

Stratum basale

Dermis

Blood vessel

Keratinocyte

Merkel cell

Tactile (Merkel)disc

Melanocyte with branching processes

Langerhans cell

Sensory neuron

Stratum lucidum

Stratum granulosum

Stratum basale

Stratum corneum

Stratum spinosum

Basement membrane

Figure 2 – 2   Structure of the epidermis

cells of this layer are large, flat, polyhedral, plate-like envelopes filled with aggregated keratin fibers. Dead cells that lack nuclei become membranous and multi-layered, resembling fallen leaves, and exfoliate sequentially, beginning with the outer layer, in what is commonly called grime. This layer is very thick in the palms and soles.

Keratinocytes account for 95% of the cells within the epidermis. The remaining 5% are melanocytes, Langerhans cells, and Merkel cells, which are involved in melanin formation, antigen presentation, and sensation respectively.

2.1.2   Melanocyte

Melanocytes take their origin from the neural crest. The majority of melanocytes are found in the epidermis of the skin, stria vascularis of the inner ear, pigmented retinal epithelium, and choroid layer of the eye. Melanocytes are melanin-producing cells located in the stratum basale of the skin's epidermis. Mela-

nin is a pigment which is primarily responsible for the color of skin. The major determinant of color is not the number but rather the activity of the melanocytes. Melanin production takes place in unique organelles known as melanosomes. Each melanocyte supplies melanin to approximately 36 nearby keratinocytes via its dendrites to form an epidermal melanin unit (EMU). Melanin protects the skin from ultraviolet light while the melanocytes also increase the production of melanin in response to sun exposure.

2.1.3   The Langerhans Cell

Langerhans cells are derived from the monocyte-macrophage-histiocyte lineage. They are normally present in lymph nodes and other organs, including the stratum spinosum layer of the epidermis. They can be found elsewhere, particularly in association with the condition histiocytosis. These cells have a dark nucleus and pale or clear cytoplasm without desmosomes or melanosomes. However, they do contain smooth vesicles, multivesicular bodies and lysosomes, but most characteristic is the Birbeck granules which are rod shaped or "tennis-racket" shaped cytoplasmic organelles with a central linear density and a striated appearance. The function of Birbeck granules is under question, but it is thought to be contributed to receptor-mediated endocytosis, similar to clathrin-coated pits, based on one theory. The Langerhans cells are part of the immune system, and like much of the immune system they have a lot of different functions. They possess surface receptors common to macrophages, the receptors for immunoglobulin Fc and complement C3 and function as antigen presenting cells to T or B lymphocytes.

2. 1. 4 *The Merkel Cell*
Merkel cells appear in the glabrous skin of the fingertip, lip, gingiva and nail bed, and in several other regions. They are associated with the sense of light touch discrimination of shapes and textures. In the skin, Merkel cell receptors are typically situated near sensory nerve endings, with each Merkel cell and each nerve ending forming what is known as a "Merkel cell-neurite complex". The Merkel cell-neurite complex acts as what is called a mechanoreceptor. When the sensation of light touch is detected, mechanoreceptors respond to a particular stimulus and react by producing electrical nerve impulses eventually reaching the brain.

2. 1. 5 *Adhesion between Keratinocytes*
Epidermal keratinocytes adhere to each other by desmosomes, hemidesmosome and structures such as adherens junctions, gap junctions and tight junctions (Figure 2 – 3).

2. 1. 5. 1 Desmosome

Desmosome is the major adhesion complex in epidermis. It is composed of an attachment plaque comprising inner and outer plaques. It's a structure that penetrates membranes to connect cells. The attachment plaque is mainly composed of desmoplakin, to which keratin fibers connect, and to strengthen the cytoskeleton. Their adhesion molecules are as follows: the desmosomal core is composed of desmoglein (Dsc) and desmocollin (Dsg). The desmoplakin (DP) links the adhesion molecules to the intermediate filaments (IFs), and the plakoglobin(PG) and plakophilin link the adhesion molecules to desmoplakin and appear to regulate desmosomal assembly and size. If the connecting adjacent

epithelial cells of the skin are not functioning correctly, layers of the skin can pull apart and allow abnormal movements of fluid within the skin, resulting in bullous diseases such as pemphigus vulgaris or pemphigus foliaceus.

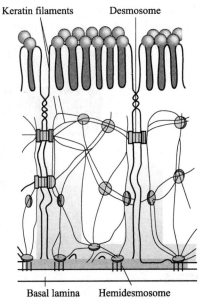

Keratin filaments   Desmosome

Basal lamina   Hemidesmosome

Figure 2 – 3   Desmosome and hemidesmosome

2. 1. 5. 2   Hemidesmosome

Hemidesmosomes are very small rivet-like structures that attached an epithelial cell to the basement membrane beneath epithelial. They are similar in form to desmosomes. At the ultrastructure level, the hemidesmosome appears as an electron dense structure whose cytoplasmic plaque serves to anchor keratin-type intermediate filaments to the cell surface. The extracellular, electron-dense lines which are parallel to the plasma membrane, subjacent to the outer plaque are termed sub-basal dense plates (SBDPs). Besides, the dense plates have proteins such as BPAG 1, BPAG2 and integrin.

2. 1. 6 *The Dermal-Epidermal Junction*
The epidermal basement membrane plays a key role in dermal-epidermal adhesion.

Basement membrane zone(BMZ)

The basement membrane zone is the anchoring complex jointing the epidermis and dermas of the skin and can be stained by periodic acid Schiff (PAS) under the light microscope. BMZ includes the lamina densa (LD) and the lamina lucida (LL), which are observed by electron microscopy. The layer close to the epithelium is called the lamina lucida. The LD membrane is about 30 - 70 nm in thickness,which consists of an underlying network of reticular collagen（type Ⅳ）fibrils. The dense layer close to the connective tissue is called the lamina densa. The LL membrane includes the component laminin-332. Type ⅩⅦ collagen bridges the lamina lucida to connect hemidesmosomes directly with the lamina densa. Besides being able to anchor down the epithelium to its loose connective tissue underneath, BMZ also has mechanical support for epithelium and act as selective barrier（Figure 2 - 4）. Some diseases resulted from improper function of basement membrane zone are associated under the name epidermolysis bullosa.

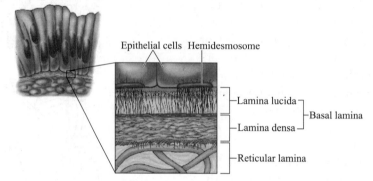

Figure 2 - 4　Basement membrane zone

2.2　Dermis

The dermis is a layer of skin between the epidermis and subcutaneous tissues. It is composed of two layers, the papillary and reticular layer. The components of the dermis are collagen fibers, reticular fibers, elastic fibers, and extra fibrillar matrix. The dermis varies in thickness depending on the location of the skin. It is 0. 3 mm thick on the eyelid and 3. 0 mm thick on the back. It contains most of the skin's specialized cells and structures, including cutaneous appendages,blood vessels,lymph vessels and nerves course（Figure 2 - 5）. Its main functions are to be responsible for the tensile strength of skin,to regulate temperature, to supply the epidermis with nutrient-saturated blood and to store water for body.

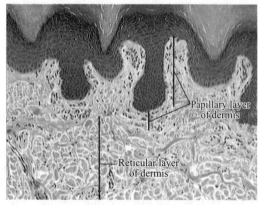

Figure 2 - 5　Dermis

2.2.1　The Papillary Layer

As the upper layer, the papillary layer, contains an arrangement of collagen fibers. It supplies nutrients to the epidermis and regulates temperature. The functions of constriction and expansion control the amount of blood that flows through the skin and detect whether the skin is hot or conserved when it is being cold.

2.2.2　The Reticular Layer

As the lower layer, the reticular layer, is made of thick collagen fibers that are arranged in parallel to the surface of the skin. The reticular layer which is thicker and denser than the papillary dermis, strengthens the skin and provides structure and elasticity. It supports other components of the skin,such as hair follicles,sweat glands, and sebaceous glands as well.

2.3　Subcutaneous Tissue

Subcutaneous tissue is used mainly for fat storage. It contains fat and connective tissue that houses larger blood vessels, nerves, eccrine glands and apocrine glands. The size of this layer varies throughout the body and from person to person.

2.4　Cutaneous Appendages

Cutaneous appendages include hair, sebaceous glands,sweat glands and nails（Figure 2 - 6）.

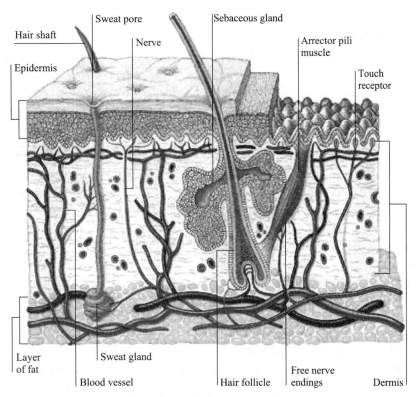

Figure 2 - 6 Cutaneous appendages

2.4.1 The Hair

Hair often refers to two distinct structures. The part beneath the skin is called hair follicle or hair bulb, located in the dermis. The part above the skin surface is called the hair shaft. A cross section of the hair shaft can be divided roughly into three zones. Starting from the outside is the cuticle which consists of several layers of keratocyte cells, the middle is cortex which contains the keratin bundles and the medulla, a disorganized and open area at the fiber's center(Figure 2 - 7). Hair has a specific growth cycle with three distinct and continuous phases: anagen (about 3 years), catagen (about 3 weeks), and telogen phases(about 3 months). Up to 80% of the hairs stay in the phase of anagen. One strand of hair may be in the anagen phase, while another is in the telogen phase. The duration of each stage varies individually, it can be affected by anatomical location, genetic influence, and a variety of environmental and physiological factors.

2.4.2 The Sebaceous Glands

Sebaceous glands are found everywhere on the body except palms, soles, top of the feet, and lower lip. They are one part of the pilosebaceous unit, and the numbers are the greatest on the face, upper neck, and chest. The function of the sebaceous glands is to produce a substance called sebum, which is responsible for keeping the skin and hair moisturized. Sebaceous glands' function is mainly under the influence of hormones called androgens.

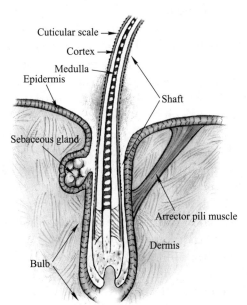

Figure 2 - 7 Hair follicle

2.4.3 The Sweat Glands

Sweat glands are divided into eccrine glands and apocrine glands according to their structures and functions.

2.4.3.1 The eccrine glands

The eccrine glands are composed of an internal epidermal spiral duct, the acrosyringium, a straight dermal portion, and a coiled acinar portion in the dermis or hypodermis. The main function of eccrine sweat gland is to regulate body temperature. They are controlled by the sympathetic nervous system. These sweat glands are found all over the body but particularly concentrated on palms, soles and forehead. These areas consequently produce sweat which is composed mainly of water along with small amounts of various minerals.

2.4.3.2 The apocrine glands

The apocrine glands are present primarily in the armpits, around the belly button, genital and anal areas of the body. Modest numbers of apocrine glands are located in the ears and aid in the formation of cerumen, more commonly known as earwax. The ducts of apocrine glands open into the canals of hair follicles. These glands produce a milky type of sweat, which causes body odor when bacteria decompose sweat on the skin surface. The stimulus for the secretion of apocrine sweat glands is a hormone known adrenaline.

2.4.4 The Nails

Nails which are made of a tough protein called keratin, a horn-like envelope covering the dorsal aspect of the terminal phalanges of fingers and toes in humans. A nail consists of nail plate, nail lunula, nail wall, nail root, nail bed and nail matrix. The nail plate is like a protective shield, covering the delicate tissues of the underlying nail bed. The nail lunula is the visible part of the matrix, which appears as whitish crescent-shaped on the base of the nail and is normally more prominent on the thumbs. The nail wall is the cutaneous fold overlapping the sides and proximal end of the nail. The nail root is the base of the nail embedded underneath the skin. The nail bed is the skin beneath the nail plate (Figure 2 - 8). They all originate from the actively growing tissue below called the matrix. In humans, nails grow at an average rate of 3 mm a month, and the growth rate depends on the age, gender, season, exercise level, diet, and hereditary factors.

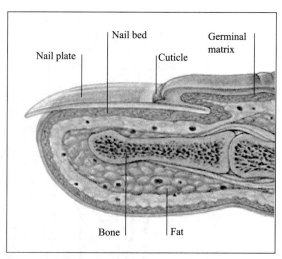

Figure 2 - 8 The structure of the nails

2.5 The Nerves, Vessels, and Muscles of the Skin

2.5.1 Nerves

The sensory nerves perceive external and internal stimuli to the skin, such as touch, tension, pain, heat and cold. Cutaneous receptors take the form of encapsulated nerve endings such as the Pacinian corpuscles which react to vibration, the Meissner corpuscles which detect touch, acting as pressure key, and being responsible for perceiving touch and pressure, and the Ruffini corpuscles. The autonomic nerves regulate the vessels, the appendages of the skin and arrector pili muscles (Figure 2 - 9).

2.5.2 Vasculature

The supply of blood to the skin generally takes the form of microscopically small loops of blood vessels coming up from the deeper layer of larger blood vessels, each supplies a small local area of skin. The blood vessels of the dermis provide nutrients to the skin and regulate body temperature.

2.5.3 Lymph Vessels

The lymph vessels parallel some important blood vessels and function to conserve plasma proteins and scavenge foreign material, antigenic substances. Blind-ended lymphatic capillaries arise within the interstitial spaces of the dermal papillae. These superficial dermal vessels drain into the deep dermal and subdermal plexuses.

2.5.4 Muscles

The arrector pili muscles are the most common mus-

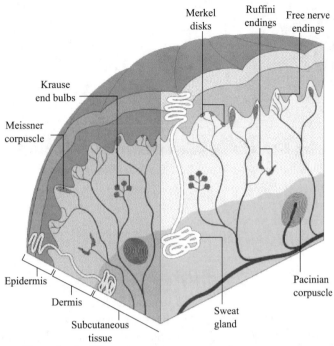

Figure 2 - 9　The major sensory nerves and sensory receptors
Most of the nerve endings are located at the junction between the dermis and epidermis skin layers

cle type in the skin. They are bundles of smooth muscle fibers, attached to the deep part of the hair follicles in humans. Contraction of these muscles causes hairs to stand on end—known as the "goose bumps". The facial muscles are a group of striated muscles innervated by the facial nerve that controls facial expression.

▪ Summary

　　The skin has three layers—the epidermis, dermis, and the subcutaneous layer. Each layer performs specific function.

　　The epidermis is the relatively thin, tough, outer layer of the skin. Most of the cells in the epidermis are keratinocytes. They originate from cells in the deepest layer of the epidermis called the basal layer. The outermost portion of the epidermis, known as the stratum corneum, is relatively waterproof. The epidermis also protects the internal organs, muscles, nerves, and blood vessels against trauma. Scattered throughout the basal layer of the epidermis are cells called melanocytes, which produce the pigment melanin. The epidermis also contains Langerhans cells, which are part of the skin's immune system.

　　The dermis, the skin's next layer, is a thick layer of fibrous and elastic tissue that gives the skin its flexibility and strength. The dermis contains nerve endings, sweat glands and sebaceous glands, hair follicles, and blood vessels. The sweat glands produce sweat in response to heat and stress. The sebaceous glands secrete sebum into hair follicles. The hair follicles produce the various types of hair found throughout the body. The blood vessels of the dermis provide nutrients to the skin and help regulate body temperature.

　　Below the dermis lies a layer of fat that helps insulate the body from heat and cold, provides protective padding, and serves as an energy storage area. The subcutaneous tissue varies in thickness, from a fraction of an inch on the eyelids to several inches on the abdomen and buttocks in some people.

▪ Questions

　　1. How many layers are there in the epidermis? What are they?

　　2. What are cutaneous appendages?

(Wei Xu 徐薇)

Chapter 3

Functions of Skin

▪ Objectives

To master the knowledge of the seven functions of the skin.

To have an intimate knowledge of the relationship between the physiological functions of the skin and the whole.

▪ Key concepts

The skin is a complex metabolically active organ, which performs important physiological functions that are summarized as follows.

Skin barrier function: The skin provides a protective barrier against mechanical, thermal and physical injury and noxious agents; prevents loss of moisture; reduces the harmful effects of UV radiation.

Skin absorptive function: The efficiency of the barrier differs between body sites. Healthy human skin with complete dense stratum corneum and sebum membrane can more easily absorb the substance with chemical property similar to sebum membrane.

Skin sensory function: The skin acts as a sensory organ. The skin is rich in nerves, particularly with hands, face and genitalia. Free sensory nerve endings lie in the dermis where they transmit pain, itch and temperature.

Skin secretion and excretion function: Skin has secretion and excretion mainly through sweet glands and sebaceous glands.

Skin temperature regulation function: The skin plays an important role in maintaining a constant body temperature through changing blood flow in the cutaneous vascular system and evaporation of sweat from the surface.

Skin metabolism function: It includes glycometabolism, protein metabolism, lipid metabolism and water-electrolyte metabolism.

Skin immunological function: Skin plays a role in immunological surveillance. It normally contains all the elements of cellular immunity, with the exception of B cells.

▪ Introduction

Skin is the body's largest organ, covering the whole body. As it is in contact with the outside world, skin is the first line of defense. Since it has rich and highly developed nerve receptors, plays a part in feeling and reflecting the internal and external environment. In addition, it possesses the functions such as barrier function, absorption function, sensation function, secretion function, excretion function, temperature regulation, metabolism, immunologic function and so on.

In consequence, skin maintains a stable environment within and without the body.

3.1　Skin Barrier Function

Skin likes a tough impermeable membrane, with elasticity and tension, covering the surface of the body completely. On the one hand, skin can prevent the loss of moisture, electrolytes and other material inside the body; on the other hand, it can prevent the body from being invaded by the outside harmful and unwanted materials. So the skin plays an important role in maintaining a stable environment within the body.

3. 1. 1　Protection of Physical Injury

The epidermis, the outermost layer of the skin, is directly contiguous with the environment. It is composed of four basic cell types: keratinocytes, melanocytes, Langerhans cells, and the Merkel cells. The basic function of keratinocyte is to synthesize keratin, a filamentous protein that serves a protection function. Skin having characteristics of tenacity and elastic, has the role to protect and buffer against the external mechanical extrusion, friction, force and collision.

The stratum corneum can reflect sunlight, and epidermal cells can absorb most of ultraviolet. Chronic sun exposure can stimulate the melanocyte to produce larger melanosomes, thereby making the distribution of melanosomes within keratinocytes resemble the pattern seen in dark-skinned individuals.

The skin, as a poor conductor of electricity, has certain impedance ability of low current.

3. 1. 2　Protection of Chemical Irritation

Stratum corneum cell possesses lipid membrane with full, rich keratin in the cytoplasm, and abundant acid glycosamine glycan resistant to weak acid and alkali between cells. Normal skin pH is 5. 5 – 7. 0, but in different parts of the skin pH since 4. 0 to 9. 6. Skin has buffer ability against acid and alkali, which can protect body from the material damage of weak acids and weak bases.

3. 1. 3　Defense Mechanism of Microorganism

Stratum corneum is a good barrier to defense microorganism. Normally bacteria and virus cannot enter the body through skin. Because some free fatty acid of the skin surface can inhibit the growth of microorganism. When the defense function is destroyed, skin is vulnerable to pathogenic microorganism.

3. 1. 4　Preventing Nutrient Loss

The unique structure of stratum corneum can prevent dehydration. Generally stratum corneum of water conservation in 10% – 20%, when below 10%, skin could be dry, coarse, or even chapped.

3.2　Skin Absorptive Function

The skin has the ability to absorb different materials. The main way is penetrating the stratum corneum, and then being absorbed by dermis through epidermis layers, the second way is penetrating through the hair follicle, the sebaceous gland and sweat gland conduit.

The efficiency of the barrier differs between body sites. The scrotum, face, forehead and dorsa of the hands may be more permeable to water than the trunk, arms and legs.

Healthy human skin with complete dense stratum corneum and sebum membrane can absorb the substance with chemical property similar to sebum membrane more easily. The material of both hydrosoluble and liposoluble could be absorbed more easily than it of only hydrosoluble or liposoluble. Secondly, skin has a very high permeability to the fat-soluble matter, such as vitamins A, E, D, and has a very low permeability of water-soluble vitamin B and vitamin C.

The order of absorption is animal fat>vegetable oil >mineral oil. The skin absorbs various metals, such as gold, hydrargyrum, and plumbum.

The barrier is affected by many other factors, such as age, environmental conditions and physical trauma, and permeability can be enhanced by various agents.

3.3 Skin Sensory Function

The skin sensation can be generally divided into two types: ① single sensation, which is transmitted by nerve endings or special small body sensors accepting the inside oneness stimulation; ② composite sensation as dry, wet, smooth, soft, hard, rough, etc. They are the common perception by several different sensors or nerve endings through the cerebral cortex analyses comprehensively.

Itch is very common in dermatology, but is not well studied, mainly because it is the subjective feeling of patient, which could not be objectively measured.

3.4 Skin Secretion and Excretion Function

Skin has secretion and excretion mainly through sweet glands and sebaceous glands.

3.4.1 The Eccrine Sweat Unit

Eccrine sweat units are found at virtually all skin sites. They are most abundant on the palms, soles, forehead, and axillae. Some eccrine glands in the axillae, especially in patients with hyperhidrosis, may have widely dilated secretary coils that contain apocrine-appearing cells. Secretion of sweat occurs as result of many factors and is mediated by cholinergic innervation. Heat is a prime stimulus to increased sweating, but other physiologic stimuli, including e-motional stress, are important as well. Increasing sweat production in response to heat is part of the thermoregulatory system of the body; together with increasing cutaneous blood flow, which can effectively dissipate excessive body heat. At friction surfaces, such as the palms and soles, eccrine secretion is thought to assist tactile sensibility and improve adhesion.

3.4.2 The Apocrine Unit

The composition of the product of secretion is only partially understood. Protein, carbohydrate, ammonia, lipid, and iron are all found in apocrine secretion. It appears milky and is odorless until it reaches the skin surface, where it is altered by bacteria, which makes it odoriferous. Apocrine gland secretion in humans serves no known function. In other species it has a protective as well as a sexual function,

and in some species, it is important in thermoregulation as well.

3.4.3 The Sebaceous Gland

Sebaceous glands are found in greatest abundance on the face and scalp, though they are distributed throughout all skin sites except the palms and soles. They are always associated with hair follicles except at the following sites: the eyelids (meibomian glands), the buccal mucosa and vermilion border of the lip (Fordyce's spots), the prepuce (Tyson's glands), and the female areolas (Montgomery's tubercles). Although sebaceous glands are independent miniorgans in their own right, they are anatomically and functionally related to the hair follicle. Cutaneous disorders attributed to sebaceous glands, such as acne vulgaris, are really disorders of the entire pilosebaceous unit. The clinical manifestations of acne, namely the comedo, papule, pustule, and cyst, would not form, regardless of increased sebaceous gland activity, as long as the sebaceous duct and infundibular portion of the hair follicle remained patent and lipid and cell debris (sebum) were able to reach the skin surface.

3.5 Skin Temperature Regulation Function

The thermoreceptor cells of the skin are distributed irregularly over the skin, including warm- and cold-sensitive thermoreceptors. High environmental temperatures, fever or strenuous exercise leads to an expansion of blood vessels in the skin and an increase of perspiration. This aids in cooling the blood and thus provides a regulatory function of body temperature and blood pressure. Low temperature leads to a reduction in perspiration, thereby reducing evaporation and preserving heat. Heat can be lost through the skin surface by radiation, convection, conduction and evaporation. Temperature regulation is important, because organs, including our brain can not operate without a certain temperature range.

3.6 Skin Metabolism Function

3.6.1 Glycometabolism

Glucose content of normal skin is 2.2 –4.45 mmol/L (44 – 81 mg/dl), approximately 1/3 – 1/2 of blood sugar. Glucose content of epidermis is more than which of dermis and subcutaneous tissue. The glucose of skin is hepatin, glucose and mucoitin, etc. The mucoitin of dermis zymolite is abundant. The most important are hyaluronic acid and chondroitin sulfate, which have close influence to water-electrolyte metabolism balance. Mucoitin has an effect upon dermis and subcutaneous tissue of sustaining, connecting and sheltering. The efficiency of glucose in epidermis is higher than in dermis.

3. 6. 2 Protein Metabolism
The protein of epidermis can be divided into the fibrin, non-fibrin. Fibrin forms keratin, such as the tonofilament of epidermis can make epidermis cell maintain certain form. The non-fibrin participates in the process of all other cell function except cornification.

3. 6. 3 lipid Metabolism
The lipid includes fat and adipoid. The former is providing energy, and the latter is main component of the biomembrane. Steroid such as cholesterol can be transformed into 7-dehydrocholesterol in epidermis cells. Then after exposed to ultraviolet radiation, it could be an active vitamin D_3 to prevent rickets. When plasma lipid and lipoprotein metabolism are abnormal, it could do clinical skin xanthoma damage. The fat of dermis and subcutaneous is abundant, which can provide energy via the β-oxidation. Fat synthesis is mainly in the epidermis cells.

3. 6. 4 Water-electrolyte Metabolism
The skin is important reservoir. The water content of children is higher than which of adults, and the water content of women is slightly higher than which of male. Skin moisture distributes mainly in the dermis, which not only provides an internal environment for various skin physiological functions, but also plays a certain role of adjusting the water of the whole body. when the body dehydrates, skin can provide 5%-7% of moisture to maintain the stability of the blood circulating capacity. The electrolyte of skin is mostly stored inside subcutaneous tissue, which includes sodium, potassium, magnesium, chlorine, calcium, phosphorus. etc.

3.7 Skin Immunological Function

The concept of skin immune system (SIS) was put forward by Bos in 1986. The immunological functions of the skin have been the subject of intense re-

search in recent years, and it is clear that the skin has an important role in immunological host defense. The skin immune system mainly consists of skin cell, functional unit, and molecular composition (Table 3 – 1).

Table 3 – 1 The skin immune system

Functional unit	Epidermis, dermis, blood vessel, lymphatics and lymph nodes
Skin cell	Keratinocyte, Langerhans cell, lymphocyte, monocyte/macrophages, granular cells and mast cells
Molecular composition	Antigen and half antigen, antibody, alexin, cytokine, adhesion molecules and histocompatibility antigen

3. 7. 1 Skin Cells of the Immune System
3. 7. 1. 1 Keratinocyte
Keratinocytes play a role in the immune function of the skin, and they participate in communication, interaction, and regulation of cell systems, collaborating in the induction of the immune response. Keratinocytes secrete a wide array of cytokines and inflammatory mediators. They also can express molecules on their surface such as ICAM-1 and MHC class II molecules, which demonstrates that keratinocytes actively respond to immune effector signals.
3. 7. 1. 2 Langerhans cell
Functionally, Langerhans cells are of the monocyte macrophage lineage and originate in bone marrow. They play a role in induction of graft rejection, primary contact sensitization, and immunosurveillance. If skin is depleted of them by exposure to ultraviolet radiation, it loses the ability to be sensitized until its population of Langerhans cells is replenished. Langerhans cells' function primarily in the afferent limb of the immune response by providing the recognition, uptake, processing, and presentation of antigens to sensitize T lymphocytes.
3. 7. 1. 3 Lymphocyte
Lymphocytes of skin are mainly $CD4^+$ T lymphocytes, then $CD8^+$ T lymphocyte. T lymphocytes with epidermotropism can be recycled, exchanging between skin blood circulation and organs, transferring different information.

3. 7. 2 Molecular Composition of the Immune System
3. 7. 2. 1 Cytokine
Intraepidermal cytokine is brought by keratino-

cyte, followed by Langerhans cell and T lymphocytes, etc. Cytokine have an impact upon cell differentiation, proliferation and activation, etc.

3. 7. 2. 2 Immunoglobulin

Excretive IgA is concerned with resisting infection and antiallergic through blocking adhesion, dissolving, regulating engulf and neutralization, etc.

3. 7. 2. 3 Alexin

Alexin is concerned with specific and non-specific immune response through dissolving cell, immune adhesion, sterilization, allergy toxin and promoting media release, etc.

▪ Summary

The skin covering the whole body is the largest organ. It has several functions. The most important function are forming a physical barrier to the environment, and providing protection against microorganisms, ultraviolet radiation, toxic agents and mechanical insults. The skin has the ability to absorb different material. The material of both hydrosoluble and liposoluble could be absorbed more easily than those only hydrosoluble or liposoluble. The order of absorption is animal fat＞vegetable oil ＞mineral oil. The skin sensation can generally be divided into two types: single sensation and composite sensation. Skin has secretion and excretion function mainly through sweet glands and sebaceous glands. The thermoreceptor cells of the skin are distributed irregularly over the skin, including warm- and cold-sensitive thermoreceptors. Skin metabolism function includes glycometabolism, protein metabolism, lipid metabolism and water-electrolyte metabolism. The skin is not only a organ with barrier function, absorption function, sensation function, secretion and excretion function, temperature regulation and metabolism, but also is an important immunological organ, which has a variety of immune cells secreting immune factors such as cytokine or chemokine to participate in immune response and play the role of the immune monitoring.

▪ Questions

1. Describe the physiology function of skin.

2. Depict briefly the factors affecting the skin absorption.

（Yanqing Gao 高艳青）

Chapter 4

Clinical Manifestations and Diagnosis of Dermatosis and Venereal Diseases

▪ Objectives

To master the contents, concepts, pathological changes and clinical manifestations of primary and secondary skin lesions.

To understand the diagnosis methods for dermatosis and venereal diseases (including the general medical history, physical examination, laboratory examination, etc.)

▪ Key concepts

The subjective symptoms are the patients' subject feelings, discomforts.

The objective symptoms that are also called physical signs or skin lesions are changes of skin, mucosa and appendages which can be objectively seen or felt, they are divided into primary lesions and secondary lesions.

The main evidence used for diagnosing dermatosis and venereal diseases is clinical manifestation, namely symptoms and signs. Furthermore, comprehensive analysis of information such as medical history, physical examination, assistant examination and so on is required.

▪ Introduction

The clinical manifestations of dermatosis and venereal diseases include symptoms and signs, which are the main diagnosis evidences for dermatosis and venerism.

4.1 Clinical Manifestations of Dermatosis and Venereal Diseases

The clinical manifestations of dermatosis and venereal diseases include symptoms and signs.

4.1.1 The Symptoms and Signs of Dermatosis

4.1.1.1 Symptoms

It is the discomfort that is subjectively feelings of patients, such as itch, ache, burning sensation, numbness, and other sharp pain, foreign body sensation, formication, etc. The above symptoms are related to the character, severity of the disease and also the patient's sensitivity.

(1) Itch

It is the most common subjective symptom of dermatosis. It's light or serious, continuous or discontinuous; it can affect the whole body or a local area. Serious itch is usually felt by contact dermatitis, eczema, lichen simplex chronicus and urticaria sufferers. Some systemic diseases, such as malignant lymphoma, diabetes mellitus, jaundice, renal inadequacy and so on can all cause itches. More itch can happen on the old people in winter, this may have something to do with the dry skin or too much washing.

(2) Pain

It can happen coupled with infection and some neuropathy. Ache caused by furuncle is confined to where is red and swollen. Herpes zoster can invade the ganglion, which will cause burning sensation or twinge in the nerve area of the affected ganglion.

Moreover, systemic symptom such as shivering, fever, fatigue, inappetence, arthrodynia and so on will happen when dermatosis affects the all organic function or general reaction associated.

4. 1. 1. 2   Signs

They are dermatic and mucosal lesions that can be objectively seen or touched. They are divided into primary lesions and secondary lesions. Sometimes the two couldn't be differentiated completely; however, pustule induced by psoriasis is primary lesion, while the one induced by eczema is from secondary infection.

(1) Primary lesion

It's brought by characteristic pathological process of dermatosis, and usually its traits contribute more to diagnosis.

1) Macule: It is the localized change of skin color, neither concave nor convex (Figure 4 – 1). Macules are divided into erythema, pigmentation macule, hypopigmentation macule and blood spots, etc. The macule whose diameter is more than one centimeter is called patch.

Erythema are mostly induced by telangiectasis or hyperemia, they are divided into the inflammatory (Color Figure 4 – 1) and the no-inflammatory. The former will lead to a higher local temperature and somewhat swelling and elevation. The no-inflamma-

tory macules are brought about by angiotelectasis or capillary increase, fading with pressure without higher local temperature. Hemangioma and rosacea and so on are all of this kind.

Pigmentation macule appear as various shade of brown or black, found in pigmentation of dermis or epidermis, chloasma (Color Figure 4 – 2) and pigmented nevus, for instance. Pityriasis Alba is one kind of hypopigmentation macule, while vitiligo belongs to depigmentation macule (Color Figure 4 – 3).

Pigmentation or hypopigmentation may sometimes follow by inflammatory reaction of skin. Fixed drug eruption often leaves characteristic gray-blue pigmentation. Scald can leave hyperpigmentation or hypopigmentation maculae. Tinea versicolor may leave transient hypopigmentation macule.

Blood spots may appear as small bleeding points, one to two millimeters or so, they are induced by dermatorrhagia, and may be found in hemorrhagic disease or trauma (Color Figure 4 – 4). It is called ecchymosis when its diameter is more than two millimeters.

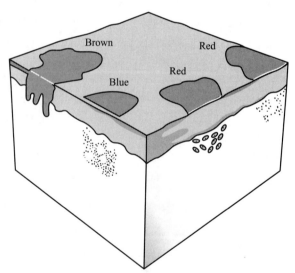

Figure 4 – 1   Ideograph macule

2) Papules: It's a localized, substantial, elevated lesion, with a diameter of less than one centimeter (Figure 4 – 2), and its surface may appear planate, like flat wart (Color Figure 4 – 5); it can also present a circular appearance, like molluscum contagiosum; or mammillary, such as common wart.

Papules can appear various colors, which contribute to diagnosis. For example, lichen planus usually appear mauve, xanthoma nankin, while pigmented nevus often presents black brown, etc.

Papule may arise because of inflammation, it appears faint red in early folliculitis (Color Figure 4 – 6); it can also be caused by metabolic product deposited, like the flavescent eyelid xanthoma; vitamin A deficiency can lead to keratotic plug with acute top, which takes shape by reason for the thicker cuticle in pilosebaceous orifice.

Maculopapules are lightly raised lesions between macule and papule. When minor blisters or little blisters form on top of papule, it is called papulovesicle or papulopustule.

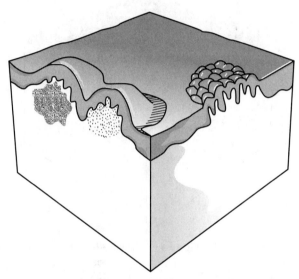

Figure 4 – 2   Ideograph papule

3) Plaque: It's a planate, elevated, infiltrating lesion, with an area of more than one centimeter or so, it is mixed together by some lager papule or some of them (Figure 4 – 3, Color Figure 4 – 7 and 4 – 8).

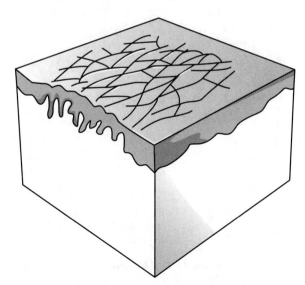

Figure 4 – 3   Ideograph plaque

4) Wheal: It's a lightly raised lesion caused by the acute edema in superficial dermis, often together with severe itch. It may appear faint red or pale, with flushing around, it has a quick attack; extends promptly; has an irregular edge which appears pseudo pod, it often disappears in several hours, with no marks left. Wheal appears in urticaria (Figure 4 – 4, Color Figure 4 – 9).

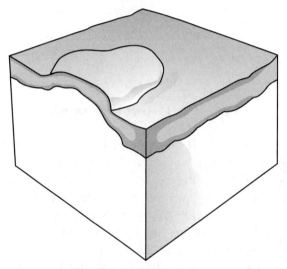

Figure 4 – 4   Ideograph wheal

5) Blister and bulla: With liquid inside, it's a lesion higher than the surface of the epidermis. It is called a litter blister when it is like a needle point to rice grains in shape; and when its diameter is less than one centimeter, it is called a blister, and when its diameter is more than one centimeter, it is called a bulla (Figure 4 – 5, Color Figure 4 – 10). The liquid in the bulla and blister can be serous fluid, which appears nankin; it is called a blood blister when it contains blood, by this, it appears red or crimson; it appears transparent if it contains lymph. High color may encircle around the blister. According to the position of the blister, its exine may be thick or thin. Its exine is thinner if the blister appears under the horny layer, it appears transparent, and will dry and desquamation easily, like miliaria Alba. While its exine is a little thicker if the blister takes place in the spinous layer and will not easily break, such as herpes simplex and varicella. The bulla that happens in pemphigus is both large and thin, and is easy to break. A bulla that happens under the epidermis owns a thicker exine and seldom breaks, like erythema multiforme, pemphigoid and so on.

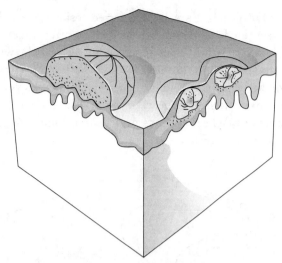

Figure 4 - 5   Ideograph blister and bulla

6) Pustule: It is a kind of blister that contains pus. The pus may appear muddy, thick or thin (Figure 4 - 6, Color Figure 4 - 11). A pustule which is under the horny layer may be a little larger; its exine can break easily, like impetigo. Pustules can be divided into the infectious like bacteria or virus infection and the non-infectious, induced by pustular psoriasis, for example. A pustule forms after blister infection is a secondary lesion.

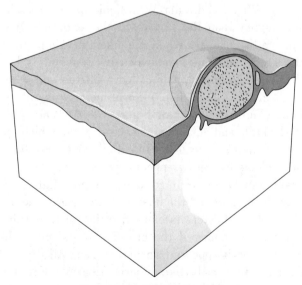

Figure 4 - 6   Ideograph pustule

7) Nodule: It's a localized, substantial lesion with a round or round-like shape and hard texture, it often occurs in dermis or hypoderm, palpation is needed to inspect, consequently. Shallower or larger ones may rise from the surface of skin (Figure 4 - 7). Nodule may be caused by several circumstances,

like inflammatory infiltration in dermis or hypoderm, deposit of metabolic product, calcification in cutaneous tissues, etc (Color Figure 4 - 12 and 4 - 13).

Sometimes because of the obvious localized thickness in epidermis, together with the inflammatory infiltration in dermis, a raised, a bit larger and hard papule may form, and it is also called a nodule, like nodular prurigo. A nodule whose diameter is more than two to three centimeters is called a mass.

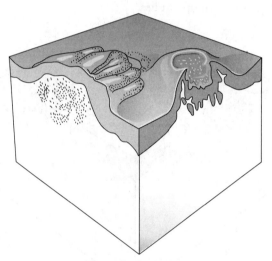

Figure 4 - 7   Nodule

8) Cyst: It's a cystoid lesion, containing ropy material and cell component in liquid, it usually lies in dermis or even deeper; can elevate or just be touched, it often has a round or oval shape, elastic sensation if touched, like cystic acne, sebaceous cyst and so on(Figure 4 - 8, Color Figure 4 - 14).

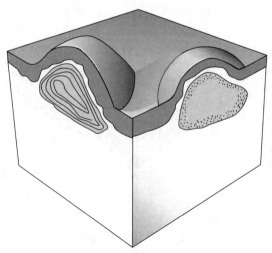

Figure 4 - 8   Ideograph cyst

(2) Secondary lesion

It develops from primary lesions spontaneously or comes into being when some lesions from scratching, infection, therapeutic treatment which are in their reparative process go to a step further.

1) Erosion: When the epidermis or mucosa falls off at their border with dermis, they will reveal red wetted surface, and this is called erosion (Figure 4 - 9, Color Figure 4 - 15). It usually comes from the break of the blister or pustule and it can also come from the falling of the epidermis when skin is macerated, a kind of itching and tingling sensation will be felt. Since the lesion is light and part of basal layer cells still exist, consequently it will heal quickly and leave no scar.

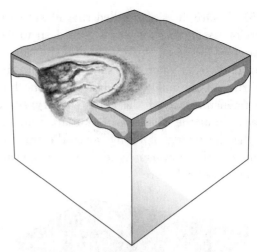

Figure 4 - 10　Ideograph ulcer

(Color Figure 4 - 17).

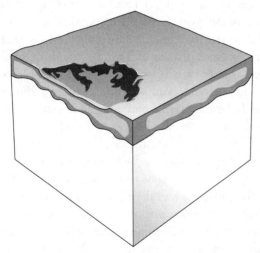

Figure 4 - 9　Ideograph erosion

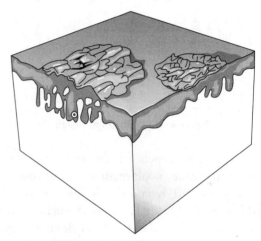

Figure 4 - 11　Ideograph scale

2) Ulcer: When an absence on the surface of the skin or mucosa goes to the dermis or even deeper, then it is called an ulcer (Figure 4 - 10). It can have a deep, intermediate, or shallow sunken bottom, necrotic tissue will be found, it has an irregular border, steep or oblique. Microbial infection, inflammatory reaction, circulatory disturbance, neoplasm necrosis (Color Figure 4 - 16), and trauma can all lead to an ulcer. It usually leaves scar after healing.

3) Scale: The accelerated formation, incomplete cornification and thickened accumulation of horny layer cells which are at pathological state can lead to the formation of the scale (Figure 4 - 11). It is hoar dry fragment with different size and thickness, it is little as scurfin, the big one appears flaky with a diameter of several millimeters or even larger, scale is usually found in dry skin, or after some lesions such as inflammatory erythema, swelling, pustule, etc.

4) Maceration: The horny layer will turn soft after soaked for a long period of time, and this is called maceration. The area where is soaked can easily appear exfoliation, erosion or fissure when rubbed (Figure 4 - 12, Color Figure 4 - 18).

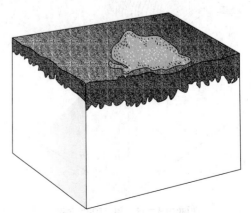

Figure 4 - 12　Ideograph maceration

5) Fissure: It is also called rhagades, the linear fissure or tissue absence which goes deep to dermis (Figure 4 – 13). It is usually found in the skin crimple at joint, areas where the skin is easy drawn like the corner of the mouth, the bottom of the breast, the circumambience of the anus, etc. Dry skin, the degradation of the elasticity of skin after inflammation, the thickening of horny layer, the fragility or hardness of the skin usually leads to the appearance of fissure (Color Figure 4 – 19).

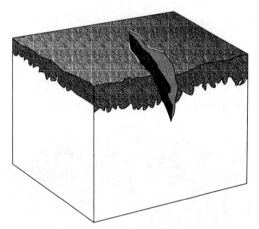

Figure 4 – 13　Ideograph fissure

6) Scar: After absence or destruction of the dermis or deep tissue, neoformative connective tissue and epidermis will repair the lesion, by this, scar forms (Figure 4 – 14). It has smooth surface, no hair or irregular shape, without normal dermatoglyph. If sweat gland and sebaceous gland suffer from destruction, hyposecretion of sweat and sebum will occur.

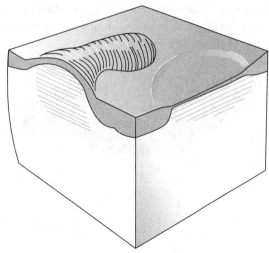

Figure 4 – 14　Ideograph scar

Scars are divided into hyperplastic scars (Color Figure 4 – 20) and atrophic scars. The former rises obviously, appears dark red gelosis, and often develops lesions like burn or chronic ulcer and so on, that usually itches. When it appears around the joint or face, joint motion will be disturbed and malformation may form. The latter is usually more concave than normal skin, and epidermis attenuation, local hemangiectasis, bagged, softer, smoother skin may appear, and that can be found in erythematosus lupus and old scar.

7) Atrophy: Degeneration of skin, it can appear either in epidermis, dermis or hypoderm, and comes about because skin component decrease (Figure 4 – 15). In epidermal atrophy, the epidermis where is damaged is thin, light red and transparent, and some ectatic blood vessels may be found. There are thin wrinkles with parchment appearance on its surface, and its normal groove of skin get shallow or disappeared, this is usually seen at skin of the old breast; in dermal atrophy, you will find that local skin is depressed, dermatoglyph may appear normal, hair may get thinner or even disappeared, and this is often found after inflammation or an injury; striae gravidarum or striae atrophicae that induced by taking steroid over a long period of time is the result of atrophy of both epidermis and dermis, and dark red and a little depressed striae atrophicae appear (Color Figure 4 – 21, 4 – 22); subcutaneous atrophy has obvious concave, it is seen in any disease that causes adipose atrophy and muscular atrophy.

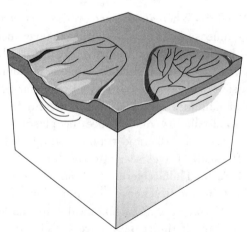

Figure 4 – 15　Ideograph atrophy

8) Crust: Seriflux, pus, blood and dropped tissue on the surface of exudative skin lesions, combined with drug produce a kind of lesion when they are dry, and this is crust. It may appear yellow brown or

dark red, and it can also appear various colors on account of mixed dyeing of drugs (Figure 4 – 16, Color Figure 4 – 23).

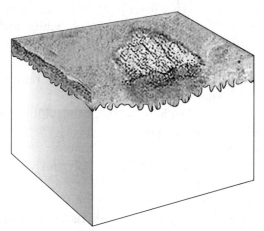

Figure 4 – 16　Ideograph crust

9) Excoriation: It is also called exfoliation. Scratching or an injury makes the epidermis damaged, and leads to the linear or snatchy defect of the shallow layer of epidermis. Blood scar may form on the surface. No scar will be left if there is a shallow lesion (Figure 4 – 17, Color Figure 4 – 24).

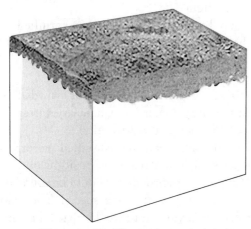

Figure 4 – 17　Ideograph excoriation

10) Lichenification: The constant scratching and rub result in thickening of the corneum layer and spinous layer; minor chronic inflammation of dermis which result in hypertrophic mottled lesion, and this is called lichenification, it appears taupe, and there may be increase of pigmentation and mild scales. The dermatoglyph deepen and the skin graves among them mostly appear small polyangle papules which cluster together, the skin thickens, rises, clear border will be found and severe itching will be felt. It is usually seen in chronic pruritic skin disease like lichen

simplex chronics and so on (Figure 4 – 18, Color Figure 4 – 25).

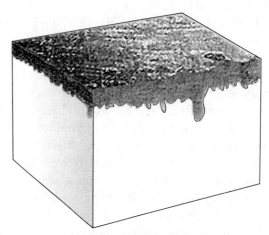

Figure 4 – 18　Ideograph lichenification

What is to be stressed out is that, dermatosis is the reaction and the recovery process of skin and organism to pathogenic factors, consequently, kinds of basic lesions are not solitary and constant. It is common to see a basic lesion developing to another, for example, macula may develop to papule, blister, erosion, crust, scale and at last it heals. Differences among the features, numbers, size, and position and conversion process of basic lesions contribute to the identification of the characteristic of all kinds of skin diseases.

4.2　Diagnosis of Dermatosis and Venereal Diseases

The diagnosis of skin and venereal diseases is the same with other diseases, which needs comprehensive analysis to medical history, physical examination, accessory examination and information and so on. Since the complicated manifestation of skin diseases, different etiological factor can lead to the same erythra, and the same can also bring about different clinical manifestation. Consequently, in the diagnostic process of skin diseases, besides the skin lesions and clinical manifestation which a doctor has found, other examinations should be got help from.

4.2.1　Medical History
4.2.1.1　General information

This includes a patient's name, age, sex, occupation, native place, race, marital status, address and so on.

4.2.1.2　Chief complaint

Records of the skin lesion, position, subjective symptom and disease time in this visit.

4. 2. 1. 3　History of present illness

The whole process from the time the patient is attacked to the time he comes to visit a doctor should be recorded completely, it ought to include the disease's inducing agent, precursory symptom, primary lesion status (including character, position, number, distribution, spread order, change regulation, etc.), local and constitutional symptom coupled with, treat course and its curative effect. The relationship between the disease and factors like diet, drugs, contactant, season, environment temperature, solar radiation and so on should be considered.

4. 2. 1. 4　Past medical history

It includes names, treatment situation, and curative effect of systemic diseases that are suffered from in the past, particularly those that are related with skin disease in being. History of allergy to drugs or other allergic history should be paid attention to.

4. 2. 1. 5　Personal history

The patient's living condition, eating habits, marital status, fertility condition and sexual life history, menstrual history and pregnancy history should be encompassed in a female patient's personal history.

4. 2. 1. 6　Family history

To have or not similar diseases or inherited diseases, as well as intermarriage which contribute a lot to the diagnosis to genetic skin diseases in the family should be asked.

4.2.2　Physical Examination

Comprehensive systemic examinations should be carried out before skin check, since kinds of skin diseases happen related to systemic diseases. When skin check is being carried out, comprehensive examinations on mucous membrane and its appendix should be done to acquire more message; to receive information close to actuality on skin lesions, enough light (natural light is best) is necessary; proper temperature is required indoor, since there may be effect on the color and character of the skin lesion when overheated or super cooled.

4. 2. 2. 1　Inspection

(1) Character

Pay attention to the character of skin lesion, primary lesion or secondary lesion, single or coexisting.

(2) Area and number

The area can either be measured or described with a real object, such as sesame, millet, soybean, pigeon egg, egg or palm; the number can be described solitary, multiple, or with figures.

(3) Color

It can be given a description of normal skin color, red, yellow, violet, brown, blue, white and so on. According to the shade of the color, further differentiation can be depicted, for example, the red can be described as light red, dark red, bright red, etc.

(4) Bound and brim

Bound may be distinct, less distinct, blurry; brim can be regular or irregular.

(5) Shape

It may appear circular, oval, polygonal, irregular shape or map-like.

(6) Surface

It may appear smooth, rough, flat, raised, central hilar depression, papillary, cauliflower, hemispheric, etc. Examine if there is erosion, ulcer, exudation, bleeding, pus, scale and crust and so on. Pay attention to the light specific changes of some skin lesions, such as Wickham lines of lichen planus, follicular keratotic plugging of DLE, etc.

(7) Base

It may be wide, narrow or pedicle-like.

(8) Content

It may be blood, mucus, sebum, cornified matter and other foreign matters, and is mainly used to observe blister, pustule and cyst.

(9) Arrange

Arrange of it may be isolated or crowded, the arrange fashion may appear linear, annular or irregular.

(10) Position and distribution

Skin diseases can be classified according to where the skin lesion happens, position of the skin lesion (exposed or shrouded) should be found out, as well as its identity with some special. The distribution fashion is divided into the localized and the systemic; whether or not it spreads along blood vessels, nerve segments or spreads symmetrically.

4. 2. 2. 2　Palpate

Mainly to find the skin lesion compact or soft, shallow or deep; whether or not it infiltration incrassate, atrophic attenuation, flabby or sunk; its local temperature normal, high or low; if it has conglutination with peripheral tissue; whether tenderness, hyper aesthesia, hypoesthesia or abnormal sensation exists; if there is intumescence, ache when touched, adhesion and so on occurs on lymph nodes around.

4. 2. 2. 3　Other physical examinations

(1) Dermatograph test

When paddling on the flexor aspect of fore arm, if the following three united reactions occur, it is called dermatograph test positive. First, 3 to 15 seconds after paddling, there will be red line left, which may be caused by angiotelectasis brought by dermis mast cell releasing histamine. Second, 15 to 45 seconds after paddling, blush appears at both sides of the red line, which is caused by arteriola expansion brought by neural axis reaction, this kind of reaction does not appear at leprosy skin lesions. Third, 1 to 3 minutes after paddling, raised, pale wheal-like line that may be caused by dropsy brought by histamine, kinin, appears. The phenomena related above are usually seen at dermography, urticaria, urticaria pigmentosa, etc(Color Figure 4 - 26).

(2) Diascopy

Place a slide or transparent tongue depressor onto skin with pressure for 10 to 20 seconds, inflammatory; erythema, hemangioma and angiotelectasis will disappear under this pressure, ecehymosis, petechiae and pigmentation exist still, granuloma nodule with apple jam-like color will be found at skin lesions of lupus vulgaris.

(3) Scale curettage

Scrape scale on the skin lesion with a dull knife, do microbiological examination to the tissue erased or observe changes of base skin erased of scale, it can be used in pityriasis simplex.

(4) Filtered ultraviolet light examination

Ultraviolet rays whose wavelength is 320 - 400 nm will be gained when the light of high pressure mercury lamp used for examination gets across color filter containing nickel oxide, its application are as following, the diagnosis and preventive treatment for tinea capitis, diagnosis for other mycotic and bacterial infection, such as erythrasma, tinea versicolor, trichomycosis axillaris and pseudomonas aeruginosa infection. Urine of porphyria cutanea tarda sufferers, teeth of erythropoietic porphyria, blood of protoporphyria appear light red, red or salmon pink fluorescence under filtered ultraviolet (Color Figure 4 - 27).

(5) Prickle-cell brisement phenomenon examination

Prickle-cell brisement phenomenon occurs in palpation for some skin diseases like pemphigus, four kinds of positive manifestation can be found. First, the blister will move along the pushing direction when one side of it is pushed by the finger; second, the fluid of blister will move all around when top of it is pressed on; third, rub the normal like skin with little pressure will lead to the epidermis peeled off. Fourth, the normal like skin around the blister will also be peeled off when the broken blister wall is pulled.

■ **Summary**

The clinical manifestation of the skin diseases and the venereal diseases include symptoms and signs which are the principal basis for diagnosis of the skin diseases and the venereal diseases.

Symptoms are the discomforts that are subjectively felt by the patient, such as itch, ache, causalgia, numbness, and other sharp pain, foreign body sensation, formication, etc. The above symptoms are related to the character, severity of the disease as well as patient's sensitivity.

Sighs are skin and mucosal lesions that can be objectively seen or touched. They are divided into primary lesions and secondary lesions.

Primary lesions are brought by characteristic pathological process of skin diseases, and usually their traits contribute more to diagnosis. They include macule, plaque, papule, wheal, blister and bulla, pustule, nodule and cyst.

The secondary lesions develop from primary lesions spontaneously or come into being when some lesions from scratching, infection, therapeutic treatment which are in their reparative process going to a step further. They include erosion, ulcer, scale, maceration, fissure, scar, atrophy, crust, excoriation and lichenification.

■ **Questions**

1. Describe primary skin lesions and secondary skin lesions as well as the concept of every skin lesion.

2. How to diagnosis a kind of skin disease (that is the essential conditions).

(Xiumin Yang 杨秀敏)

Chapter 5

The Dermatopathology

▪ Objectives

Have an intimate knowledge of commonly used descriptive terms in histopathology.

5.1 Terms of the Disorders in the Epidermis

5.1.1 Hyperkeratosis

Hyperkeratosis is thickening of the stratum corneum. It may occur in various disorders of keratinization, such as the keratodermas and ichthyosis (Color Figure 5-1).

5.1.2 Parakeratosis

Parakeratosis is an abnormal formation of horn cells of the epidermis characterized by the persistence of nuclei, incomplete formation of keratin. It is observed as scales in many conditions such as psoriasis (Color Figure 5-2).

5.1.3 Follicular Plug

Follicular plug is formed by excessive keratin in an inactive hair follicle. It often occurs in lupus erythematosus and lichen sclerosus atrophicus (Color Figure 5-3).

5.1.4 Dyskeratosis

It is abnormal keratinization occurring prematurely within individual cells or groups of cells below the stratum corneum. It often occurs in malignant and premalignant epithelial lesions, such as squamous cell carcinoma and Bowen's disease (Color Figure 5-4).

5.1.5 Hypergranulosis

This term describes an increased thickness of the stratum granulosum. It is often seen in chronic lichenification, lichen planus and related disorders (Color Figure 5-5).

5.1.6 Hypogranulosis

This term describes a decreased thickness of the stratum granulosum. It is often seen in ichthyosis vulgaris and psoriasis (Color Figure 5 – 6).

5.1.7 Acanthosis

An abnormal but benign thickening of the prickle cell layer of the epidermis. It is often seen in psoriasis (Color Figure 5 – 7).

5.1.8 Acantholysis

Acantholysis is the loss of intercellular connections resulting in loss of cohesion between keratinocytes, seen in diseases such as pemphigus vulgaris, its variants, and Darier's disease(Color Figure 5 – 8).

5.1.9 Spongiosis

Spongiosis is mainly intercellular edema between the keratinocytes in the epidermis, and is characteristic of eczematous dermatitis(Color Figure 5 – 9).

5.1.10 Kogoj Spongiform Pustule

An epidermal pustule formed by infiltration of neutrophils into necrotic epidermis in which the breaked cell walls persist as a spongelike network, seen in pustular psoriasis (Color Figure 5 – 10).

5.1.11 Munro Microabscess

A microscopic collection of polymorphonuclear white blood cells found in the stratum corneum in psoriasis (Color Figure 5 – 11).

5.1.12 Pautrier Microabscess

A microscopic lesion in the epidermis, formed by histiocytes and lymphocytes, often seen in mycosis fungoides (Color Figure 5 – 12).

5.2 Terms of the Disorders in the Dermis

5.2.1 Collagen degeneration

It refers to the deposition of extracellular homogeneous gelatinous material of variable composition. It is typically seen in colloid milium (Color Figure 5 – 13).

5.2.2 Fibrinoid Degeneration

Degeneration of tissues such as connective tissue or blood vessels, in which deposits of an acidophilic homogeneous material accumulated, which resembles fibrin when stained (Color Figure 5 – 14).

5.3 Other Terms in Dermatopathology

5.3.1 Necrosis

This term describes the death of cells or decay of tissues (Color Figure 5 – 15).

5.3.2 Granuloma

This term describes an organized inflammation of monocytes, macrophages, lymphocytes and epithelioid cells (Color Figure 5 – 16).

5.3.3 Vasculitis

This term refers to a heterogeneous group of disorders which are characterized by inflammatory destruction of blood vessels (Color Figure 5 – 17).

5.3.4 Neoplasm

This term refers to an abnormal mass of tissues, the growth of which exceeds and is uncoordinated with that of the normal tissues, and persists in the same excessive manner after the stimulus which evoked the change stopped (Color Figure 5 – 18).

5.3.5 Atypia

An abnormality of cell appearance, which may or may not be associated with later malignancy (Color Figure 5 – 19).

5.3.6 Papilloma

This term refers to a benign epithelial tumor growing exophytically (outwardly projecting) in fingerlike form (Color Figure 5 – 20).

(Lin Ma 马琳)

Chapter 6

Laboratory Tests

▪ Objectives

To master common laboratory tests and their indications.

To have an intimate knowledge of the meaning of the results especially for the results of hypersensitivity and syphilis.

▪ Key concepts

Fungal tests, including KOH test, fungal cultures and histological biopsy, are used to help detect and diagnose a fungal infection, to help guide treatment, and/or sometimes to monitor the effectiveness of treatment.

Allergy testing involves having an in vivo (skin puncture test and intracutaneous test) or in vitro tests to find out what allergen, may trigger a type I allergic reaction in a person. Patch test is a classical method of identifying whether a substance causes a type IV allergic reaction. These investigations are useful tools in the diagnosis and management of allergic diseases and can provide aids to diagnose and assess disease activity.

Serological tests for syphilis may be classified into two groups—nontreponemal tests (VDRL, USR and RPR) and treponemal tests (TPHA, TPPA and FTA-ABS). These tests can be helped to diagnose and monitor effectiveness of treatment.

▪ Introduction

Besides common laboratory tests, numerous special investigations can refine a dermatological diagnosis, or for diseases or therapy monitoring. In this chapter, the tests for fungal infections, allergic diseases, parasitic infection and sexually transmitted infections (STIs) are discussed.

6.1 Laboratory Tests of Fungi

Fungal tests are not only used to help to diagnosis and differential diagnosis of fungal infections, but also help to guide treatment and monitor the effectiveness. KOH test, fungal cultures and histological biopsy are methods to screen fungi infections.

6.1.1   The Methods of Obtain the Specimen
The correct way to obtain specimen is critical for tests. The skin area needs to be cleaned if there is some ointment on it. If the lesion has an edge, specimens should be taken from the margin. If the blisters are present, it should be cut off to obtain the samples. To obtain specimens from nail is more difficult than from skin. It is the debris under nail but not the superficial material of nail has more diagnostic value, except in case of superficial white onychomycosis. The specimens from the mouth, glans penis and angina are used swabs, and should be examined immediately. The hairs should be removed with the roots.

6.1.2   KOH Test
The standard for diagnosing fungus infections relies first on direct examination—the KOH test. For routing examination, the specimen should be placed on a slide, 10%– 15% KOH solution was dropped on the slide, covered with cover slip and heated on alcohol burner for a while (beware not boiling). Then observe with a light microscope. The positive result is found viridescence hyphae and/or spores (Color Figure 6 – 1). The specimen of vaginal secretion should not add KOH, so as not to destroy white blood cells.

The advantage of KOH test is simple and high specificity, the disadvantage is that results are operator dependent and cannot identify the specific organism.

6.1.3   Fungal Cultures
Fungal cultures are always used to obtain higher sensibility, identify the specific organism and sensitive of antifungal agents. Sabouraud agar is the ordinary one. Sometimes, the nutrient media should be used typically inhibits bacterial growth and must support fungal growth for several weeks. Multipoint inoculation and microculture can elevate sensibility. Broth microdilution testing is the recommended method of susceptibility test. And disk diffusion and "Etest" provide convenient for application in the routine laboratory tests.

6.1.4   Histological Biopsy
The histological biopsy is critical and reliable meth-od in diagnosis of deep mycosis. The routine HE and periodic acid-Schiff (PAS) stain is the classical method to identify fungi in infected tissues. In recent years, Immunostaining, based on the development of biotechnology, is also a reliable method, shows a good prospect in the diagnosis of deep mycosis.

6.2   Laboratory Tests of Allergen

Some dermatoses such as atopic dermatitis, eczema, allergic contact dermatitis can be induced by exogenous factors. Based on the allergic theory, numerous tests are used to identify the etiological factors and could be helpful to the therapy. Skin puncture test, intracutaneous test are in vivo test to determine causal factors of immediate hypersensitivity. Patch test is the in vivo test for delayed hypersensitivity. Some in vitro tests used immunoassay to detect IgE and sIgE levels.

6.2.1   The Tests for Type I Hypersensitivity
The tests for type I hypersensitivity are based on major pathological changes of the degranulation and histamine releasing of mast cells induced by IgE antibody and it's levels. Numerous testing are used to refine the diagnosis, but direct testing by puncture test, intracutaneous test and serologic testing for IgE are used commonly.

6.2.1.1   The in vivo tests

The characteristic reactions of type I hypersensitivity including erythema and wheal, the peak is at 15 – 20 minutes. Puncture test is the preferred method to diagnose exogenous factors of atopic diseases, which attempts to provoke a small, controlled, allergic response. Despite of kinds of antigen solutions, the test kit contains histamine and physiological saline solution for positive and negative control. The intracutaneous test is the most common method to screen of drug allergy.

As the routing testing of puncture test, a droplet of solution is dropped on the inside of forearm. Then the skin is punctured with a special needle. The results of immediate-phase response (IPR) will be observed after 20 minutes, and the late-phase response (LPR) after 1 – 2 hours. The intensity of reaction of antigens is divided into 5 grades based on experience of erythema and wheal compared with positive and negative results. If the appearance of erythema and wheal is the same as positive control, the grade of the reaction should be marked as (+++);

if the appearance likes the negative control, it should be marked as (−).

The clinician must pay attention to some details. First, the patient who has extensive dermatitis should avoid skin testing. Second, some interfering factors which could depress the sensitivity should be avoided. For example, patients should not use any antihistamine agents, at least 3 biological half-life periods. The other medications, tricyclic antidepressant (TCA), chlorpromazine should be avoided either. At last, epinephrin and other emergency drugs should be gotten ready for patients who were extremely sensitive to allergens.

6.2.1.2   The in vitro tests

When patient suffers from severe allergies, or has a high sensitivity level to suspected allergen which might result in potentially serious side effects, or uses allergy medication, in vivo tests are contraindicant and in vitro tests (the methods of blood testing) are alternative methods to indicate causal allergens.

The in vitro testing, for example, radio allergosorbent test (RAST) which was marked in 1970's and replaced with a superior test named the ImmunoCAP in 1980's is now recognized as one of the effective methods to measure total IgE and specific IgE (sIgE), with specificity and high sensitivity.

The levels of total IgE antibody provide an overview of the patient's atopic status. High levels of circulating total IgE antibodies are usually associated with allergy. But the serum concentration of total IgE is age-related and sometimes cannot correlate with the symptom and skin tests. Compare with the total IgE antibody, it is the fact that the sIgE antibodies are associated with allergic disease is well established. The high level of sIgE antibodies is a result of sensitization to an allergen which is exposed by an individual. However, the amount of specific IgE present does not necessarily predict the potential severity of a reaction.

To interpret the relevance of tests, either positive or negative, a skillful and experience clinician is needed. Elevated levels of sIgE antibodies usually can indicate an allergy, but this result must be interpreted under the patient's history. If a patient who was asymptomatic but had a positive result, he/she might be exposed to that substance before, predict the risk of developing allergy in the future.

Too many substances can induce allergic reaction. Negative results can only indicate that a person probably does not have an IgE-mediated response to such specific allergen. Over hundreds of different allergens are available for determinations today. Further testing might be needed if necessary.

6.2.2   The Test for Type IV Hypersensitivity (Patch Test)

Patch test is not only a classical method used to identify if a specific substance causes type IV allergic reaction in the skin but also the only acceptable method to provide scientific evidences of allergic contact dermatitis. It is the indication to the patient who has eczematoid lesions which needs to exclude allergic factors, the patient has treatment resistance or recurrence eczema, and the patient who has eczema on face, hands or feet.

A patch test kit contains chemicals frequently used in metals, rubber, leather, hair dyes, formaldehyde, lanolin, fragrance, preservative and other additives. For routing examination, tiny quantities of allergens in individual square plastic or round aluminium chambers are applied to the upper back, and are kept in place with special hypoallergenic adhesive tape. The patches stay in place undisturbed for at least 48 hours. After 48 hours, the patches will be removed. A preliminary reading is done, and another 24 – 48 hours later (72 – 96 hours after application), it should be checked again if the testing area has some changes. The characterized manifestations of the results are classified as 4 grades: no erythema and itch as the reaction of the negative control should be (−), faint or homogenous erythema and no infiltration should be (±), erythema, discrete papules infiltration and itch should be (+), erythematous-edematous, discrete vesicles and papule should be (++), and the coalescing vesicles, bulla should be (+++). If the lesions appeared as patchy or homogenous erythema and burn-like reactions, it should be the irritant reactions.

As the in vivo test, clinicians must pay attention to some details as the puncture test. For example, steroid creams need to be stopped for 3 – 4 weeks prior testing. The patients should keep his back dry, and vigorous exercise which may disrupt the tests should be avoided.

6.2.3   How to Explain the Testing Results

Any professional interpreting of tests must first interpret the results in the light of the patient's history, and should not be read in isolation. It is critical to the correct diagnosis. A positive testing result might not be the causal factors to explain the present skin problem, it might only indicate that the individual encounters with those chemicals at some point in his life and became allergic. To establish by determining the casual relationship between the positive result and the diseases not only based on the history but also on further observation: the patient has avoided exposure to the material and after that his dermatitis was improvement or clearance. If results are negative, and there are not any factors to induce false negative results during test procedure, the disease is probably not due to an allergic reaction to the antigens we tested. It is possible, however, that you were not tested by other antigens, and further investigation might be required.

6.3　Laboratory Tests of Sexually Transmitted Diseases

6.3.1　Laboratory Tests of Neisseria Gonorrhoeae

(1) Indication

Direct smears: to detect rapid infection.

Isolating culture: to detect chronic and non-symptomatic infection.

(2) Procedure

For male patient, insert cotton swab 1 to 2 cm into the urethra and gently rotate the swab. For female patient, using a cotton swab, remove external vaginal secretions from the cervix before collection of endocervical secretions. Then using a clean collection swab, insert and rotate the swab and allow several seconds for absorption. Other areas, using a cotton swab, collect secretions from the area under examination.

Smear, heat-fix the specimen and use Gram staining the smear. Then use the oil immersion objective examining it under the microscope directly.

Subcultivate the specimen and incubate the culture for 24 to 48 hours before identification.

(3) Result and clinical prompt

Positive result of direct smears examination provides initial diagnosis. Positive result of culture can give definitive diagnosis.

6.3.2　Laboratory Tests of Chlamydia

There are direct smears, cell culture, antibodies-detect and immunofluorescence methods to detect the specimen.

6.3.2.1　Direct smears

The method of collection is same as examination of *Neisseria gonorrhoeae*. Smear the specimen, then heat-fix and Gram stain the smear and using microscope to examine. Lyons blue inclusion bodies inside epithelial cells can be found in positive specimen.

6.3.2.2　Cell culture

(1) Procedure

Inoculate the specimen in the culture tube. 3 to 4 days later using Gram or direct immunofluorescence stain it and examine under the microscope.

(2) Result and clinical prompt

Red inclusion bodies can be found in positive specimen (Gram stain). Those having urethral symptoms with positive result of definitive culture can be diagnosed.

6.3.2.3　Clearview chlamydia

(1) Procedure

The method of collection is same as examination of *Neisseria gonorrhoeae*. Using commercial kit to detect the specimen.

(2) Result and clinical prompt

Those having clinical symptoms with positive result can be diagnosed. While negative specimens need cell culture to determine.

6.3.2.4　Immunofluorescence

The method of collection is same as examination of *Neisseria gonorrhoeae*. Drying-fix the specimen and stain with specific fluorescein-labeled antibody. Then drying-fix again and examine under the microscope directly. Positive granules inside epithelial cells can be found in positive specimen.

6.3.3　Laboratory Tests of Urealytium

The method of collection is same as examination of *Neisseria gonorrhoeae*. Inoculate the specimen in the fluid culture media. Incubate 24 to 72 hours and observe the color changing. Changing to pink prompts the growth of mycoplasma. Inoculate the specimen on the solid culture media and examine after 48 hours under microscope. "Fried egg" colony prompt positive.

Result and clinical prompt

Positive culture results are diagnostic.

6.3.4　Laboratory Tests of Syphilis

6.3.4.1　Direct smears

(1) Indication

To detect initial infection.

(2) Procedure

Specimens are effusion from lesions, pucture fluid from lymph nodes and mashed tissue fluid. Darkfield microscopy is used to demonstrate. Also the specimen can be examined with silver-stain, Gram-stain or Indian ink-stain. In addition, direct immunofluorescence is another method to examine.

(3) Result and clinical prompt

Positive findings on dark-field examination permit a primary diagnosis of syphilis. A negative dark-field finding does not exclude the diagnosis of syphilis. Positive results, unsure sexual contact and clinical presents constitute a definitive diagnosis.

6.3.4.2　Nontreponemal serological tests

Following tests are considered nontreponemal serological tests: VDRL, USR and RPR.

These nontreponemal tests can be used as qualitative tests for initial screening or as quantitative tests to follow treatment.

(1) Venereal disease research laboratory test (VDRL)

This test is measuring antibody to a nonspecific cardiolipin, lecithin or cholesterol antigen. The antilipoidal antibodies are not only produced as a consequence of syphilis and the other treponemal diseases, but also may be produced in response to nontreponemal diseases. Without some other clinical evidence, a reactive nontreponemal test can not confirm infection.

(2) Unheated serum regain test (USR)

The USR test is a modification of the VDRL test. It has similar sensitivity and specificity.

(3) Rapid plasma regain test (RPR)

The RPR test is a modification of the USR test. The result is easily readout and plasma can also be used as specimen. It has higher sensitivity and lower specificity. False-positive reactions occur in diseases associated with immunoglobulin abnormalities, leprosy, and few pregnancy or aged people. Patients with very high antibody titers(for example, secondary syphilis patients), may have false-negative results. This phenomenon is called as "prozone" and will be overcome by diluting the serum specimen.

6.3.4.3　Treponemal serologic tests

Treponemal serologic tests are specific test to confirm *T. pallidum* infection. All of these tests use *T. pallidum* as the antigen and measure immunoglobulin G (IgG) antibodies. Three tests are currently considered standard treponemal tests: FTA-ABS, Treponema pallidum hemagglutination assay (TPHA), and *T. pallidum* particle agglutination

test (TPPA). The Treponemal tests become positive early, before the nontreponemal tests, and remain positive for life. Therefore a positive result means that the patient had or still has active syphilis, but no assessment about the activity of the disease or the result of therapy.

Fluorescent treponemal antibody absorption test (FTA-ABS)

The FTA-ABS test is an indirect fluorescent-antibody technique. It has both highly sensitivity and specificity. Especially the specificity is much higher than the TPHA test.

6.3.5　*Laboratory Tests of Trichomonas Vaginalis*

Scrape secretions of posterior fornix, vaginal wall and cervix. For male, use urethral secretions, prostatic fluid and urinary sediment as specimen. Detect the specimen in saline under microscopy. Trichomoniasis is usually diagnosed by visualization of motile trichomonads.

6.4　Laboratory Tests of *Sarcoptes Scabie*

Whenever possible, the diagnosis of scabies should be confirmed by identifying the mite or mite eggs or fecal matter (scybala). The following tests have no difficulty to be done and have more availability. However several factors may influence the level of sensitivity, e.g. the clinical presentation (unscratched lesions are more valuable), the number of sites sampled and/or repeated scrapings, and the sampler's experience.

6.4.1　*Ink Test*

The burrows of scabies mites can be highlighted by using an ink test. The suspicious area can be rubbed with ink then wiped off using an alcohol pad. If this area was infected with scabies, some of the ink will remain and will have tracked into the burrows, the characteristic zigzag or S pattern of the burrow across the skin will appear.

6.4.2　*Microscope Examination*

To confirm the diagnosis, a sample of skin may be gently scraped from the affected area, for examination under a microscope. The sample will be used to look for the mites, their eggs, and their feces. There are two ways to obtain the specimen. ① One or two drops of glycerol or mineral oil are applied to the suspicious area, which is then scraped several times with scalpel. The surface scrapings can be placed on a slide. ② The suspicious area could be sterilized by alcohol pad, the blister, papulovesicle or burrow can be punctured with syringe needle, the off-white punctiform can be placed on a slide. Drop some physiological saline on the slide, cover with cover slip and observe with a light microscope under low power.

6.5 Laboratory Tests of Pediculus Pubis

Microscopic examination of a nit or louse of *Pthirus pubis* may be undertaken if the diagnosis is uncertain. Lice and nits can be removed either with forceps or by cutting the infested hair with scissors (with the exception of an infestation of the eye area). The specimen can be fixation by ethanol solution 70% or formaldehyde solution 5%–10%, and then a magnifying glass or a stereo-microscope can be used for the exact identification. The presence of a single live louse is adequate for the diagnosis of active infestation. The presence of nits only does not necessarily indicate active infestation. The further observation for viable embryos should be examined microscopically.

▪ Summary

Besides clinical features, many laboratory tests can provide a dermatological diagnosis, or therapy monitoring. Knowing the indications and the meanings of the results will be useful for clinical dermatologists.

▪ Questions

1. Describe the common laboratory tests and their indications.
2. Describe 3 frequent laboratory tests of syphilis.

(**Liyuan Sun** 孙立元, **Xiaoyang Wang** 王晓阳, **Xiaoling Chu** 褚晓玲)

Chapter

7

Treatment of Skin Diseases and Sexually Transmitted Diseases

▪ Objectives

To master the kinds of systemic agents.

To master the knowledge of the principles of selecting topical agents.

To have an intimate knowledge of the pharmacological mechanism of antihistamines and glucocorticoids.

To have an intimate knowledge of the vehicles and kinds of topical agents.

To have an intimate knowledge of the physical treatment including electrotherapy, phototherapy, microwave therapy, cryotherapy, hydrotherapy, radiotherapy.

To have an intimate knowledge of the kinds of dermatologic surgery.

▪ Key concepts

Systemic therapies include a series of agents which can be given systemically by the form of oral medicine, intramuscular medicine or intravenous medicine. Take care of the side effects of glucocorticoids.

Topical therapies are used widely in treating skin diseases. Topical therapies involve the application of a topical agent on affected sites of skin. Topical agents are compounds of a main agent and a vehicle (base). The main agent acts on lesions, whereas the vehicle acts supplementarily to increase the absorption of the agent.

Electrotherapy, phototherapy, microwave therapy, cryotherapy, hydrotherapy and radiotherapy are common methods used to treat a variety of skin problems.

Dermatologic surgery is now a major component of dermatology, with an increasingly complex skill set and knowledge base required for contemporary practice.

Dermatologic surgery encompasses a wide variety of methods to remove or modify skin tissue for healthy or cosmetic benefit.

▪ Introduction

Dermatological treatments are largely divided into systemic therapies（oral administration of drugs，injections），external application of drugs，physical therapies，laser therapies and surgical therapies. Among these treatments, topical therapies are the most frequently used treatments in dermatology. Physical therapies，including irradiation and warming/cooling of affected sites，are also frequently applied. It is essential for dermatologists to have full knowledge of various therapies and combinations of effective treatments.

Topical agents more readily permeate places where the horny cell layer is thin，such as the face and scrotum，than places where the horny cell layer is thick，such as palms and soles. The absorption of a topical agent increases at a site where horny cell layer is injured by erosion，ulceration or the like. Oleaginous ointments are fairly slow to show effects on these types of lesions. A topical agent's absorption tends to increase with the duration of contact. This characteristic is taken advantage of occlusive therapy.

7.1　Systemic Treatment

7.1.1　Antihistamine Agents

Histamine，a chemical mediator released from mast cells，could cause a serials skin disorders. Antihistamine agents are drugs that could bind to histamine receptors to inhibit histamine's functions.

There are several types of antihistamine agents，including H_1 receptor inhibiting agents and H_2 receptor inhibiting agents. H_1 receptor inhibiting agents are the most effective in treating inflammational and allergic disorders and are widely used in treatments of dermatological diseases. The contraindications of antihistamine agents：patients with glaucoma and enlarged prostate should avoid taking antihistamines.

7.1.1.1　First-generation antihistamines

The effects of first-generation antihistamines include sedation，anticholinergic activity，local anesthesia，antiemetic activity，and anti-motion sickness effects. Of course，they have anti-inflammatory and antiallergic properties which are widely used to treat allergic dermatosis.

Side effects of first-generation antihistamines：first-generation antihistamines are also called sedating antihistamines. Therefore they might make patients feel sleepy，though this may improve after patients have been taking the medicine for a few days. Other side effects are included in Table 7 − 1.

7.1.1.2　Second-generation antihistamines

Second-generation antihistamines，such as loratadine，cetirizine，and fexofenadine，have a mild depressant action on the central nervous system and have a long serum half-life. Therefore they are also called non-sedating antihistamines. These agents have little sedative and anticholinergic side effects. They are less lipid-soluble，minimally cross the blood brain barrier，and preferentially bind to peripheral H_1 receptors. Therefore they are widely used in the treatment of allergy in recent years. The contraindications and usage of second-generation antihistamines are included in Table 7 − 2.

Table 7 − 1　First-generation antihistamines

First-generation antihistamines	Usage	Side effects
Chlorpheniramine	12 − 48 mg/d，tid 5 − 20 mg，im	Sedating Headaches Difficulty in passing urine Dry mouth Blurred vision Feeling sick or vomiting Constipation or diarrhea
Diphenhydramine	50 − 150 mg/d，tid 20 − 40 mg，im	
Doxepin	75 mg/d，tid	
Cyproheptadine	4 − 12 mg/d，tid	
Promethazine	50 mg/d，q6h 25 mg，im	
Ketotifen	2 mg/d，bid	

Table7 - 2 Second-generation antihistamines

Second-generation antihistamines	Usage	Contraindications
Astemizole	10 mg/d, qd	Patients with glaucoma and enlarged prostate
Fexofenadine	120 mg/d, bid	
Terfenadine	120 mg/d, bid	
Loratadine	10 mg/d, qd	
Cetirizine	10 mg/d, qd	
Mequitazine	10 - 20 mg/d, bid	
Acrivastine	8 - 24 mg/d, qd to tid	
Mizolastine	10 mg/d, qd	

7.1.2 Glucocorticoid

Corticosteroids afford anti-inflammatory and anti-immune effects. They are administered orally for long periods in serious connective tissue diseases (dermatomyositis, systemic lupus erythematosus, mixed connective tissue disease, eosinophilic fasciitis, relapsing polychondritis), blistering diseases (pemphigus, bullous pemphigoid, cicatricial pemphigoid, linear IgA bullous dermatosis, epidermolysis bullosa acquisita, herpes gestationis, erythema multiforme, toxic epidermal necrolysis), vasculitis, neutrophilic dermatosis, and type I reactive leprosy.

Short-term systemic uses of corticosteroids include: drug eruptions, auto-sensitization dermatitis, acute urticaria/angioedema, and severe dermatitis (contact dermatitis, atopic dermatitis, photodermatitis, exfoliative dermatitis, erythroderma).

The initial dosage of steroids is determined according to the severity of the disease. The dosage should be reduced gradually to a maintenance dose and then stop. Pulse therapy (500 mg to 1,000 mg of methylprednisolone intravenous injection per day for 3 successive days) should be performed if necessary. Various corticosteroids could take the same effects with different doses (Table 7 - 3).

Table 7 - 3 Various corticosteroids: comparison of the dose for the same effects

	Glucocorticoid	Dose needed for the same effect
Weak	Hydrocortisone	20
Mild	Prednisone	5
	Prednisolone	5
	Methylprednisolone	4
	Triamcinolone	4
Potent	Dexamethasone	0.75
	Betamethasone	0.5

Side-effects of corticosteroids: If patients have to take a high dose of oral or injected corticosteroids long-term, the following side-effects should be considered:

Central nervous system: Pseudotumor cerebri and psychiatric disorders.

Musculoskeletal: Osteoporosis with spontaneous fractures, aseptic necrosis of bone, and myopathy.

Ocular: Glaucoma and cataracts.

Gastrointestinal: Peptic ulceration, intestinal perforation, and pancreatitis.

Cardiovascular and fluid retention: Hypertension, sodium and fluid retention, hypokalemic alkalosis, and atherosclerosis.

Endocrinologic: Suppression of hypothalamic-pituitary axis (HPA), growth failure, and secondary amenorrhea.

Metabolic: Hyperglycemia and unmasking genetic predisposition to diabetes mellitus, nonketotic hyperosmolar states, and hyperlipidemia. Alterations of fat distribution (typical cushingoid appearance) and fatty infiltration of the liver.

Fibroblast inhibition: Inhibition of wound healing, subcutaneous tissue atrophy (striae, purpura, ecchymoses).

Immunosuppression: Effects on phagocyte kinetics and function and increased incidence of infections.

Other relatively mild side effects of corticosteroids include: moon face, central obesity, hyperphagia, leukocytosis, skin streaks, subcutaneous hemorrhage (purpura), steroid acne, and hypertrichosis.

7.1.3 Antibiotics

Antibiotics are used to treat cutaneous and subcutaneous infections, such as cellulitis and impetigo contagiosa. Serious acne and folliculitis are often treated by antibiotics, such as minocycline, penicillins, cephalosporins, and erythromycin are used to treat streptococcal and staphylococcal infections, and erythromycin for bacillary angiomatosis(Table 7 - 4).

Table 7 - 4   Common antibiotics and their indications

Antibiotics	Sensitive bacteria	Indications	Note
Phenoxymethylpenicillin (penicillin V)	Gram positive infections	Erysipelas	
Flucloxacillin	Infections due to penicillinase producing organisms	Impetigo and cellulitis	
Ampicillin	Broad spectrum		Destroyed by penicillinase
Cephalosporins	Gram positive and Gram negative infections		
Ciprofloxacin	Gram positive and Gram negative infections		
Erythromycin	Gram positive infections	Acne	Resistant strains of staphylococcus appeared
Metronidazole	Anaerobic infections and trichomonas infections	Rosacea	

We should pay attention to drug resistant. Some bacteria such as MRSA have been frequently found in community-acquired infections in recent years. In order to avoid the possible drug resistant, cultivation tests (on exudate, pus or the like) should be performed before administration of antibiotics. When antibiotics are not effective enough, the drug may be changed according to the results of laboratory culture test.

For patients with severe liver disorder or kidney dysfunction, the dosage and times of administration should be reviewed in consideration of the metabolic pathway of the drugs.

7. 1. 4 Antifungal Agents

Antifungal agents are used to treat fungal infections on skin and nail. They are also used to treat more serious fungal infections that can affect the tissues and organs, such as systemic candidiasis, pulmonary aspergillosis (infection of the lungs) and cryptococcal meningitis (infection of the brain).

Itraconazole, terbinafine and fluconazole are widely applied in many types of skin diseases, such as kerion celsi, sycosis trichophytica, or mycosis profunda. They have a broad antifungal spectrum, highly keratinophilic (drugs are known to concentrate in a skin lesion) and fewer side effects. Other antifungal agents, including potassium iodides, griseofulvin, amphotericin B, nystatin, flucytosine and miconazole, which have a narrow antifungal spectrum, and side effects, have not been used commonly.

For tinea unguium, pulse therapy of itraconazole (400 mg per day, 1 week per month for 4 cycles) is common used. Potassium iodide is only used to treat sporotrichosis.

The mechanism of antifungal agents: Some antifungals, such as amphotericin and terbinafine, work by killing the fungal cells. They may do this by interfering with the cell membrane (the outer layer of the cell), which causes the contents of the cell to leak out, or by producing toxic chemicals inside the fungal cells. Other antifungals, such as itraconazole and fluconazole, work by stopping the fungal cells from growing and multiplying.

7. 1. 5 Antiviral Agents

Antiviral agents are often used to treat skin diseases with viral infection. There are three types of medicines often used to treat viral infection, including aciclovir (valaciclovir, famciclovir and ganciclovir), ribavirin and ara-A (adenine arabinoside). They are effective against herpes viruses, including herpes simplex and varicella zoster. Aciclovir may be administered orally or by injection. Ganciclovir is effective against cytomegalovirus, and some kinds of anti-HIV drugs.

Adverse Effects: Acyclovir is generally well tolerated. The major toxicity caused by acyclovir is renal. It may be crystallized in renal tubules when it is administered with high dosage, dehydration, or rapid intravenous administration. Interstitial nephritis associated with acyclovir has also been reported.

7.1.6   Vitamins

Skin diseases caused by vitamin deficiency are aribo-flavinosis (vitamin B deficiency), pellagra (niacin deficiency), and biotin deficiency (vitamin H deficiency). Vitamin replacement therapy is administered.

Some vitamins are administered as second line drugs in the treatment of skin disorders.

Vitamin A is given in cases of keratinized diseases, such as ichthyosis, keratosis pilaris, and vitamin A deficiency.

Vitamin C is given in cases of allergic diseases, such as urticaria and eczema, melasma and post-inflammatory pigmentation.

Vitamin E is given to treat vascular diseases, pigmentation, and porphyria.

7.1.7   Retinoids

Retinoids are vitamin A derivatives. They control the proliferation and differentiation of epithelial tissues. Retinoic acid is a metabolite of vitamin A, including acitretin, isotretinoin and all-trans retinoic acid.

Vitamin A administration could increase the ex-foliation of the horny cell layer. Therefore retinoids are useful against various disorders of keratinization, such as ichthyosis, palmoplantar keratosis, Darier's disease and severe psoriasis.

Side effects and contraindications: Retinoids could cause teratogenesis and bone defects. Therefore patients are strictly advised to avoid pregnancy after the administration of retinoids within 2 years for women and 6 months for men. Other side effects are epidermal exfoliation, nail fragility, liver disorders and abnormal lipid metabolism.

7.1.8   Immunosuppressants

Immunosuppressants are often used to treat systemic lupus erythematosus (SLE), dermatomyositis, pemphigus, bullous pemphigoid and Behcet's disease. When it is difficult to reduce the steroid dosage, immunosuppressants may be used in combination with steroids. Azathioprines (AZP), methotrexates (MTX), cyclophosphamides (CTX), cyclosporine A (CsA) and tacrolimus are known to be immunosuppressants. Cyclosporines may be used alone in intractable psoriasis; however, they tend to cause dose-dependent kidney disorders and high blood pressure. Therefore, blood concentration monitoring is necessary when cyclosporines are administrated. The usages of immunosuppressants are included in Table 7 - 5.

Table 7 - 5   Usage of immunosuppressants

Immunosuppressants	Usage
Cyclophosphamides	2 - 3 mg/(kg · d), 10 - 14 days, total 6 - 8 g
Azathioprines	50 - 100 mg/d, increasing to 2.5 mg/(kg · d)
Methotrexates	5 - 10 mg/d, 1 - 2 times/week
Cyclosporine A	12 - 15 mg/(kg · d), decreasing to 5 - 10 mg/(kg · d)
Tacrolimus	0.3 mg/(kg · d), bid

7.1.9   Biologic (Molecular-targeted) Therapies

Biologic agents are including molecular-targeted agents and immuno-regulators. Molecular-targeted agents are monochrome antibodies such as infliximab, adalimumab, etanercept and alefacept. They have recently been used to treat lymphoma, collagen diseases, autoimmune bullous diseases and psoriasis. Immuno-regulators are including interferon (IFN), Bacillus Calmette-Guerin (BCG), transfer factor, thymosin, intravenous immunoglobulin (IVIG), which are used to treat eczema, vitiligo and some viral infectious diseases.

In contrast to immunosuppressants, biologics have less side effects. Therefore the widespread use of biologic therapies is expected in the future. However, we should pay attention to secondary infections such as tuberculosis. Tuberculosis and fever are the contraindication of biologic agents.

7. 2　**Topical Treatment**

7. 2. 1　*Vehicles for Topical Agents*

Vehicles help main agents permeate the skin. The agents have various actions, including hydration, cooling, lubrication, drying (removal of exudate), protection, softening, purification, and itch relief. A vehicle can be applied without a main agent in many cases. Vehicles should be non-stimulating, colorless and scentless, stable (non-denaturing), able to retain the main agent evenly, moderately viscous, appropriately firm, and moderately absorbable.

The same main agent may be mixed into various vehicles for various types of topical agents with different applications. Typical vehicles and their characteristics are listed below with brief explanations.

7. 2. 1. 1　Ointments

Ointments are the most frequently used topical agents. They are less stimulative than other vehicles and are highly protective.

They are transparent or translucent semisolids.

(1) Oleaginous ointments

Various oils such as olive oil, vaseline, paraffin, and plastibase are the most frequently used vehicles for oleaginous ointments. These ointments are free of water, absorb little water, and are insoluble in water. They are also called water-repellant ointments. The vehicle itself protects and softens the skin and works as an anti-inflammatory. Oleaginous ointments are the least stimulative, and are applied on all kinds of eruptions.

(2) Emulsified ointments

These are water-in-oil ointments containing emulsifiers such as polyethylene glycol. Because of the cooling sensation they bring with when applicated, emulsified ointments are commonly called cold creams. They are more protective and less sticky than creams (see below) and are easily washed off with water. They are mostly applied on dry lesions.

7. 2. 1. 2　Creams

Creams, also called oil-in-water emulsive vehicles, are semisolid mixtures of oil suspended in water containing emulsifiers. Creams are less sticky than ointments, and the color disappears when they are applied thinly (vanishing cream). Since they do not stain clothes, creams are readily accepted by patients, and the compliance with application is ensured. However, they may be irritating, and less

protective than ointments. Although creams are useful for erythema and papules, they should not be used on eroded or moist sites.

7. 2. 1. 3　Lotions

Lotions are liquids (usually water) with an agent mixed in. When applied topically, the liquid vaporizes, bringing cooling, astringent and protective effects. The agent remaining on the skin acts pharmacologically. In addition to water, the following are often used as liquid vehicles for lotions: alcohol, propylene glycol, glycerin, and zinc oxide oil (a 1 : 1 mixture of zinc oxide and olive oil). Some lotions require shaking prior to application. They are known as shake lotions.

(1) Emulsive lotions

Emulsive lotions are emulsions of oil in water. They are more permeable in skin than shake lotions (see below). They are used for non-moist lesions and are often applied on the hairy scalp.

(2) Shake lotions

Shake lotions are liquids with powdered agents mixed in. The powder settles, so these need to be shaken before use. When applied, a cool sensation is produced as the liquid evaporates; shake lotions are effective on lesions that are accompanied by fever and evaporable moisture, such as erythema and papules. They are unsuitable for intensely exudative lesions, such as erosions, because they may cause irritation.

(3) Other topical agents

Tinctures: agents dissolved in alcohol or in alcohol and water aerosols: vaporized liquid agents gels are transparent agents that are solid to semisolid. Gelatine is dissolved in water or acetone, yielding a gelatinous product.

7. 2. 1. 4　Gels

Gels are transparent agents that are solid to semisolid. Gelatine is dissolved in water or acetone, yielding a gelatinous product. After application, it dries to become a thin adhesive film on the skin. Gels with high solvent content are called jellies. These are used on mucous membranes to protect lesions from friction.

7. 2. 1. 5　Powders

The main ingredients of powders are zinc oxides, talc (magnesium silicate), and starches. Powders dry affected sites by absorbing moisture. They also cool the skin, reduce friction, and smooth the skin surface. They are effective in preventing miliaria and intertrigo.

7. 2. 1. 6 Liniments

Liniments are mixtures of water and zinc oxides, phenol or glycerin. They dry fast on the skin. They are effective in cooling the skin and relieving itching. Carbonic acid liniments are used for erythema and papules, for instance, varicella; however, they must be avoided for lesions with moist surface, because of their water solubility.

7. 2. 1. 7 Pastes

Pastes are highly viscous mixtures of oil-based substances and microparticles of powder. In this they resemble oleaginous ointments; however, pastes contain more powder than oleaginous ointments do.

7. 2. 1. 8 Plasters

Plasters are cloth, paper, or plastic film spread with topical agents. One example is 30% salicylic acid plaster. They are applied to lesions such as callus and clavus. Adhesive plasters containing steroids are also useful. Adhesive plasters with nitroglycerine or fentanyl are used for systemic administration in non-dermatological medical departments, utilizing the transdermal absorption of the skin.

7. 2. 1. 9 Other vehicles for topical agents

These include compresses, soaps, shampoos and bath additives.

7. 2. 2 Main Topical Agents

The main agents are the components that have therapeutic effects on skin. Frequently used agents are listed below.

7. 2. 2. 1 Corticosteroids (steroid)

The main purpose of steroid topical application is to fight inflammation. Vasoconstriction, diminution of membrane permeability, liberation and inhibition of inflammatory chemical mediators, arachidonic acid reduction by phospholipase inhibition, immunosuppression, and cell division inhibition combine to inhibit inflammation.

Steroids for topical application are classified by strength: strongest, very strong, strong, mild and weak.

Steroid topical application may have side effects. Particular care should be taken in facial application, because of the high absorptiveness of the skin there. As long as the dosage and usage of steroids are appropriate, systemic side effects are rare. However, when strong steroids are applied on a large area for a long period or when they are used in occlusive therapy, side effects similar to those caused by steroid systemic administration may be produced. More-over, special care should be taken in administering steroids to infants, since the effects tend to be systemic. Topical corticosteroids induce and aggravate cutaneous atrophy, striae atrophy, telangiectasia, purpura, hypertrichosis, steroid acne, rosacea-like dermatitis and infectious diseases (tinea incognito and candidiasis in particular).

7. 2. 2. 2 Immunosuppressants

Tacrolimus (FK-506: molecular weight = 822Da), a topical calcineurin inhibitor, selectively inhibits T-cell functions, making it effective against atopic dermatitis as an immunosuppressant. It is also useful as a treatment for chronic actinic dermatitis and lichen planus.

7. 2. 2. 3 Antifungal agents

Various types of topical antifungal agents, such as those containing imidazole, benzylamine or morpholine, are used. They act by attaching to the cellular walls of fungi and inhibiting biosynthesis. These agents are used topically (as creams, lotions, or ointments) for superficial mycosis; however, they may be used orally for tinea unguium and deep fungal infections.

7. 2. 2. 4 Antibiotics

Topical agents containing antibiotics are used against superficial bacterial infections. Antibiotics should be effectively antibacterial against the targeted bacteria and have transdermal sensitization capability. Macrolide or new quinolone antibiotics are effective against folliculitis, including acne vulgaris. As antibiotic resistance among bacteria has been increased in recent years, ointments containing antibiotics are not always effective in treating superficial infectious diseases.

7. 2. 2. 5 Vitamin D analogues

Activated vitamin D_3 is used to treat hyperkeratotic and proliferative diseases such as psoriasis, ichthyosis, and palmoplantar keratosis, because of its ability to induce differentiation of the epidermis and antiproliferation. It is the first choice of treatment for psoriasis. Nevertheless, a prolonged large dosage of activated vitamin D_3 may lead to hypercalcemia; the dosage should be carefully decided.

7. 2. 2. 6 Urea

Urea is used as a moisturizer for its water retentivity. Hydrophilic ointments containing 10% to 20% urea are frequently used to treat senile xerosis, ichthyosis, palmoplantar keratosis, keratodermia tylodes palmaris progressiva, and atopic dermatitis. Urea may produce irritation on cracked or moist sites.

7. 2. 2. 7 Zinc oxide

Zinc oxide is frequently used not only as a vehicle but also a main agent for its actions of desiccation, astringency, anti-itching, cooling, and radiation blocking.

7. 2. 2. 8 Sulfur, resorcinol

Sulfur and resorcinol are antibacterials and antifungals with keratin-exfoliating action. They are effective on treating acne vulgaris.

7. 2. 2. 9 Salicylic acid

Salicylic acid is keratolytic and is used to treat keratoderma in the soles. A plaster containing 30% to 40% salicylic acid is used to soften and remove callosity and clavus.

7. 2. 2. 10 Phenol

Phenol has anti-itching and antibacterial effects. Because of its corrosive effect, it may also be used in treating verruca vulgaris and ingrown nails, and for chemical peeling.

7. 2. 2. 11 Tars

Tars such as coal tar, wood tar and Pityrolum have been applied topically for moist eruptions and lichenified lesions. Because of peculiar odor, color, and their carcinogenicity, they are rarely used now. Tars may also cause photosensitive diseases. As tars have a cellular antiproliferative effect, they have been used in the past in combination with ultraviolet rays (UVB) against psoriasis, this treatment is called Goeckerman therapy.

7. 2. 2. 12 Other agents

Antihistamines, retinoids (isotretinoin and adapalene), antitumor drugs, sunscreen, psoralen, vitamins, sex hormones, and nonsteroidal anti-inflammatory drugs (NSAIDs) are used as topical agents.

7. 2. 3 Application

Topical agents are applied as described below. Care should be paid in the application of agents for which there are restrictions on dosage and frequency. For agents whose dosage is not specified, it is necessary to determine the daily dosage for each patient.

Direct application: A topical agent is applied directly for a skin lesion. This is the most common application method.

Plaster: A cloth spread with the agent is applied to a lesion. It is effective in removing crusts and protecting erosions and ulcers.

Occlusive dressing therapy (ODT): A topical agent is directly applied, and the site is tightly sealed with polyethylene film. Steroid adhesive plasters are sold commercially. They are useful for treating infiltration, acanthosis, lichenified plaques, and hyperkeratosis. However, ODT is much more absorptive than other topical agents; therefore, the patient should be monitored for side effects such as systemic symptoms.

Chemical and mineral bath: Chemicals and minerals are dissolved in warm water, for systemic or topical soaking. The bath may also be used for disinfecting burns. Hot spring water is rich in minerals and has a thermo-therapeutic effect. In UV therapy, the patient is radiated with UV rays after a chemical bath of psoralen (PUVA-bath therapy).

7.3 Physical Treatment

7. 3. 1 Electrotherapy

7. 3. 1. 1 Electrolysis

Electrolysis is used to destroy living skin tissues by means of an electric current applied with a needle-shaped electrode. It is one of ways of removing telangiectasia and individual hairs from the face or body. Electrolysis is very safe. Sometimes, a slight reddening of the skin occurs during or immediately after treatment, but this will only last for a short time.

7. 3. 1. 2 Electrodesiccation

Electrodesiccation is a method to desiccate skin tissue by dehydration. It is used to destroy skin cancerous tissue and control bleeding. A highly or moderately damped alternating electrical current is radiated through a monoterminal active electrode that is applied directly to the lesion, the procedure of electrodesiccation is performed under local anesthesia. It is primarily used for eliminating small superficial growths in the skin, such as verruca vulgaris, pyogenic granuloma, et al.

7. 3. 1. 3 Electrocoagulation

Electrocoagulation is the therapeutic use of a high-frequency electric current to bring about the skin tissue coagulation and destruction. The electrical energy generates heat to destroy tissue by coagulation necrosis in the deep and big skin lesion, it is usually used to destroy the warts and skin tumors.

7. 3. 1. 4 Electrocautery

Electrocautery is used to destruct skin tissue by tips, which temperature can be adjusted by controllable power output of the machine. A variety of tips are available according to the clinical needs. It is usually used to treat warts and other benign skin neoplasma.

7.3.2   Phototherapy

7.3.2.1   Infrared ray therapy

Infrared ray is a ray of infrared radiation which produces a thermal effect. Infrared radiation is used to relieve pain, increase circulation to a particular area of the skin, promote inflammation subsided and tissue repair. It can be used to treat skin infection, chronic skin ulcer, frostbite, erythema multiforme and scleroderma.

7.3.2.2   Ultraviolet light therapy

Ultraviolet ray is an invisible band of radiation at the upper end of the visible light spectrum. According to wavelengths, it could be divided into ultraviolet A(UVA, wavelength from 320 to 400 nm), ultraviolet B(UVB, wavelength from 280 to 320 nm), and ultraviolet C(UVC, wavelength from 180 to 280 nm). UV light treatment can employ one of two bands of the ultraviolet spectrum: UVA and UVB. Another new development in UV therapy is the use of a laser as the source of the UVB radiation. The type of laser that is used is known as a 308 - nm excimer laser, which uses a specific mixture of gases to produce high-intensity, short pulses of UVB light. It can be used alone or in combination with other medications to treat psoriasis and a variety of other skin diseases, such as vitiligo, atopic dermatitis. UVB phototherapy usually does not require additional medications or topical preparations. The intensity of the UV applied will depend on the patient's skin type. A small area of skin will first be exposed to UVB to determine the minimum erythema dose (MED), MED is the minimum amount of UVB that produces redness 24 hours after exposure. It is better to reach the "sub-erythemic dose" (SED) in treatment, which is the maximum amount of UVB your skin can receive without burning.

Side-effects may include itching and redness of the skin due to UVA exposure, it can also cause cataracts and other eye damage, so the patient's eyes must be adequately shielded during the treatments. Cataracts can frequently develop if the eyes are not protected from UVB light exposure.

7.3.2.3   Photochemotherapy

PUVA is the exposure to UVA light while the skin is hyper-photosensitive by taking psoralens, which is an effective treatment for some skin diseases such as psoriasis. Psoralens are photosensitizing agents, which can be taken systemically or can be applied topically to the skin. The psoralens allow a relatively lower dose of UVA to be used. PUVA is a treatment for psoriasis, vitiligo, mycosis fungoides, alopecia and atopic eczema, et al. The reason of clearing psoriasis remains unclear, it is speculated that there may be effects on cell turnover and the skin's immune response.

In PUVA treatments, the 8 - methoxypsoralen (8 - MOP) is usually taken two hour before the treatment with the dosage of 0.6mg/kg. Or 0.5 - 1 hours before the treatment with 0.1%- 0.5% topical 8 - MOP. Choosing the proper dose for PUVA is very important. A small area of the patient's skin will be exposed to UVA after ingestion of a psoralen to decide the minimum phototoxic dose (MPD), 0.3 - 0.5 times of MPD becomes the starting dose for treatment, generally 0.5 - 1 J/cm^2. And it will gradually increase over time. Typical treatment regimes involve PUVA therapy 3 times a week.

The psoralen is applied or taken orally to sensitize the skin. Patients who receive psoralens must take care to avoid exposure to sunlight, Long term use has been associated with higher rates of skin cancer. Some patients may experience nausea and itching after ingesting the psoralen, for these patients, topical psoralens use may be a good option. Due to the potential damage to the liver caused by psoralens, PUVA may be used only a limited number of times over a patient's lifetime.

7.3.2.4   Photodynamic therapy

Photodynamic therapy (PDT) is a treatment for skin cancer such as basal cell carcinoma (BCC), et al, and also being used for treatment of genital warts and acne.

PDT is involving three key components: a photosensitizer, light, and tissue oxygen. Photosensitizers may be chosen which are selectively absorbed at a greater rate by targeted cells. Photosensitizer precursor, aminolevulinic acid (ALA) is the most common used, it is taken up much more rapidly by metabolically active cells. ALA will be converted by the cells to protoporphyrin IX, which is a photosensitizer. After 3 - 4 hours, bright red light is delivered on the area to be treated. A photosensitizer can be excited by light of a specific wavelength. When the photosensitizer and an oxygen molecule are in proximity, an energy transfer can take place that allows the photosensitizer create an excited singlet state oxygen molecule. Singlet oxygen is a very aggressive chemical species and will kill cells through apoptosis or necrosis.

Since malignant cells tend to be growing and dividing much more quickly than healthy cells, the ALA targets the unhealthy cells, within a few days, the exposed skin and carcinoma will scab over and flake away.

7. 3. 2. 5　Laser

Laser has the characteristics of monochromaticity, coherence and collimation. Since the theory of selective photothermolysis was postulated in 1983, a various of new laser technology has been applied to skin disorders treatment and cosmetic surgery. Major advances in laser technology have expanded their use in the treatment of many skin conditions, including vascular and pigmented lesions, and the removal of tattoos, scars and wrinkles. In recent years there is a wide spectrum of laser and light technologies available for skin resurfacing and rejuvenation.

The operator and patient should wear appropriate protection for the eyes (dense filter spectacles) in case of accidental or reflected exposure, and the laser beam should never be directed at the eyes. Laser treatments are basically burns, the major adverse effects include temporary pain, redness, bruising, blistering, crusting, pigment changes (brown and white marks) and scarring. Some pigment changes may be permanent but scarring is luckily rare.

The uses of laser are described as following:

(1) CO_2 laser surgery

Skin disorder treated with photothermal excision and ablation, a number of skin disease have been treated by CO_2 laser, including periungual and plantar warts, genital warts, benign skin neoplasma.

(2) Laser physical treatment

Certain wavelengths of light at certain intensities delivered by laser will aid tissue regeneration, resolve inflammation, relieve pain and boost the immune system.

(3) Treatment of vascular lesions

Oxyhemoglobin was used in treatment of vascular lesions, which has its main absorption peaks at 418, 542, and 577 nm, the most common used laser devices are Nd; YAG laser (532 nm), pulsed-dye lasers (585 –600 nm) and the alexandrite laser (755 nm). They are used to treat hemangiomas, port-wine stains, telangiectases and leg veins.

(4) Treatment of pigmentary disorders and tattoos

Melanin in the skin was used to treat pigmented lesion which absorbs light in the ultraviolet – 1200 nm range. The most common used devices are Q-switch Nd; YAG laser (1046 nm) and frequency-doubled Nd; YAG laser (532 nm)

(5) remove of hair

The mechanism for light assisted hair reduction remains incompletely understood. Light is probably absorbed by melanin in the hair shaft and matrix. Follicles in early anagen are thought to be most susceptible to laser treatment. The most common use devices are the normal ruby laser (694 nm), alexandrite laser (755 nm), diode laser (800 nm) and Nd; YAG laser (1046 nm).

7. 3. 3　*Microwave Therapy*

Microwave is an electromagnetic wave with a wavelength between that of infrared and short waves (one millimeter to one meter). Microwave device could be used to destroy skin tissue by dielectric heating, which accomplished by using microwave radiation to heat polarized molecules within the tissue. Microwave treatment could be used to treat warts and benign skin neoplasma.

7. 3. 4　*Cryotherapy*

Cryotherapy is a medical treatment in which skin lesion is subjected to cold temperatures and causes cell death. The mechanism of cell death caused by cryotherapy include: ice crystals formed in cell damage cellular components, osmotic difference arising causes cell disruption. Small blood vessels injury results in ischemic damage, immunological stimulation produced by releasing of antigenic component.

The common used cryogens include liquid nitrogen(– 196℃) and carbon dioxide snow(– 79℃). The former is the most widely used cryotherapy agent. Liquid nitrogen can be applied using cotton-wool swab or liquid nitrogen spray. After cryotherapy, tissue swelling is common, then blisters may occur, pain is usually transient. Hypopigmentation or hyperpigmentation is common after liquid nitrogen cryotherapy.

Cryotherapy has been used to a wide range of skin lesions, such as varies of warts, pyogenic granuloma, keloid and benign skin neoplasma.

7. 3. 5　*Hydrotherapy*

Hydrotherapy is the treatment of certain skin diseases by the external use of water, especially by warm water and drug to treat some skin diseases such as psoriasis, eczema, pruritus, et al. It could be also used in order to mobilize stiff joints or strengthen weakened muscles. The common materials used in hydrotherapy include starch, mineral water, Potassium permanganate and Chinese medicine, et al.

7.3.6 Radiotherapy

Radiotherapy is the treatment of skin disease with radiation, especially by selective irradiation with X-rays or other ionizing radiation. Radiation therapy works by damaging the DNA of cells. The most common used radiotherapy sources are X-ray and electron beam. Radiotherapy could be used to treat skin cancer which is in critical sites, particularly around eyes, ears and nose. Radio therapy is used much less in the management of benign skin conditions than formerly, the keloid is the most common benign skin condition now treated with radiotherapy.

7.4 Surgical Treatment

The acquisition of basic dermatological surgery skills is an important component of dermatological training. This section covers simple excisional surgery and provides an introduction to more advanced techniques.

Dermatologic Surgery encompasses a wide variety of methods to remove or modify skin tissue for healthy or cosmetic benefit. These methods provide high-quality, cost-effective skin surgery and include scalpel surgery, laser surgery, chemical surgery, cryosurgery (liquid nitrogen), electrosurgery, aspiration surgery, liposuction, injection of filler substances, and Mohs micrographic controlled surgery (a special technique for the removal of growths, especially skin cancers). The skin is susceptible to many diseases, discolorations, and growths. It may also be damaged by excessive exposure to the sun and the effects of aging. In most cases, skin problems requiring dermatologic surgery can be addressed in the dermatologist's office or in an outpatient setting, usually under local anesthesia, with minimal pain, and low risk of complications.

7.4.1 Indications for Skin Surgery
To establish a definite diagnosis(a skin biopsy).

To remove benign and malignant skin growths that may interfere with the body's normal function,

or may cause symptoms such as pain, itching, or bleeding.

To improve the skin's cosmetic appearance by removing growths, discolorations, or skin damage caused by aging, sunlight, or disease.

7.4.2 Removal Methods
Treatment options for removal of malignant or benign growths include:

7.4.2.1 Biopsy

Removing a piece of the skin for examination under the microscope for diagnosis.

7.4.2.2 Curettage and electrodesiccation

Scraping away malignant or benign growths with a sharp surgical instrument called a curette. An electrosurgical unit may be used to stop bleeding (cauterize).

7.4.2.3 Surgical excision

Cutting into the skin, removing the growth, and closing the wound with stitches.

7.4.2.4 Cryosurgery

Applying or spraying liquid nitrogen onto the skin to freeze and destroy the tissue.

7.4.2.5 Laser surgery

Destroying skin growths or breaking blood vessels by modifying tissue with powerful light waves.

7.4.2.6 Mohs micrographic controlled surgery

Removing a tumor and examining the tissue under the microscope to determine the extent of malignant cells before more tissue is removed. While the procedure is time-consuming, it yields a very high cure rate and conserves as much normal tissue as possible. It is used for large or aggressive tumors and tumors located in areas of high risk for recurrence, such as on and around the nose.

7.4.2.7 Photodynamic therapy

Applying a chemical called aminolevulinic acid to the skin and exposing the skin to a special light source.

7.4.2.8 Topical chemotherapy

Applying a chemical such as 5 – fluorouracil, diclofenac sodium, or imiquimod to destroy pre-cancerous growths and some cancerous lesions.

7.4.2.9 Radiation therapy

Using X-rays to destroy tissue in certain types of skin cancer, as well as in selected individuals for whom surgery is not possible.

7.4.2.10 Dermabrasion

Removing the outer layers of skin and softening irregular edges. After the skin is frozen with a spray medication, a high-speed, rotary abrasive wheel is used.

Tumescent liposuction: Removing and recontouring the body of excess fat with little blood loss and exceptional safety.

▪ Summary

Dermatological treatments are largely divided into external application of drugs, systemic therapies (oral administration of drugs, injections), physical therapies, laser therapies and surgical therapies. Among these treatments, topical therapies are the most frequently used treatments in dermatology. Physical therapies, including irradiation and warming/cooling of affected sites, are also frequently applied. It is essential for dermatologists to have full knowledge of various therapies and combinations of effective treatments.

▪ Questions

1. What are the usually used therapies for treating skin diseases?

2. What are the side effects of glucocorticoids?

3. What's the pharmacological mechanism of antihistamine?

4. What are the often used vehicles for topical agents?

5. How to choose topical agents?

6. What is Photodynamic therapy (PDT)?

7. What kinds of skin conditions are suitable for laser treatment?

8. What are the main kinds of dermatological surgery?

(**Shaowei Cheng** 程少为,**Fang Liu** 刘方,
Wenhui Lun 伦文辉,**Yanling He** 何焱玲)

Chapter

8

Skin Care and Cosmetic Dermatology

▪ Objectives

To master the knowledge of the skin care and cosmetic dermatology.

To have an intimate knowledge of characteristics of four skin types and technological approaches in skin-rejuvenation therapies.

▪ Key concepts

Skin aging is a natural process, but scientific and effective skin care can delay skin aging. Skin type classification is the basis of skin care, skin care products and approaches should be based on skin types.

▪ Introduction

Cosmetic dermatology, a branch of medical cosmetology, is a combination of dermatology and cosmetology. In recent years, advances in cosmetic approaches have drastically improved aesthetic treatment for skin. Non-surgical methods have become the majority of cosmetic procedures performed in china.

8. 1   Skin Care

Ageing, a basic biological process seen in all living creatures, is not preventable. Intrinsic, environmental, and lifestyle factors contribute to the pace of skin aging. Skin is the body's largest organ and the mirror of the internal organs. If the body functions well, the skin will look radiant and remain healthy. Many skin and hair disorders reflect some system disturbance within the body. Everything from hormonal imbalance, immune deficiency, to gastric disease can affect skin. Topical treatment and cosmetics can be very dramatic but the body functions as a whole complete complex unit which includes the skin.

8. 1. 1 *Characteristics of Healthy Skin*

Skin is one of the most powerful indicators of health. Skin color, texture, moisture, and elasticity all are signs of internal health.

8. 1. 1. 1　Skin color

There are three types of pigments in the normal skin that affect its color: melanin, hemoglobin and carotene. Homogeneity and distribution of skin color across the face contributes to perceptions of health, age, and attractiveness of human faces.

(1) Melanin

In humans, melanin is the primary determinant of skin color. Health benefits of melanin include providing protection from harmful UV radiation, reducing the incidence of skin cancer and sunburn, and reducing the photolysis of folate. Melanin also plays a role in immune defense in humans.

(2) Hemoglobin

When hemoglobin is combined with oxygen, a bright redness is formed, and this in turn results in the rosy complexion associated with good health in humans. A reduced concentration of hemoglobin gives the skin a bluish appearance. Physiologically relevant cues of increased skin blood perfusion and oxygenated hemoglobin enhance the healthy appearance of faces.

(3) Carotene

Carotenoid is obtained from consumption of fruits and vegetables, and dietary supplements and it causes yellowish discoloration of the skin. Carotenoid supplementation is associated with improved development of the immune system in human.

8. 1. 1. 2　Texture

Dermal collagen fiber bundles are the major constructional element in the dermis. Skin texture is formed by contraction of the dermal collagen fiber bundles. Compared with normal skin, photoaged skin is rough, and exhibits deep wrinkles and lichenification.

8. 1. 1. 3　Moisture

Skin needs moisture to stay smooth and supple. In general, healthy skin retains an appendage called sebum cutaneum that covers the skin with oily secretion. The less sebum cutaneum secretes, the weaker water-holding capacity of the skin is. Simple routine activities, such as showering, may remove sebum from the skin. Therefore, retaining moisture becomes difficulty as we age.

8. 1. 1. 4　Elasticity

The ability of skin to stretch and then return to its original state afterwards is called elasticity. Water content and adipose layer thickness determine the elasticity of the skin.

8. 1. 2 *Skin Type*

Skin type is determined by water content, sebum content, PH value and reactivity to external allergens.

8. 1. 2. 1　Dry skin

Dry skin feels tight, especially after cleansing. Dry skin has a tendency to develop fine wrinkles, flaking and red patches. Characteristic signs of dry skin occur when the water loss exceeds the water replacement, and water content of stratum corneum falls below 10% and pH of which is greater than 6. 5.

8. 1. 2. 2　Oily skin

Oily skin tends to look shiny with enlarged pores, and is prone to acnes and blemishes, because of excessive oil secretion from the sebaceous glands. The stratum corneum's water content is approximately 20% and pH is lower than 4. 5.

8. 1. 2. 3　Normal skin

Normal skin type has medium-sized pores, a smooth and even texture, good circulation and healthy-looking color. Normal skin has an adequate amount of water and lipids and a moderate sensitivity level.

8. 1. 2. 4　Combination skin

Combination skin means a blend of oily and dry skin. This skin type may tend to be dry on the cheeks while oily in the T-zone. Combination skin is the most common type of skin.

8. 1. 2. 5　Sensitive skin

Sensitive skin tends to be thin-layered and delicate with fine pores. It flushes easily and is prone to broken capillaries, frequently allergic and can be prone to rashes. Sensitive skin shows continuous hyperactivity to environmental factors and exhibits a reduced tolerance to frequent or prolonged use of cosmetics. The skin suffers discomfort such as itching, burning and stinging. These conditions are becoming even more pronounced after exposure to dry and cold climates. Sensitivity can also increase with age.

8. 1. 3 *Skincare Regimen*

While we cannot stop or even slow down the intrinsic aging process, we can prevent signs of premature aging by protecting our skin from the sun, quitting smoking, and so on. We should start taking care of skin when we are young and make it a habit.

8.1.3.1 Emotion and mood

There is an intimate relationship between inner health and external beauty. Anxiety, fear, and stress may cause darkening of the skin while peace of mind helps maintaining the healthy appearance of facial skin.

8.1.3.2 Adequate sleep

Adequate sleep will refresh your skin and your mind as well. 7 – 8 hours of restful sleep is essential for good healthy skin.

8.1.3.3 Healthy diet

A healthy diet (plenty of green vegetables and fresh fruits) can improve skin texture and quality. Vegetables and fruits that are rich of vitamin C and vitamin E, all of which are very good for skin because they reduce wrinkles and fine lines. Besides vitamins, minerals and other nutrients can give skin a more radiant, healthy glow. Cigarette smoking causes biochemical changes in our body that result in deeply wrinkled, leathery complexion. These signs can be diminished by stopping smoking.

8.1.3.4 Skin massage

Skin massage helps blood circulation, which carries away wastes and helps keep skin clear and healthy looking.

8.1.3.5 Facial cleaning

Wash your face with warm water and facial cleanser. A gentle facial cleaner will help to remove dull skin cells and reveal radiance. However, excessive washing or chemical content of water draws moisture from the skin.

8.1.3.6 Prevention of photoaging

Intrinsic aging is an irreversible and inevitable process that occurs with the passage of time. It is characterized by cellular senescence and decreased proliferative capacity and gene mutations. Extrinsic aging is the result of exposure to environmental factors, primarily ultraviolet irradiation. Without protection from the solar rays, just a few minutes of exposure each day over the years can cause noticeable changes to the skin. Freckles, spots and leathery skin are associated with sun exposures. Repeated UV exposure breaks down collagen and impairs the synthesis of new collagen. UV rays also attack another important content of extracellular matrix, elastin. Therefore, sunscreen cream is recommended to be applied all year round. Broad spectrum sunscreen (SPF of 30 or higher) should be applied 30 minutes before going outdoors and should be reapplied after sweating.

8.2 Cosmetic Dermatology

Skin is the largest and outmost organ of human body. The same with the other organs, skin will age gradually over time. The signs of aging skin include the loss of elasticity and flexibility of the dermis, as well as wrinkles and the thinning of the epidermis. Skin aging has been defined as the accumulation of molecular damages over time, caused by both intrinsic and extrinsic factors. Intrinsic aging (natural aging) process is a continuous process that normally begins in our mid-20s. The accumulation of damages provoked by environmental factors (e.g. exposure to sunlight) can be defined as extrinsic aging. We will give an account of technological approaches in skin-rejuvenation therapies.

8.2.1 Laser and Light Based Technologies

There has been a significant progress in clinical application of laser and light based technologies in aesthetic dermatology in recent years. Laser with wavelength of 510 nm and 532 nm are used for treatment of pigment disorders in epidermis, such as freckle, seborrheic keratosis. Laser with wavelength of 1064 nm is used for treatment of pigment disorders in dermis, such as nevus of ota. Laser with wavelength of 694 nm and 755 nm are used for treatment of pigment disorders between epidermis and dermis. Laser with wavelength of 595 nm is used for treatment of nevus flammeus and facial telangiectasia. Semiconductor laser is used for depilation. A noncoherent, broadband, intense pulsed light(IPL) source is being used for the symptoms of photoaging skin as a nonablative method. IPL is used for treatment of fine wrinkles, telangiectasia, acne, rosacea, pachylosis and pigmented stain. Radio frequency (RF) is electromagnetic radiation in the frequency range of 3 to 300 Hz. The primary effects of RF energy on living tissue are considered to be thermal. RF has been used successfully for nonablative skin rejuvenation, atrophic scar revision and vascular lesions and inflammatory acne.

8.2.2 Photodynamic Treatments

Photodynamic treatments are another group of promising therapies for acne, photoaging, non-melanoma skin cancers and condyloma acuminatum. The application of porphyrin cream to the skin followed by illumination of blue or red light activates the drug and inhibits cells in the skin.

8. 2. 3　Chemical Peel

Chemical peel uses a chemical solution to improve and smoothen the texture of the facial skin by removing its damaged outer layers. In this treatment, a caustic chemical agent is applied on the surface of skin lesion. Skin damages are cured after local epidermis or dermis is corroded. Commonly used corrosive chemicals are trichloroacetic acid and phenol. Chemical peels can help adult acne blemishes, wrinkles, freckle, seborrheic keratosis, xanthelasma palpebrarum and sun-damage.

8. 2. 4　Dermal Filler and Cosmetic Botulinum Toxin Injections

Soft-tissue augmentation of the face is an increasingly popular cosmetic procedure. Patients in different age groups have diverse treatment needs ranging from the correction of fine lines and wrinkles in younger patients to volume restoration in older patients. In recent years, the most popular fillers are those made from cross-linked hyaluronic acid (HA), collagen, calcium hydroxylapatite, and injectable poly-L-lactic acid to improve facial volume changes and contour irregularities. Botulinum toxin is a neurotoxin produced by the bacterium *Clostridium botulinum*. The cosmetological applications include correction of lines, creases and wrinkling all over the face, chin, neck, and chest to dermatological applications such as hyperhidrosis.

8. 2. 5　Aesthetic Surgery

The surgical and aesthetic branch of dermatology has undergone a complete transformation in recent years. Mohs micrographic surgery is now a well-known and established modality for the treatment of various skin cancers, deformity and defects. There are various other aesthetic procedures, such as brow-lift, blepharoplasty, lateral canthoplasty, midface-lift, rhytidectomy, cheek augmentation, lip vermillion advancement, hair removal, fat removal and mentoplasty.

▪ Summary

Skin is the body's largest organ and the body's natural protective cover. Healthy and beautiful skin is not only able to complete a variety of complex physiological functions, but also an important aesthetic feature. As people's living standards rise, people have increasingly strong demand for beauty. Therefore, the discussion on skin care and cosmetic dermatology is of particular importance.

▪ Questions

1. Describe the characteristics of four skin types.
2. Describe technological approaches in skin-rejuvenation therapies.

(**Hui Chen** 陈慧, **Wei Zhu** 朱威)

Chapter 9

Viral Skin Diseases

▪ Objectives

To grasp the knowledge of the causes and clinical features of viral skin diseases.

To understand the knowledge of the diagnosis and management of viral skin diseases.

▪ Key concepts

Viral skin diseases are caused by viruses.

Herpes simplex is a viral disease caused by both Herpes simplex virus type 1 (HSV-1)and type 2 (HSV-2).

A wart is generally a small, rough growth, typically on a human's hands or feet but often other locations. They are caused by human papilloma virus(HPV).

Molluscum contagiosum (MC) is caused by a DNA poxvirus called the molluscum contagiosum virus(MCV).

HFMD (hand-foot-mouth disease) is a contagious viral illness that commonly affects infants and children.

▪ Introduction

Viral skin diseases are mucocutaneous lesions caused by virus. Different viruses have different organization tropisms, such as herpes virus causing herpes zoster due to the characteristics of epidermal and neurotropic, human papilloma virus addicted to skin, which can cause all kinds of warts, and the pan-tropic measles virus causing skin lesions in addition to extensive tissue damage. Skin lesions caused by different viruses have big differences, which can be presented as a new vegetation type(such as a variety of warts), herpes type(such as herpes simplex)and red rash type(such as measles).

9.1   Herpes Simplex

Herpes simplex is caused by herpes simplex virus(HSV), clusters of painful inflamed papules and vesicles are often seen on the mucosa or skin. The infection is self-limited but apt to recurrence.

9.1.1 Etiology

HSV is a double-stranded DNA virus of two major types: HSV-1 and HSV-2. HSV has a genome size of 150 kbp, and codes for about 80 proteins. It has an almost universal distribution. Transmission occurs through mucous membranes or small cracks in the skin when a susceptible person has direct physical contact with an infected individual. These infections are asymptomatic in up to 90% of patients. HSV carriers can transmit virus asymptomatically. HSV-1 is mostly responsible for herpes labialis and herpetic gingivostomatitis, HSV-2 is usually associated with herpes genitalis.

HSV enters through small defects in skin or mucosa and starts to replicate locally; then ascends via axons to sensory ganglia where further replication occurs. After the primary infection, HSV becomes latent in the sensory ganglia.

Virus could be reactivated by various trigger factors (physical trauma, UV light, fever, systemic infections) as well as local or systemic immunosuppression, which leads to spreading of the virus into area served by the sensory ganglia and thus to the recurrent herpetic lesion.

9.1.2 Clinical Features

Primary infection with HSV is often asymptomatic. Both HSV-1 and HSV-2 infections have similar clinical manifestations that most commonly develop on skin and mucosa junction. The Incubation period is about 6 – 8 days. The severity of the lesions in primary infection is generally greater than that in recurrences. Usually, erythematous macules or patches are preceded by a day or two of local prodrome of unlikable feeling, where clusters of small blisters occur (Color Figure 9 – 1). These blisters change into superficial ulcers with crusts. The lesions are accompanied by severe pain and tender lymphadenopathy. Most lesions heal within 1 to 2 weeks without leaving scars. High fever and pustules may indicate bacterial infections.

(1) Herpetic gingivostomatitis

Herpetic gingivostomatitis is the most common clinical type of primary infection with HSV-1. It is most often seen in early childhood. Small painful vesicles appear on pharyngeal and oral mucosa, soon ulcerate, and increase in number to involve buccal mucosa, tongue, soft palate, floor of mouth, lips and cheeks. Primary infection may be accompanied with systemic symptoms, involving fever, headache and lymphadenopathy. Patients may have trouble with eating.

Infection at other cutaneous sites.

(2) Herpetic whitlow

HSV infection of the fingers may be develop from primary oral or genital herpes by autoinoculation, or may occur through occupational exposure. Edema, erythema and local tenderness of the infected finger appear. Lesions at the finger tip may be confused with suppurative bacterial paronychias.

(3) Eczema herpeticum

HSV infection of the skin is much more severe in patients with pre-existing skin lesions including eczema, burns, or other blistering skin diseases. HSV infection may become disseminated.

(4) Genital herpes: See "Genital Herpes"

(5) Neonatal herpes simplex

Majority of cases are caused by HSV-2, and often acquired by vaginal delivery of infected mother. Incubation is 4 – 7 days usually. Neonatal HSV infection may occur as lesions on the skin, eye, and mouth, or as encephalitis or disseminated splanchnic infection. Congenital infection may be accompanied with jaundice, hepatosplenomegaly, disseminated intravascular coagulation, encephalitis and seizures with or without mucocutaneous lesions. Without treatment, visceral infection has a high mortality.

9.1.3 Diagnosis and Differential Diagnosis

Diagnosis is made mainly depending on the typical clinical presentations. Change in specific antibody titer can be used to diagnose primary infection but not to recurrent lesions. A cytological smear of the base of the vesicle, looking for giant cells and inclusion bodies, is helpful.

The differential diagnosis can be any of the following: herpes zoster, chicken pox and impetigo. Cutaneous HSV infection may be confused with herpes zoster, although herpes zoster is usually easy to diagnose by its typical unilateral dermatomal distribution.

9.1.4 Treatment

9.1.4.1 Antiviral therapy

(1) Primary mucocutaneous infection

Acyclovir 200 mg 5 times daily need to be given orally for 7 to 10 days from the onset. If patients have difficulty in swallowing, intravenous acyclovir (5 mg/kg 8 hourly)may need to be given. Famciclovir 250 mg 3 times daily or valaciclovir 500 mg twice daily are alternatives.

Symptomatic reactivation of mucocutaneous infection.

The same dosage as above for primary infection can be given for 5 days.

(2) Long-term suppressive therapy

This can be considered in patients who have frequent reactivation episodes (more than six occurrences per year). A dose of acyclovir 400 mg twice daily remarkably reduces the frequency of viral attacks.

(3) Neonatal herpes simplex

Intravenous acyclovir[30 – 60 mg/(kg • d)]need to be given for 10 to 21 days.

9. 1. 4. 2   General measures

Cleansing mouthwashes with benzalkonium bromide 1 : 1000 clean the involved mucous membranes. Apply topical antibacterials such as mupirocin or povidone-iodine ointment to prevent bacterial superinfection.

9.2   Herpes Zoster

Shingles(herpes zoster) is caused by the varicella-zoster virus(VZV), which is characterized by small blisters clusters along the peripheral nerve in zonal distribution by unilateral side, often accompanied by significant neuralgia.

9.2.1   Etiology

VZV has been named human herpes virus 3(HHV-3), a brick-shaped virus, three-dimensional symmetry capsid, containing double-stranded DNA molecule, only one serotype. VZV resistance in vitro is weak and quickly loses activity in the dry callus.

Human is the only host of VZV. The virus may enter blood through the respiratory tract mucosa to form viremia, presented by chicken pox or talent infection, then the virus can become latent in the spinal cord root ganglia or nerve sensory ganglion; After certain stimuli such as trauma, fatigue, cancer, or weakness after illness which may decrease the host immune response, the latent virus is activated resulting in downstream along the sensory nerve axon, to reach the region dominated by the nerve and replicate locally, resulting in blisters, and the nerve is involved reducing inflammation, necrosis, accompanied by neuropathic pain. Obtained lasting immunity after

recovering from the disease, preventing recurrence.

9.2.2   Clinical Features

The disease often occurs in adults, the incidence increasing as age increasing significantly.

9. 2. 2. 1   A typical manifestation

Mild fatigue, fever, anorexia and other systemic symptoms are the earliest symptoms, soon followed by skin lesions. Skin burning or burning conscious, touch-sensitive obvious pain in the affected area, persisting for 1 – 5 days, or without any prodromal symptom. Intercostal nerve, cervical nerve, the trigeminal nerve and sacral nerve area are often involved. The lesion often appears erythema, soon to form soybean size miliary papules by clustered distribution without fusion, becoming blisters quickly, shiny blister filled with clear fluid, peripheral around to flush; Lesions are in zonal distribution along the peripheral nerve, just occurring in unilateral side, generally do not exceeding the midline(Color Figure 9 – 2). One of the characteristics-based disease neuralgia may occur before and during the onset of lesions, often more severe in elderly patients. The course of the disease often lasts for 2 – 3 weeks, 3 – 4 weeks among the elderly, leaving a temporary redness or pigmentation.

9. 2. 2. 2   Special performance

(1) Eye shingles(herpes zoster ophthalmicus)

The ophthalmic of the trigeminal nerve are involved, common in the elderly, severe pain, the cornea can result in formation of ulcerative keratitis.

(2) Ear shingles(herpes zoster oticus)

The facial nerve and hearing nerve are involved, manifested by herpes in ear canal or tympanic membrane. Geniculate ganglion of facial nerve are involved while violating the motor and sensory nerve fibers, which may result in facial paralysis, earache, and ear canal triad of herpes, known as the Ramsay-Hunt syndrome.

(3) Post-therapeatic neuralgia(PHN)

Before, during or after herpes zoster, often accompanied by nerve pain, called as zoster-associated pain(ZAP), if the pain persists for more than 4 weeks after the skin lesions heal, which is known as PHN.

(4) Others

According to the different resistance, the clinical types are classified into frustrated type(only neuralgia without rash), incompetence type(only erythema, papules without blisters), bullous type, blood type, gangrene type and the Pan-onset type(more than 2 ganglions are involved), the virus spread through blood into the lung, brain and other organs, known as disseminated herpes zoster.

9.2.3 Diagnosis and Differential Diagnosis

The disease can be diagnosed based on typical clinical presentation, multinucleated giant cells and intranuclear inclusions in blister fluid. PCR detection of VZV DNA and viral culture contribute to the diagnosis.

Herpes zoster should be differentiated from intercostal neuralgia, pleurisy, appendicitis, sciatica, urinary tract stones, migraine, cholecystitis during the prodromal stage or among the patients without rash. Sometimes this disease should be differentiated from herpes simplex infection and impetigo.

9.2.4 Prevention and Treatment

The disease is self-limited, the principles of therapy including anti-viral, pain relief, anti-inflammatory and preventing complications.

9.2.4.1 Drug therapy

(1) Antiviral drugs

Early, adequate antiviral therapy, especially in patients over 50 years old, used to relieve the nerve pain and shorten the course. Rash usually occurs within 48 – 72 hours after starting antiviral therapy. Acyclovir 800 mg, orally, 5 times daily; or valaciclovir 1000 mg, orally, 3 times a day; or famciclovir 250 mg, 3 times a day orally. Course of treatment is 7 days.

(2) Pain relief

Indomethacin and neurotrophic drugs, such as oral or intramuscular vitamin B_1, B_{12} can be applied.

(3) Corticosteroids

Studies of the benefits of corticosteroid therapy together with acyclovir in the treatment of shingles have given conflicting results. Early and rational application can inhibit inflammatory process and shorten the course of acute phase of herpes related pain, but efficacy for prevention of PHN is not as definitive. Prednisone 30 – 40 mg/d should be taken during 7 days post-infection in elderly patients without other related diseases, for 7 – 10 days orally.

9.2.4.2 Topical therapies

(1) Drug for external use

Calamine lotion, acyclovir cream or penciclovir cream are given for patients without broken blister; 3% boric acid solution or 1:5000 nitrofurazone solution can be chosen with broken blister.

(2) Eye care

3% acyclovir eye ointment or iodine monophosphate eye drops topically, glucocorticoid preparations are forbidden.

9.2.4.3 Physical therapy

The pain can be relieved by using of therapy such as ultraviolet light, spectrum therapy, infrared or local irradiation to facilitate making the blisters dry up.

9.3 Warts

Warts are new benign growths on the skin and mucous membrane, caused by viruses from the HPV family. Four types of warts including verruca vulgaris, verruca plantaris, verruca plana and genital wart are common in clinical practice. Verrucous epidermal dysplasia has a close relationship with HPV infection.

9.3.1 Etiology

The source of infection may be patients and healthy carriers of the pathogens. The disease is transmitted primarily by direct or indirect contact. Through the broken skin and tiny abrasion in the mucosa, HPV enter and replicate inside the cell, inducing abnormal differentiation and proliferation of epithelial cells, causing benign epithelial neoplasms. The general population is susceptible, with the peak age of 16 to 30 years old. Immunocompromised patients and those who experience trauma are easy to suffer from this disease.

9.3.2 Clinical Features

9.3.2.1 Verruca vulgaris

Verruca vulgaris commonly occur in the back of the hand, fingers, feet and skin around nails, and other parts of the body. A typical lesion size is like soybean or larger, grayish brown, brown or skin colored papules, with a rough surface, hard texture, and may presented as papilloma hyperplasia. The lesion around the nails is called periungual wart, beneath the nail plate called subungual wart. Wart with protruding thin filaments on the top is called verrucal filiformis, often occurring on the neck, forehead and eyelids. Wart with irregular surface is called digitate wart, commonly occurring in the hair and toes(Color Figure 9 – 3).

9.3.2.2 Verruca plantaris

Verruca plantaris commonly occur on the sole of the foot. Early lesions are like small shiny papules, then gradually grow up to a size of soybean and form pale yellow or brown flat-surfaced corpus callosum-like papules or plaques under pressure, with a round or oval shape, and a rough hard surface surrounded by a slightly protruding keratin ring. After removing the layer of stratum corneum, keratinal soft core can be seen, with black dots formed by capillary bleeding.

The lesion containing several soft cores is called mosaic wart. The patients may feel pain or have no symptoms (Color Figure 9 – 4).

9.3.2.3　Verruca plana

Typical lesions are flat-topped elevations with the size from rice to soybeans, in a round or oval shape, smooth surface, hard texture, normal color or light brown. Most of the lesions may suddenly appear, with large number and concentrated distribution. The lesions can be arranged in a string of beads after scratching, which is called self-inoculation response (Color Figure 9 – 5).

9.3.2.4　Genital warts

Genital warts also called condyloma acuminatum (see Chapter 27).

9.3.3　Histopathology
The common features are characterized by vacuolization of cells in granular layer and spinous layer and virus particles in nuclear under electron microscope.

9.3.4　Diagnosis and Differential Diagnosis
The disease can be diagnosed by history and typical skin lesions, if necessary, combined with pathological examination, HPV DNA test is required in a few patients for diagnosis.

9.3.5　Treatment
The most effective treatment is topical medications and physical therapy. Internal medication is suitable to a large number of lesions and patients fails to a long-term treatment.

9.3.5.1　Topical medication

(1) 0.05% – 0.1% Vitamin A acid cream or adapalene cream, administered topically 1 or 2 times per day for flat wart.

(2) 5 – fluorouracil ointment, 1 or 2 times per day for external use, used with caution in the face due to pigmentation.

(3) Bleomycin 10mg with 1% procaine dilution 20ml injected in the wart root, 0.2 – 0.5 ml each wart, once per week for refractory common warts

and plantar warts.

9.3.5.2　Physical therapy

Including freezing, electrocautery, curettage, and laser surgery, which are suitable to treat small lesions.

9.3.5.3　Internal medication

There are no specific anti-HPV drugs. Immunomodulatory agents (such as interferon, levamisole) can be tried. Traditional Chinese medicine may get better effects in some patients.

9.4　Molluscum Contagiosum

Molluscum contagiosum is a contagious skin disease caused by molluscum contagiosum virus (MCV) infections.

9.4.1　Etiology
MCV is a pox virus, the most common type is MCV-1. Almost all children patients are caused by the MCV-1 type, however, approximately 60% immunocompromised persons (especially HIV infection) are caused by MCV-2. Close contact is the main routine of transmission, which can also be transmitted through sex or indirectly routine in swimming pools and other public facilities.

9.4.2　Clinical Features
The disease mostly occurs in children, the sexual active population and immunocompromised persons. Incubation period is 1 week to half a year. Lesions can occur in any part of the back, limbs, trunk or face among children. In adult patients through sexual contact, the rash can be found in the genitals, buttocks, lower abdomen, pubic or thigh medial and so on. A typical lesion is a hemispherical papules in 3 – 5 mm size, pearl gray, the wax-like luster, umbilical concave (see figure), cream cheese-like substance that contains molluscum bodies.

9.4.3　Diagnosis and Differential Diagnosis
The disease can be diagnosed based on typical clinical manifestations, if necessary, combined with pathological examination. Sometimes the disease should be differentiated from keratoacanthoma and basal cell carcinoma.

9.4.4　Prevention and Treatment
Scratching usually should be avoided to prevent the spread of this disease. Clothes and towels should not be shared in kindergarten.

Therapy topically such as Victoria A acid ointment or cantharidin can be used. Removing molluscum bodies using curved forceps in sterile conditions is very effective and topical iodine to prevent bacterial infection. Topical mupirocin ointment is given for the patients with bacterial co-infection.

9.5 Hand,Foot and Mouth Disease

HFMD(hand,foot,and mouth disease)is a viral skin disease characterized by blisters occurring in hand, foot and mouth, mainly in children. The disease is mainly transmitted through the fecal-oral route. It can also be spread by droplets through the respiratory tract. The virus can be isolated from the blister fluid,pharyngeal secretions and feces.

9.5.1 Etiology
The disease is related with Coxsackie virus.

9.5.2 Clinical features
The disease is commonly seen in children under 5 years. Incubation period ranges from 3 to 7 days. Fever, headache, anorexia and other prodromal symptoms may occur before 1 to 3 days of red spots appear on the hand,foot and mouth,which develop into 2 – 4 mm blisters with thin wall and clear liquid,surrounded by a pink areola. Pale erosion surface or shallow ulcers occur after rupture of the blisters. Sometimes only the mouth or the hands are involved. The lesions heal within a week and the recurrences are rare(Color Figure 9 – 6).

9.5.3 Diagnosis and Differential Diagnosis
The diagnosis is confirmed by the characteristic skin lesions occurring on the hand,foot,mouth and other parts, and epidemiological history. The disease should be differentiated from erythema multiforme, herpes pharyngitis and chicken pox,etc.

9.5.4 Prevention and treatment
The patients should be isolated to prevent the spread of the disease in nursery. Supportive and symptomatic measures are needed. Ulcer plaster can be used for dental damage,and topical lidocaine mouthwash can be used to ease mucosal pain.

■ Summary

Herpes Simplex is an infection caused by the virus called herpes simplex virus. It usually occurs as small painful vesicles in clusters on skin or mucosa. The lesions can be self-limited. Recurrent infections are common. Depending on the typical manifestations, clinically diagnosis can be made. Treatment is with acyclovir, valacyclovir,or famciclovir.

Warts are small benign growths on the skin and mucous membrane,caused by viruses of the Human papilloma virus(HPV)family. There are four types of warts classified by affected sites and clinical features. Diagnosis depends on clinical features. The effective treatment is topical medicines.

HFMD is a viral skin disease caused by the Coxsackie virus which is characterized by blisters occurring in hand,foot and mouth, mainly in children. It can be diagnosed according to characteristic skin lesions and epidemiological history. Only symptomatic measures are available.

■ Questions

1. What is the clinical feature of herpes simplex and how to diagnose and treat it?

2. What is the clinical feature of herpes zoster and how to manage it?

3. What is the cause of all kinds of warts and how to treat it?

4. What is the cause of molluscum contagiosum and how to treat it?

5. What is the cause of hand-foot-mouth disease and how to treat it?

(**Yingxue Song** 宋映雪,**Xiaojie Huang** 黄晓婕)

Chapter 10

Bacterial Infectious Diseases

▪ Objectives

To master the knowledge of the cause, typing, clinical manifestation, diagnosis and treatment of impetigo.

To have an intimate knowledge of way of infection in impetigo.

To master the knowledge of the cause, clinical manifestation, diagnosis and treatment of erysipelas.

To have an intimate knowledge of provocative factors and predilection locations of erysipelas.

To handle the knowledge of the clinical features of tuberculosis of the skin, how to diagnosis and heal the disease.

To have an intimate knowledge of patterns of tuberculosis of the skin.

To have an intimate knowledge of patterns of leprosy.

▪ Key concepts

Impetigo is a purulent skin infection characterized by pustules and purulent crusts. Folliculitis and furunculosis are bacterial inflammatory diseases involving follicles and perifollicular tissues. Erysipelas is an acute hemolytic streptococcal infection of the skin involving the superficial dermal lymphatics.

Tuberculosis of the skin is a chronic skin disease caused by *Mycobacterium tuberculosis* (*M. tuberculosis*). Lesions appear in normal skin as a result of direct extension of adjacent tuberculous focus, of hematogenous or lymphatic spread; they can also be caused by an infection of the mucous membranes from minor injuries.

Lesions of cutaneous TB demonstrate typical histopathologic characteristics of tuberculosis. "Morning, full dosage, rule, affiliation and to apply antituberculosis drugs in the whole range" is the principle.

Leprosy is a chronic infectious disease caused by *Mycobacterium leprae*, principally affecting peripheral nerves and skin.

Diagnosis should be made prudently and comprehensively on the basis of the medical history, clinical manifestation, smear test and pathological examination of the patient. Defining signs of leprosy are included.

10.1 Impetigo

Impetigo, prone to epidemic infection among children, is transmitted by contact and autoinoculation.

10.1.1 Etiology

The most frequent cause of infection is coagulase-positive *Staphylococcus aureus*, secondarily *Streptococcus hemolyticus* or a combination of both pathogens.

10.1.2 Clinical Features

Impetigo is divided into four types according to clinical manifestation.

10.1.2.1 Impetigo contagiosa

Impetigo contagiosa occurs most frequently on the face, mouth and nose in early childhood. The typical lesion presents as a cluster of thin-walled pustules with peripheral erythema. Then the pustules rupture and leave red moist surface that dry to form golden-yellow crusts (Color Figure 10 – 1). The lesion can spread to trunk and limbs by self-inoculation after scratching. Constitutional symptoms are not universal but rare including swelling of lymph nodes, fever, septicemia and nephritis.

10.1.2.2 Bullous impetigo

The variety of impetigo is caused by phage type 71 group Ⅱ *Staphylococcus aureus*, occurring most in child. The lesion is about 1 – cm discrete pustules in which there is half-moon pus. As the wall of pustules is thin, these pustules are liable to rupture and become erosions or crusts. Bullous impetigo, occurring characteristically in newborn infants is called neonatal type bullous impetigo, which is highly contagious and develops rapidly. The disease presents as multiple, generalized, large, purulent bullae, surrounded by erythema, which rupture to red erosions. Nikolsky sign is positive. Constitutional symptoms with fever and other infectious toxic manifestations are common. Septicemia and pneumonia may be present, with fatal termination.

10.1.2.3 Ecthyma

Ecthyma is an ulcerative impetigo caused by *Streptococcus hemolyticus* and a rare disease, which typically occurs in primarily malnourished children and elders and most commonly shins and hips. Ecthyma begins with a vesicopustule, which enlarges to become erythematous necrosis covered with oyster shell-like black thick crust. When the crust is removed, there is a saucer-shaped ulcer with elevated edge and pain. The lesions may be solitary or multiple and leave scars after healing. Regional adenopathy may be present.

10.1.2.4 Staphylococcal Scalded Skin Syndrome

Staphylococcal scalded skin syndrome (SSSS) occurs most commonly in neonates and is due to the exfoliative exotoxin elaborated by coagulase-positive phage type 71 group Ⅱ *Staphylococcus aureus*. The disease begins abruptly with haematose erythema around mouth, which spread to the whole body after 24 – 48 hours. On the erythema there present as flabby bullae. Nikolsky sign is positive. Bullae quickly exfoliate and leave fresh erosion like scalded skin. Large sheets of desquamated epidermis are seen on hands and soles. Constitutional symptoms present as fever, anorexia and vomiting etc. SSSS sometimes complicates with septicemia and cellulitis, whose mortality rate is high.

10.1.3 Laboratory Test

The number of leukocytes and neutrophil leukocytes in SSSS are more than normal. When the pus is cultured, *Staphylococcus aureus* or *Streptococcus hemolyticus* can be obtained.

10.1.4 Diagnosis and Differential Diagnosis

Diagnosis can be made easily according to clinical manifestations and bacteriology tests. Impetigo contagiosa must be differentiated from popular urticaria and varicella. SSSS should be differentiated from non-staphylococcal toxic epidermal necrolysis (TEN).

10.1.5 Treatment

The patient should be insulated and treated in time to avoid other infections. Keeping skin clean, bathing frequently and improvement of nutrition condition are as prophylactic measure in high-risk persons against impetigo. Topical therapy is advised primarily, however systemic therapy is applied only when clinical disease is severe.

10.1.5.1 Topical therapy

The basic principle of topical therapy is sterilization, anti-inflammatory and dryness. Lotion is applied to the non-ruptured pustules and solution to the ruptured pustules. Applying mupirocin or erythromycin ointment to the lesion is effective. In SSSS, eyes, mouths and perineums are emphatically nursed.

10. 1. 5. 2 Systemic therapy

Applying antibiotics in time is indicated in cases with diffused lesions and severe constitutional symptoms. The preferred antibiotics is penicillinase-resistant penicillin or cephalexin, if necessary antibiotics directed according to the susceptibility of the recovered organism.

10. 2 Folliculitis and Furunculosis

Folliculitis and furunculosis are bacterial inflammatory diseases involving follicles and perifollicular tissues. Folliculitis locates the infection in follicles; however, furunculosis invades the tissues around and under follicles.

10. 2. 1 Etiology

The pathogen is mainly coagulase-positive *Staphylococcus aureus*, rarely *S. epidermis*, *streptococcus*, *pseudomonas*, *escherichia coli* etc. sole or combined. The predisposing factors include hot, sweaty, scratching, poor sanitation, systemic illnesses such as diabetes, organ transplantation, and long-time application of glucocorticoid.

10. 2. 2 Clinical Features

10. 2. 2. 1 Folliculitis

Folliculitis occurs most frequently in scalp, face, neck, hip and vulvae. The lesion begins with red papules in hair follicles. In a day or two, pinhead-sized pustules develop on the central papules. After these rupture, there leave yellow crusts which desquamate without scars. The rashes are multiple and non-confluent with light itching, tender, no constitutional symptoms. In general, symptoms that folliculitis occurs in different body parts are named with different terminologies. Specifically, folliculitis decalvans occurs in scalp, healed with alopecia and scars; Folliculitis vulgaris occurs in the bearded region; Folliculitis keloidalis nuchae occurs in the neck with papillary hyperplasia and forming scars and scleromas.

10. 2. 2. 2 Furunculosis

The favorite locations are the scalp, face, neck and hip. The initial lesion is inflammatory papule in hair follicles with infiltrated fundus, which develops into hard, heat, tender, red, swelling nodule. Several days later the central becomes soft with fluctuation

and yellow-white head, forming abscess. After it ruptures, the lesion discharges purulent, necrotic debris, leaving ulcer and healing gradually. Regional adenopathy may appear (Color Figure10 - 2). Constitutional symptoms present as fever, even seriously bacteremia or septicemia. Furunculosis is always solitary, however, when the lesion is multiple, recurrent and refractory, it is called chronic furunculosis, which is usually caused by immunodeficiency with underlying illnesses such as diabetes, nephropathy and tumor.

10. 2. 3 Laboratory Test

The pathogen may be discovered by the smear of the pus following Gram stain. In addition, the pus can be cultured to take the identification and drug sensitivity test.

10. 2. 4 Diagnosis and Differential Diagnosis

Diagnosis of folliculitis depends on the inflammatory papules and pustules in hair follicles. Furunculosis is diagnosed by the deep nodule in hair follicle, central purulent core accompanied with redness, swelling, heat and tender.

10. 2. 5 Treatment

Routine precautions include keeping skin clean, avoiding trauma and enhancing immunity etc. Topical treatment is indicated chiefly. Multiple folliculitis and severe chronic furunculosis are suggested systemic therapy.

10. 2. 5. 1 Topical therapy

Primitive follicle and furunculosis are treated with one of those topical drugs: ichthammol ointment 20%, iodine tincture 3% - 5%, mupirocin and neomycin 5%. Ruptured terminal diseases should be cut and drained.

10. 2. 5. 2 Systemic therapy

Penicillin, cephalexin, macrolides or quinolones is recommended. Sometimes antibiotics directly according to the susceptibility to the recovered organism is needed. Physical therapies are also adviced, such as ultrashort wave, far infrared ray, or ultraviolet ray. It is necessary for chronic furunculosis to confirm the underlying illness or predisposing factors and administer immunomodulators.

10. 3 Erysipelas

Erysipelas is an acute skin infection involving the dermal lymphatics. The pathogen invades skin or membrane through tiny trauma to cause infection.

10. 3. 1 *Etiology*

Erysipelas is induced by group A *beta-hemolytic streptococcus*. The predisposing factors are nose infection, digging nose dung, picking ears, tinea pedis and chronic eczema. The provocative factors are those immunocompromised illnesses: diabetes, chronic liver disease, undernourishment. The causative organism always hides inside lymphatics, which results in erysipelas recurrence.

10. 3. 2 *Clinical Features*

Dorsum pedis, legs and face are the most frequent site affected. Erysipelas occurs acutely and usually unilateral. The distinctive lesion is sharply defined, brawny, swollen erythema with hot to the touch, pain. Erysipelas may be accompanied by a constitutional reaction with enlargement of adjacent lymph nodes, chills, tenderness and high fever. Secondary septicemia can occur in the infants, aged and weaklings. Pathogenetic conditions achieve the peak at the fourth or fifth day from the onset and leave slight pigmentation and desquamation after the lesions fade away.

The skin lesions may be divided into several types by different clinical features. The eruption begins at erythematous patch and develops into blisters, bullae or pustules, which is separately called erysipelas blistosum, erysipelas bullosum, erysipelas pustulosum. The eruption invades subcutaneous tissue and results in gangrene, which is called gangrenous erysipelas. The eruption is extending on one side as vanishing on other side, which is called erysipelas ambulans. The eruption relapses many times, which is called recurrent erysipelas. Recurrent erysipelas in lower limbs causes obstruction of lymphatic channels of the skin and lymphedema. The final result is a permanent hypertrophic fibrosis or elephantiasis nostras(Color Figure 10 – 3).

10. 3. 3 *Laboratory Test*

There is an increase in the number of leukocyte, mainly neutrophilic leukocyte in which shifting to the left and toxic granulation can be discovered.

10. 3. 4 *Diagnosis and Differential Diagnosis*

Erysipelas can be recognized not difficultly by the predilection site, acute onset, sharply defined edematous erythema with accompanied symptoms of pain, fever and increase of blood leukocyte. It may be differentiated from contact dermatitis, erysipeloid, and dermatophytid.

10. 3. 5 *Treatment*

Predisposing factors of recurrent erysipelas should be found as soon as possible and taken active treatment to the factors. Treatment is mainly on systemic therapy, secondarily on topical therapy.

The basic principle of systemic therapy is to use antibiotics with nonage, full dose, and high performance. Systemic application of penicillin is first advised, which is administered in the usual dose of 4 800 000 – 8 000 000 U/d in intravenous transfusion. The general condition will improve in 2 – 3 days, but resolution of the cutaneous lesion may require two weeks in order to prevent recurrence. Erythromycin or quinolones can be adopted if the patient is hypersensitive to penicillin.

Furacillin solution or berberine solution is hydropathic compressed on ruptured lesions and mupirocin ointment on the non-ruptured lesions. Physical therapy such as ultrashort wave, far infrared ray, ultraviolet ray or soundfrequency electrotherapy is advised. Suppurated lesion should be cut and drained.

10. 4 Tuberculosis of the Skin

Tuberculosis of the skin is a chronic skin disease caused by *Mycobacterium tuberculosis* (M. *tuberculosis*).

10. 4. 1 *Etiology*

Tuberculosis of the skin is caused by *Mycobacterium tuberculosis* (human tuberculosis and bovine tuberculosis). Its sources of infection can be exogenous and endogenous. For the former, the bacillus enters the skin through abrasions and minor injuries; for the latter, the tuberculosis existing in certain body organ or tissue spread to the skin through hematogenous or lymphatic system.

10. 4. 2 *Clinical Features*

10. 4. 2. 1 Major categories

There are four major categories of tuberculosis of the skin:

(1) Inoculation forms an exogenous source (such us tuberculosis verrucosa cutis, primary inoculation tuberculosis).

(2) Endogenous cutaneous spreads contiguously

or by autoinoculation(such us scrofuloderma, tuberculosis cutis or oncialis).

(3) Hematogenous spreads to the skin(lupus vulgaris, acute miliary tuberculosis).

(4) Tuberculids(lichen scrofulosorum, papulonecrotic tuberculid, erythema induratum).

10.4.2.2　Clinical features of major categories of tuberculosis of the skin

(1) Lupus vulgaris(LV)

LV is the most common form of tuberculosis of the skin, taking up $50\%-75\%$ of all cases, and commonly occurs among children or adolescents. LV lesions mainly occur on the head and neck, particularly around the nose; they also occur on the buttocks and exposed skin of extremities. LV typically is single plaque composed of grouped soft, red-brown papules, whose appearance on diascopy, have a pale brownish yellow or "apple-jelly" color. LV lesions usually sharply marginated. The edges of the lesion tend to heal slowly in one area and progress in another. They diffused in the infiltrated dermis, expanding by the development of new plaques at the periphery, which coalesce with the main plaque, and often are covered by adherent scales, and causes ulceration. Reappearance of new nodules within previously atrophic or scarred lesions is characteristic. The disease is chronic and slowly spreads peripherally over the years. Patients usually do not feel pain or itchy as the disease develops(Color Figure 10-4).

(2) Tuberculosis verrucosa cutis

Tuberculosis verrucosa cutis is a less common form of tuberculosis of the skin, taking up about $4\%-5\%$ of all cases, and commonly occurs among adult males(70.8%). It occurs from exogenous inoculation of bacilli into the skin, and mostly occurs on trauma-sites. Lesions mostly occur on the dorsa of the hands, and fingers in adults, and then feet, ankles and buttocks are involved. The lesion usually starts as a small, purplish, red or brown, indurated, warty papule, which becomes hyperkeratotic. It enlarges by peripheral expansion, resembling a wart. Fissuring of the surface may occur, discharging purulent exudate. The lesion may show central involution with a white atrophic scar, or the whole lesion may form a massive papillary excrescence covered with adherent crusts or superficial ulcers. The lesions are persistent for many years(Color Figure 10-5).

10.4.2.3　Laboratory examination

(1) Histopathology

The common characteristic of tuberculosis of the skin is clumped epithelioid and multinucleated giant cell forming typical tubercles with caseation-like necrosis within it.

(2) Purified protein derivative(PPD)

A positive test can result from clinical or latent tuberculosis infection or vaccinate bacille Calmette-Guerin(BCG).

(3) Microphytology

Direct smear or tissue sections help to find *Mycobacterium tuberculosis* and diagnose.

10.4.3　Diagnosis and Differential Diagnosis

According to clinical features, histopathology of tuberculosis of the skin, normally it is not very difficult to diagnose.

(1) Lupus vulgaris must be differentiated from a number of other diseases such as discoid lupus erythematosus, nodular syphilid and tuberculoid leprosy.

(2) Tuberculosis verrucosa cutis must be differentiated from verrucous naevus and chromomycosis.

10.4.4　Treatment

Give patient active treatment to treat the tuberculose focus on the other part, at the same time, to have an inoculation of bacille Calmette-Guerin is the key to prevent tuberculoderma. The basic principle of therapy is applying systemic antituberculosis on a timely, full dosage, and regular medication. Standard triple antituberculosis therapy should be given for 6 months at least.

10.4.4.1　System therapy

(1) Isoniazid, 300 mg daily.

(2) Ethambutol, dosage 15 mg/kg body weight daily or 750 mg daily.

(3) Pyrazinamide, 15-30 mg/kg, up to 2 g daily for 2 months.

(4) Rifampin: 450-600 mg daily.

10.4.4.2　Topical therapy

Ointment of $5\%-20\%$ pyrogallic acid is effective for the treatment of lupus vulgaris and tuberculosis verrucosa cutis. Skin lesions that show an impact on the patient can be removed by surgery.

10.5 Leprosy

Leprosy is a chronic infectious disease caused by *Mycobacterium leprae* (*M. Leprae*), principally affecting peripheral nerves and skin. Leprosy patients are the natural hosts of *M. Leprae* and the only source of infection for leprosy. *M. Leprae* spreads mainly from person to person in respiratory droplets. It is also likely to be transmitted by close contact with a leprosy patient. Men are different in their susceptibility to *M. Leprae*; men's resistance to the bacillus usually grows as they get older. Leprosy occurs mainly in Asia, Africa and Latin America.

10.5.1　Etiology

Mycobacterium leprae is a Gram-positive(G^+) bacterium, $2-6$ μm in length and $0.2-0.6$ μm in width. In size and shape, it is a rod-shaped or slightly curved bacillus with no flagella, capsules and spores. The acid-fast stain of *M. leprae* is red. *M. Leprae* demonstrates a strong resistance to the external environment. It can live in vitro for $2-9$ days in secretions in dry air, or $3-4$ weeks under 0 ℃; but it may lose fertility if boiled for 8 minutes or exposed to direct sunlight for $2-3$ hours.

10.5.2　Clinical Features

The disease is classified into five types: early and indeterminate leprosy, tuberculoid leprosy, lepromatous leprosy, lepra reaction, and histopathology.

10.5.2.1　Early and indeterminate leprosy

The onset of leprosy is insidious usually. The disease is not recognized because of the prodromal symptoms are generally so light until the appearance of a lesion. The lesion is solitary or more hypopigmented or erythematous macules, without or with defined margins. Such lesions are most commonly to occur on the cheek, extensor surface of the arms, thighs, buttocks or trunk. Sensory functions are minimally altered or normal. Peripheral nerves are not enlarged. Lepromin test reveals positive or negative. In addition, indeterminate leprosy has not been classified into the five-classified type, which type of leprosy they may progress to depends on their immune status. Indeterminate leprosy can autotherapy.

10.5.2.2　Tuberculoid leprosy(TT)

The lesions are few in number, often solitary, and are likely to occur on the face, limbs, or trunk. The typical lesion is the large, erythematous plaque with well-defined elevated border and flattened atrophic center. The surface is dry, hairless, insensitive, and sometimes scaly. Superficial peripheral nerves proximal to the lesion may be enlarged and thickened. Loss of sensation may occur at site of

some lesions; patients in the late stage of the disease may suffer from muscular paralysis in the form of "clawed hand", "dropped foot" and "Lagophthalmos" (eyes cannot be closed). The skin smears of TT patients are negative. The lepromin test is strong positive in advanced stage. There is often remission may result sooner with treatment, or spontaneous remission of the lesions (Color Figure $10-6$).

10.5.2.3　Lepromatous Leprosy(LL)

This type of leprosy may be evolved from downgrading of the BB or BL type or develop following indeterminate leprosy. Lesions are numerous, widespread and symmetrical, with numerous bacilli in them. There is a negative reaction to lepromin. The cutaneous lesions mainly consist of pale lepromatous macules or infiltrations, causing patients to have "leonine facies" in some cases. The plaques are pale and smooth with ill-defined borders, and may appear red, reddish yellow or brown. Loss of eyebrow hair may occur symmetrically. Peripheral nerve becomes large and tender with noticeable sensory deficit. Sweating may be lost in lesions. In the mid and late period of the disease, patients may suffer from amyotrophy, deformation or physical disability. Lymph nodes, visceral and internal organs become severely damaged (Color Figure $10-7$).

10.5.2.4　Lepra reaction

It refers to the state when patients develop rapidly progressive new skin lesions or nerve damages comparing with their existing lesions or neuritis with symptoms such as chills, fever, fatigue, general malaise, loss of appetite, etc during the course of disease.

10.5.2.5　Histopathology

In TT, groups of epithelioid cells with giant cells are found around the small blood vessels or nerves of dermis. Acid-fast bacilli are rare; In LL, granulomas are composed of lepra cells or foam cells in the dermis. Acid-fast bacilli are typically abundant. The infiltrate is localized in the dermis and is separated from the epidermis by a well-defined grenz zone.

10.5.3　Diagnosis and Differential Diagnosis

Diagnosis should be made prudently and based on the medical history, clinical, bacteriologic, immunologic, and histopathologic features. Defining signs of leprosy include:

（1）Sensory deficit, sweating difficulty or

numbness in skin lesions;

（2）Thickened peripheral nerve trunks with functional disorders;

（3）*Mycobacterium leprae* can be found in tissue section or film preparation; leprae are found on skin smears or biopsy material;

（4）Characteristic alterations are observed pathologically.

Diagnosis can be established when two or more of the above four signs are determined, or when the third sign is confirmed with the patient.

Skin lesions of leprosy are varied. So the differential diagnosis must take into account a large number of other skin diseases (e. g. lupus vulgaris, erythema nodosum, sarcoidosis, primary cutaneous T-cell lymphoma and granuloma annulare); as the sensory deficit caused by leprosy is similar to that by some neurologic diseases (e. g. multiple neuritis, facioplegia), it should be differentiated as well.

10.5.4 Treatment

Principle: good results can usually be obtained by intervening as early and timely as possible; treating the patient regularly in full dosage during the entire course of treatment.

10.5.4.1 MDT

MDT is a treatment regimen for leprosy recommended by WHO.

（1）Multi-bacillary leprosy(LL, BL, BB and a few BT cases)

Treat with rifampicin (RFP): 600 mg once a month; dapsone (DDS): 100 mg/day; B663: 300 mg once a month or 50 mg/day; treatment lasts for 24 months.

（2）Pauci-bacillary leprosy(TT, some BT and indeterminate cases)

Treat with rifampicin (RFP) 600 mg once a month and dapsone(DDS) 100 mg/d for 6 months. Patients should continue to receive regular visits from the prevention agencies subsequent to the treatment. Smear test should be performed once per year for at least five years.

10.5.4.2 Treatment of lepra reaction

Steroid is the drug of choice for the treatment of lepra reaction. Treat with prednisone 30 - 60 mg/d PO multiple times. Reduce the dose gradually if treatment is effective. Thalidomide is also useful in treating lepra reaction. Treat with thalidomide 300 - 400 mg/d PO, administered 3 - 4 times per day. It

usually takes 1 - 3 days to control the symptoms. Reduce the dose gradually to 25 - 50 mg/d afterwards.

■ Summary

Impetigo is a purulent skin infection characterized by pustules and purulent crusts. The pathogen is primarily coagulase-positive *Staphylococcus aureus*, secondarily *Streptococcus hemolyticus*. Impetigo is divided into four patterns. Diagnosis depends on epidemic season, age of onset, favorite location and representative pustule. The topical antibacterial drugs are advised firstly to be applied on lesions. Folliculitis and furunculosis are bacterial inflammatory diseases involving follicles and perifollicular tissues. Folliculitis locates the infection in follicles; however, furunculosis invades the tissues around and under follicles. The main pathogen is coagulase-positive *Staphylococcus aureus*. They can be diagnosed not difficultly by the onset sites and rash appearance. Topical antibacterial therapy is applied primarily. Systemic therapy is advised to multiple folliculitis and severe chronic furunculosis. Erysipelas is an acute skin infection induced by streptococcus hemolyticus. The typical lesions present rush onset, edematous erythema with clear boundary and pain, fever and leukocyte more than normal. Systemic penicillin applied in early stage and full dose is indicated. Tuberculosis of the skin is a chronic skin disease caused by *Mycobacterium tuberculosis(M. tuberculosis)*. Lesions appear in normal skin as a result of direct extension of adjacent tuberculous focus, of hematogenous or lymphatic spread; they can also be caused by an infection of the mucous membranes from minor injuries. Lesions of cutaneous TB demonstrate typical histopathologic characteristics of tuberculosis. "Morning, full dosage, rule, affiliation and to apply antituberculosis drugs in the whole range" is the principle. Leprosy is a chronic infectious disease caused by *Mycobacterium leprae*, principally affecting peripheral nerves and skin. Diagnosis should be made prudently and comprehensively on the basis of the medical history, clinical manifestation, smear test and pathological examination of the patient.

▪ Questions

1. Describe the cause and clinical manifestation of folliculitis and furunculosis.

2. Describe the clinical manifestation and therapy of erysipelas.

3. Describe the clinical feature of main patterns of tuberculosis of the skin.

4. Describe the clinical feature of 5 patterns of Leprosy.

(Yadi Li 李娅娣,Jing Tian 田晶)

Chapter 11

Fungal Diseases of the Skin

▪ Objectives

To master the causes and clinical features of the fungal disease of the skin.

To have an intimate knowledge of diagnosis and management of tinea capitis, tinea corporis, tinea cruris, tinea manuum, tinea pedis, pityriasis versicolor, onychomycosis and candidiasis.

▪ Key concepts

Tinea capitis refers to a cutaneous fungal infection that involves the hair and scalp. Clinical diagnosis can be confirmed by clinical manifestations, examination of fungi under direct microscopy, and Wood's lamp examination.

Tinea corporis refers to the cutaneous fungal infection of hairless (glabrous) skin usually of the scalp, but also the hands, feet, and nails. Tinea cruris refers to the cutaneous fungal infection of the inguinal, perineal, and perianal areas; it is a type of tinea corporis at specific sites.

Tinea manuum and tinea pedis refer to a cutaneous fungal infection that involves the hands and the feet. Clinical diagnosis can be confirmed by clinical manifestations, examination of fungi under direct microscopy and fungal cultures. Treatment strategy is multifold, including oral medication, topical medication and patient education.

Pityriasis versicolor is a common skin condition in which flaky discolored patches appear mainly on the chest and back. Clinical diagnosis can be confirmed by clinical manifestations, examination of fungi under direct microscopy, and Wood's lamp examination. Treatment strategy is multifold, including oral medication and topical medication.

Onychomycosis is a term used to describe all fungal infections of the nail plate and nail bed. Diagnosis depends on KOH examination and tissue culture. The effective treatment contains system and topical medicines.

Candidiasis is the normal colonizer of the individuals. While, it is also the most common opportunistic pathogens, which primarily attack the immunocompromised individuals. Diagnosis depends on clinical signs and symptoms and a positive culture of the tissue.

▪ Introduction

Tinea capitis is a cutaneous fungal infection of the hair and scalp. Clinically, according to the pathogenic fungi and clinical presentation, it can be classified into white tinea capitis, black-dot tinea capitis, and crusted tinea capitis, whereas pustular tinea capitis is usually secondary to white or black-dot tinea capitis. Tinea corporis is fungal infection of glabrous skin of the scalp, hands, feet, and nails. Tinea cruris, considered to be a type of tinea corporis at specific sites, refers to the cutaneous fungal infection of the inguinal, perineal, and perianal areas. Tinea manuum is a dermatophyte infection of the hand, one or both. In this form, the palms become diffusely dry, scaly and erythematous. Tinea pedis as known as Athlete's foot is a common fungal infection of the feet, characterized by fissures, scales and maceration in the toe web, or scaling of the soles and lateral surfaces of the feet. The diagnosis is confirmed by microscopy and culture of skin scrapings. Pityriasis versicolor which is also known as tinea versicolor is an infection of the skin caused by the yeast Malassezia furfur. The disease is characterized by the occurrence of multiple macular patches of all sizes and shapes, and varying in pigmentation from fawn-colored to brown. Onychomycosis is a term used to describe all fungal infections of the nail plate and nail bed. Tinea unguium is the invasion by species of dermatophytes. Candidiasis is an infection caused by some of the genus *Candida*. *Candida* is the normal colonizer of the individuals, which is inclined to attack individuals with a compromised immune system, such as patients with malignancies and diabetes mellitus, and those requiring antibiotics and oral cortisone for prolonged periods.

11. 1　Tinea Capitis

Tinea capitis is a cutaneous fungal infection of the hair and scalp. Clinically, according to the pathogenic fungi and clinical presentation, it can be classified into white tinea capitis, black-dot tinea capitis, and crusted tinea capitis, whereas pustular tinea capitis is usually secondary to white or black-dot tinea capitis.

11. 1. 1　Etiology

Common pathogens for tinea capitis in China include *Trichophyton schoenleinii*, *Microsporum ferrugineum*, *Microsporum canis*, *Trichophyton violaceum*, and *Trichophyton tonsurans*. In Canada and the United States, *Microsporum audouinii* is also a common cause of white tinea capitis, and, occasionally, *Trichophyton rubrum* results in black tinea capitis. These pathogenic fungi usually infect growing hairs(anagen phase) and rarely involve hairs in the resting phase(telogen phase).

11. 1. 2　Clinical features

In clinical settings, tinea capitis is most often seen in children who have a history of direct contact with pets or individuals with the infection. According to the pathogen and clinical presentation, it can be further classified into white tinea capitis, black-dot tinea capitis, and crusted tinea capitis, whereas pustular tinea capitis usually develops secondary to white or black-dot tinea capitis.

11. 1. 2. 1　White tinea capitis

White tinea capitis is caused by Microsporum spp. infection. It presents with white or grey scaling patches in round or oval shape without any inflammatory reaction (Color Figure 11 - 1). The hair growing in the infected areas breaks off at 2 - 4 mm from the root, where a white fungal sheath can be seen surrounding the hair shaft. There may be mild itchiness in some cases. This type is prone to develop into pustular tinea capitis.

11. 1. 2. 2　Black-dot tinea capitis

This type of tinea capitis is caused by *Trichophyton* spp. The infected hair breaks off at the scalp surface. The residual hair at the follicular opening creates the appearance of black dots(Color Figure 11 - 2).

11. 1. 2. 3　Pustular tinea capitis

This type of tinea capitis often develops from white or black-dot tinea capitis. The patient first presents with clusters of follicular pustules, followed by skin elevation(Color Figure 11 - 3). The affected area later develops into a dark red infiltrated plaque covered by honeycomb-like pitted follicles, sometimes accompanied by mild pain and tenderness. Scar tissue may remain after the healing of the lesion, which is likely to destroy the hair follicles and results in permanent hair loss. The occurrence of pustular tinea capitis may be related to the body's intrinsic reaction to the pathogenic fungus. Recently, *Candida* spp. has been reported to cause this type of tinea capitis.

11.1.2.4 Crusted tinea capitis

Crusted tinea capitis is caused by *Trichophyton schoenleinii*. The patient first presents with butterfly-shaped red patches covered by a yellow crust (Color Figure 11-4). The lesions may expand, fuse with each other, and thereby create a large area of dirty crust, which is often accompanied by rodent-like odor. The infected hair seldom breaks but turns to be withered, yellow, and lack of gloss. Prolonged infection can result in permanent hair loss in large areas. This disease is also characterized by a lack of subjective symptoms or only mild itchiness.

11.1.3 *Diagnosis and Differential Diagnosis*

The diagnosis of tinea capitis is mainly based on characteristic history, age of onset, and a history of contact with pets prior to disease onset. Broken hairs can be found through physical examination, and endothrix or ectothrix spores, sometimes accompanied by hyphae, can be discovered by direct microscopy. Fungus culture using infected hair can confirm the pathogenic fungi. In addition, the use of Wood's lamp can also facilitate diagnosis. However, in the clinical setting, tinea capitis should be differentiated from other diseases: scalp psoriasis, pityriasis capitis, seborrheic dermatitis and pyodermia of the scalp. If it is difficult to establish the diagnosis clinically, fungal culture and Wood's lamp examinations should both be employed.

11.1.4 *Treatment*

Treatment for tinea capitis requires a combined treatment plan composed of five steps: oral medication, topical medication, hair washing, hair cutting, and sterilization.

(1) Griseofulvin is the first choice for oral medication followed by itraconazole and terbinafine. The criteria of cure are negative results from microscopic examination and/or culture.

(2) Topical application of 5% sulfur gel, 2% iodine tincture, or other topical anti-fungal medications are recommended.

(3) The patient's head should be washed with soap every evening before applying topical medication. The patient's hair should be kept short or shaved if possible.

(4) Towels, hats, pillowcases, and combs used

by the patient should be boiled and sterilized.

(5) In China, hair removal by the way manual plucking can be taken into consideration for a patient with an infected area smaller than a nickel and fewer than three lesions. X-ray epilation is indicated for patients with white or crusted tinea capitis. Once the hair starts to fall out, usually 14-18 days after X-ray radiation, all hair should be removed within 2-3 days and the affected area treated with application of topical 5% sulfur gel and 2% iodine tincture. Generally, new hair will grow back within 4-6 months. For patients with pustular tinea, antibiotic should be considered with the presence of excessive suppuration, and small amounts of cortical steroid can also be used as needed.

11.2 Tinea Corporis and Tinea Cruris

Tinea corporis is fungal infection of glabrous skin of the scalp, hands, feet, and nails. Tinea cruris, considered to be a type of tinea corporis at specific sites, refers to the cutaneous fungal infection of the inguinal, perineal, and perianal areas.

11.2.1 *Etiology*

The common pathogens of tinea corporis in our country include *Trichophyton rubrum*, *Trichophyton mentagrophytes*, *Trichophyton schoenleinii*, *Trichophyton violaceum*, *Epidermophyton floccosum*, *Microsporum ferrugineum*, *Microsporum gypseum*, and *Microsporum canis*.

Tinea cruris is often caused by *Epidermophyton floccosum*, *Trichophyton mentagrophytes*, and *Trichophyton rubrum*.

11.2.2 *Clinical Features*

Tinea corporis and tinea cruris are similar in clinical presentation. A typical lesion is characterized by annular papules, papulovesicles, or blisters, accompanied by scaling(Color Figure 11-5, 11-6).

The lesion begins with papules, blisters, or papulovesicles. As the lesion grows, it develops an annular appearance, hence it is also named tinea circinata or tinea glabrosa. Several lesions may start singly but may fuse and overlap with one other as they expand. In some cases, the lesions may even be so widespread that the whole body is involved, particularly in immunocompromised patients or users of immunosuppressants, cortical steroids, or antineoplastic agents. Due to the body's defense mechanism, the lesion center can spontaneously heal with scaling, while its periphery appears elevated and circular. Sometimes the lesion may present with active erythematous plaques, papules, blisters, or scaling, whereas the central area is flat with scaling or pigmentation. Tinea corporis in children can present with special morphology, including multiple ring-shaped lesions(ringworm) overlapping with one another and forming a rosette-like appearance.

11. 2. 3　Diagnosis and Differential Diagnosis

The diagnosis of tinea corporis and tinea cruris is established on the basis of history and appearance. These diseases arise in summer or during hot and humid weather. The lesion presents as scaling erythematous plaques with well-defined borders. Hyphae or spores can be observed in skin scales taken from the lesion border under direct microscopy. Fungus species is determined by fungal culture, and a positive result can confirm the diagnosis. Major differential diagnoses include chronic eczema, lichen simplex chronicus, and pityriasis rosea.

11. 2. 4　Treatment

The prevention and treatment of tinea corporis and tinea cruris are similar. The key to prevention is to actively treat the existing tinea manus, pedis, unguium, and capitis in the patient and to avoid close contact with other patients and fungus-infected animals such as sick cats and dogs. Indirect contact with bath tubs and towels used by infected individuals should be avoided; meanwhile, such items should be sterilized regularly. Individuals taking cortical steroids and immunosuppressants that may affect immune system function should consult their physicians about appropriate dosage to help avoid secondary infection due to lowered immunity. Timely and appropriate treatment for existing chronic diseases such as diabetes should also be given.

The primary treatment for tinea corporis and tinea cruris is topical medication, including compound salicylic acid tincture, compound benzoic acid ointment, compound resorcinol liniment, 1% econazole or clotrimazole cream, 2% miconazole cream, bifonazole, ketoconazole and terbinafine, and naftifine cream.

Treatment for patients with widespread tinea corporis, particularly when infection is caused by *Trichophyton rubrum*, can include short-term oral griseofulvin, as appropriate, in addition to topical medication. The griseofulvin dosage for treating tinea corporis is the same as that for treating tinea capitis. Short-term oral fluconazole, itraconazole, or terbinafine can also be administered when needed.

11.3　Tinea Manuum and Tinea Pedis

Tinea manuum is a dermatophyte infection of one or both hands. In this form, the palms become diffusely dry, scaly and erythematous. Tinea pedis as known as Athlete's foot is a common fungal infection of the feet, characterized by fissures, scales and maceration in the toe web, or scaling of the soles and lateral surfaces of the feet. The diagnosis is confirmed by microscopy and culture of skin scrapings.

11. 3. 1　Etiology

Tinea pedis is a foot infection due to a dermatophyte fungus. Most common agents are *T. rubrum*, *T. mentagrophytes var interdigitale*, *E. floccosum*. Other agents: *M. persicolor*, *T. raubitschekii*, *T. violaceum*. Tinea manuum is the name given to infection of one or both hands with a dermatophyte infection. It is much less common than tinea pedis. Most common agents are *T. rubrum*. Other agents: *E. floccosum*, *M. canis*, *M. gypseum*, *T. mentagrophytes*, *T. verrucosum*. There are some risk factors such as hot, humid environment, sweating or maceration of the skin, occlusive footwear, diabetes mellitus, immunosuppression (e. g. AIDS), tropical environment, etc. It is contagious which can be spread by direct skin-to-skin contact. If anyone who is suffering from the fungal infection such as tinea pedis, he is more prone to get tinea manuum. "One hand, two feet disease" is a common clinical presentation of tinea pedis involving one hand and both feet.

11. 3. 2　Clinical Features

Tinea pedis is thought to be the world's most common dermatophytosis and has no predilection for any racial or ethnic group. It affects all ages but is more common in adults than in children. Tinea manuum can occur as an acute inflammatory rash and is usually a raised border and clearing in the middle. More frequently, tinea manuum causes a slowly extending area of peeling, dryness and mild itching on the palm of one hand(Color Figure 11 - 7). Tinea pedis can take several forms: a dry, scaly form that forms a ring around the sides and bottom of the foot is called a "moccasin" pattern, and cracked and reddened areas between the toes that can occasionally have a white scaly area(Color Figure 11 - 8). Tinea manuum and pedis are often divided into three clinical types as following:

(1) Interdigital type

It is the most characteristic type of tinea pedis. Macerated, scaly plaques in toe web spaces, can be portal of entry for cellulitis of the foot, especially in diabetics.

(2) "Moccasin" type

It is also called hyperkeratotic type which is characterized by dryness, scaling and erythema of the plantar and/or lateral foot with slight scaling to diffuse hyperkeratosis.

(3) Vesicular type

Vesicles, pustules, or bullae are most often on the instep or anterior plantar surface of the feet. Cellulitis, lymphangitis, and adenopathy can complicate this type of tinea pedis.

11. 3. 3　Diagnosis and Differential Diagnosis

It is not difficult to diagnose the disease based on typical skin lesions. Potassium hydroxide(KOH) microscopy can detect hyphae and conidia in skin scrapings. Fungal cultures are necessary for the identification of the organism. The differential diagnoses must be included diseases such as eczema, pompholyx, granuloma annular and psoriasis.

11. 3. 4　Treatment

(1) Topical medication

It can be treated locally with antifungal creams, sprays, liquids and powders such as imidazole, which is most effective, clotrimazole and miconazole as well. Other antifungals include zinc undecenoate, terbinafine and tolnaftate .

(2) Oral medication

Itraconazole(200 mg once a day for 2 weeks) or terbinafine(250 mg once a day for 2 to 4 weeks). Treatment is usually successful within 2 to 4 weeks. Antibiotics are necessary when patient gets secondary infection.

(3) Patient education

Avoid factors which predispose to infection, absorbent powders in intertriginous areas. Avoid using of tinea pedis-shower -shoes in public facilities.

11.4　Pityriasis Versicolor

Pityriasis versicolor which is also known as tinea versicolor is an infection of the skin caused by the yeast *Malassezia furfur*. The disease is characterized by the occurrence of multiple macular patches of all sizes and shapes, and varying in pigmentation from fawn-colored to brown.

11. 4. 1　Etiology

Pityriasis versicolor is caused by the yeast *Malassezia furfur* (Pityrosporum). *Malassezia* has an oil requirement for growth, accounting for the increased incidence in adolescents and preference for sebum-rich areas of the skin. Three serotypes(A, B and C serotype) have been characterized. The disease onset is associated with excessive sweating, increased sebum secretion, synthetic clothing, the application of oils, and topical or systemic glucocorticoids. Other risk factors such as genetic predisposition, Cushing's syndrome, diabetes and immunodeficiency are important as well.

11. 4. 2　Clinical Features

The disease is manifested by very thin, scaly plaques that can be hyperpigmented, hypopigmented or erythematous(Color Figure 11 - 9). The lesions are generally asymptomatic and the color of the lesions varies from almost white to reddish brown or fawn-colored. They may be mildly itchy . It commonly affects the trunk, neck, and/or arms, but it can be found on the entire body . The fungus grows slowly and prevents the skin from tanning normally.

11. 4. 3　Diagnosis and Differential Diagnosis

It is not difficult to diagnose the disease based on typical skin lesions. The diagnosis can be established by KOH staining of scales obtained from affected scaly plaques. Under Wood's light examination pityriasis versicolor fluoresces a light yellow or golden color. Culture is not necessary as its' technique is difficult and not readily available.

Clinical examination usually leads to the correct diagnosis of pityriasis versicolor. However, vitiligo, pityriasis alba and other forms of postinflammatory hypopigmentation, seborrheic dermatitis, pityriasis rosea and secondary syphilis may mimic the disease.

11. 4. 4　Treatment

(1) Topical medication

Most topical treatments are used to treat pityriasis versicolor such as imidazole antifungal creams or shampoos, zinc pyrithione shampoos, selenium sulfide shampoos, and sulfur/salicylic acid shampoos.

(2) Oral medication

Ketoconazole(200 mg daily for 7 days) or itraconazole(200 – 400 mg daily for 3 – 7 days).

11.5 Onychomycosis

Onychomycosis is a term that refers to all fungal infections of the nail plate and nail bed. Diagnosis depends on KOH examination and tissue culture. The effective treatment contains system and topical medicines.

11. 5. 1 Etiology

Dermatophytes have been reported as the major cause of onychomycosis. Infections of *Candida* and other non-dermatophytes could also be the causes, such as *Scopulariopsis breviaulis* and *Scytalidium hyalinum*. *T. rubrum* is the most common causative dermatophyte. *T. mentagrophytes* and *T. tonsurans* are also concerned.

11. 5. 2 Clinical Features

Onychomycosis can be long-lasting, often without any complaint of discomfort. In most cases, onychomycosis are associated with tinea pedis or tinea manus. Four patterns have been described according to the point of entry for fungus into the nail.

11. 5. 2. 1 Superficial white onychomycosis (SWO)

Some adherent white patches can be seen on the surface of the nail plate, some striate banding may also be seen(Color Figure 11 – 10).

11. 5. 2. 2 Distal and lateral subungual onychomycosis(DLSO)

DLSO is the most common pattern of infection. Thickening, fraying and cloudy of the nails are usually presented. The infected nails may break easily (Color Figure 11 – 11).

11. 5. 2. 3 Proximal and lateral subungual onychomycosis(PSO)

This is an uncommon pattern. Destroy of the nail root and demilune can be seen(Color Figure 11 – 12).

11. 5. 2. 4 Total dystrophic onychomycosis (TDO)

The whole surface of the nail plate is completely destroyed, thickening, crumbing and exfoliation easily(Color Figure 11 – 13).

11. 5. 3 Diagnosis and Differential Diagnosis

Diagnosis depends on the typical symptoms and the positive results of KOH examination and tissue culture.

While many diseases could affect the nails, some primary destroy(such as onychodystrophy, subnail warts), and secondary destroy(such as psoriasis and lichen planus) should be considered. The differential diagnosis can be done according to the lesion and the KOH examination result.

11. 5. 4 Treatment

(1) Topical therapy

Patient with onychomycosis alone may be treated with topical medicines to remove the infected areas. One routine consists of applying topical glacial acetic acid 30% or iodine tincture 3%– 5%, twice a day. Also topical ciclopirox olamine cream 8% or amorolfine lotion 5% has been employed, once a week for 3 to 6 months(finger nails), or 9 to 12 months(toe nails).

(2) System therapy

Patients with multiple abnormal nails need oral antifungal treatment. For example, itraconazole, 200 mg bid for 1 week, then a break of 3 weeks as a course. The infection of finger nails needs 2 – 3 courses, while the infection of toe nails needs 3 – 4 courses. Terbinafine is also effective, 250 mg qd, 4 – 6 weeks for infection of finger nails, 6 – 12 weeks for infection of toe nails. Association of system and topical treatment is considered to be more effective.

11.6 Candidiasis

Candidiasis is an infection caused by some of the genus *Candida*. *Candida* is the normal colonizer of the individuals. *Candida* is capable to cause diseases when host defenses are compromised. For example, patients with malignancies and diabetes mellitus, patients requiring antibiotics and oral cortisone for prolonged periods.

11. 6. 1 Etiology

C. albicans is the most common species. Other species of *Candida*, for example, *C. glabrata*, *C. Tropicalis*, *C. Krusei* and *C. parapsilosis* are also occasional causes of human candidiasis.

11. 6. 2   Clinical Features

11. 6. 2. 1   Cutaneous and mucosal candidiasis

Mucocutaneous candidiasis has a wide spectrum of clinical presentations.

Oral candidiasis often presents as oral thrush (white patches curd-like pseudomembrane in the mouth) as well as angular cheilitis. Other presentations include vulvovaginitis and balanoposthitis.

Cutaneous candidiasis present with markedly erythematous, often accompanied by satellite inflammatory papules and pustules. The most common sites of involvement are intertriginous zones (sub-mammary, inguinal creases, intergluteal fold and finger spaces) and the scrotum, as well as the diaper area in infants. *Candida* can also infect the nail and periungual areas.

11. 6. 2. 2   Systemic candidiasis

The most common sites of systemic candidiasis are gastrointestinal tract, bronchus and lungs. In severe conditions, candidal septicemia may be evoked.

11. 6. 3   Diagnosis and Differential Diagnosis

The diagnosis of mucocutaneous candidiasis depends on the clinical symptoms and the positive results of KOH examination and tissue culture. The diagnosis of systemic candidiasis requires repeated culture.

11. 6. 4   Treatment

11. 6. 4. 1   General principles

The general principles is to strengthen and boost the immune system, reduce or stop using broad-spectrum antibiotics, keep the skin clean and desiccation, and removal predisposing factors. Regular examination of discharge and skin is required for those taking antibiotics and oral cortisone for long periods.

11. 6. 4. 2   Pharmacotherapy

Superficial cutaneous and mucosal candidiasis could be treated with topical therapy. For the severe general cutaneous and mucosal candidiasis, *Candida* onychomycosis and systemic candidiasis, critically and long-term oral antifungal chemotherapy is necessary.

▪ Summary

Tinea capitis refers to a cutaneous fungal infection of the hair and scalp. In our country, the common pathogens of tinea capitis are *Trichophyton schoenleinii*, *Microsporum ferrugineum*, *Microsporum canis*, *Trichophyton violaceum*, and *Trichophyton tonsurans*. According to the identified pathogen and clinical presentation, the infection can be further classified as white tinea capitis, black-dot tinea capitis, and crusted tinea capitis, whereas pustular tinea capitis is usually secondary to white or black-dot tinea capitis. The diagnosis of tinea capitis is based on the clinical presentation, direct microscopy examination for fungus, and Wood's lamp examination. A combined treatment plan is recommended, including oral medication, topical medication, hair washing, hair cutting, and sterilization.

Tinea corporis constitutes the cutaneous fungal infection of glabrous skin, usually of the scalp, but also of the hands, feet, and nails. Tinea cruris refers to a special type of tinea corporis that infects the skin of the inguinal, perineal, and perianal areas. Their diagnosis can be confirmed by clinical presentation of lesions, detection of fungus under direct microscopy, and fungal culture. Topical medication is the mainstay of treatment for tinea corporis and tinea cruris. An array of antifungal agents can be applied for a treatment course of 2 – 3 weeks. Patients with widespread lesions or poor response to topical medication alone can be given oral antifungal drugs.

Tinea manuum and tinea pedis refer to a cutaneous fungal infection that involves the hands and the feet. Tinea pedis is most frequently due to *T. rubrum*, *T. mentagrophytes var interdigitale*, *E. floccosum*. Other agents: *M. persicolor*, *T. raubitschekii*, *T. violaceum*. The most common agents of tinea manuum are *T. rubrum*. Other agents: *E. floccosum*, *M. canis*, *M. gypseum*, *T. mentagrophytes*, *T. verrucosum*. Tinea manuum and pedis are often divided into three clinical types, which are interdigital type, "Moccasin" type and vesicular type. Treatment strategy is multifold, including oral medication, topical medication and patient education.

Pityriasis versicolor is an infection of the skin caused by the yeast *Malassezia furfur* which has an oil requirement for growth, accounting for the increased incidence in adolescents and preference for sebum-rich areas of the skin. It commonly affects the trunk, neck, and / or arms. Diagnosis can be confirmed by clinical manifestations, examination of fungi under direct microscopy, and Wood's lamp examination. Topical treatments are wildly used.

Onychomycosis is a term used to describe all fungal infections of the nail plate and nail bed. Dermatophytes are the major cause. According to the point of fungal entry into the nail, four patterns have been described. With the typical symptoms, the positive KOH examination and cultural results, diagnosis of onychomycosis can be determined. Proper treatment contains system and topical therapy.

Candidiasis is an infection of the immunocompromised individuals caused by some of the genus *Candida*. Candida infection has a wide spectrum of clinical presentations. Diagnosis depends on the clinical symptoms and the positive results of tissue culture. Critically and longterm oral antifungal therapy is necessary for severe infections.

▪ Questions

1. Describe the clinical presentations of the four types of tinea capitis.

2. List the treatment options for tinea capitis.

3. Describe the clinical presentation, diagnosis, and treatment of tinea corporis and tinea cruris.

4. List the characteristics of skin lesions of tinea corporis and tinea cruris.

5. Briefly describe the clinical presentation and treatment of tinea manuum and tinea pedis.

6. What are the differential diagnoses of tinea manuum and tinea pedis?

7. Briefly describe the clinical presentation and treatment of pityriasis versicolor.

8. What are the differential diagnoses of pityriasis versicolor?

9. Describe the clinical feature of all onychomycosis patterns.

(**Junying Zhao** 赵俊英,**Xiaoyang Wang** 王晓阳,
Xiaoling Chu 褚晓玲)

Chapter 12

Parasitic Worms and Protozoa

- **Objectives**

To master the knowledge of the clinical feature diagnosis therapy methods of scabies, insect bite dermatitis and lice.

To have an intimate knowledge of the etiology and the pathogenesy.

- **Key concepts**

Scabies is a dermatosis caused by itch mite and often involves the tender and thin skin.

The insect bite dermatitis is skin anaphylaxis and inflammatory reaction which is caused by insects such as acaridan, mosquito, bedbug, flea and bee through pricking into human skin and sucking blood with buccal appendages, or injecting venom into human body.

Pediculosis are encountered because of louse parasitize on the human body, which divide into head louse, clothes louse, crab louse.

12.1 Scabies

Scabies in humans and other animals is caused by mites of family sarcoptidae. Human scabies has played a significant role in history.

12.1.1 Etiology

Burrowing mite also called by sarcoptic mite, includes big itch mite and animal itch mite. Scabies is usually transmitted by sleeping together with scabies patients, usually couples transmit each other and sons and daughters at the same time. People in the dormitory also can transmit each other by sitting and sleeping on the same bed and wearing patients clothing. Mankind can be infected by animal mite in rabbits, sheep and dogs, but symptom is milder.

12. 1. 2   Clinical Features

Scabies often involves the tender and thin skin, such as the finger web spaces, the wrists, the triangle of elbow, the axillary space, under-breast area, the ambi-bellybutton, the waist, lower abdomen, femoribus internus and external genitalia(Color Figure 12 - 1, 12 - 2). Skin lesions are papule or papulovesicles of about foxtail millet size, sometimes burrows . They are less frequently found on the palms, the head and the face in adults, but except in infants. Pisiformis nodules sometimes occur, particularly on the scrotum(Color Figure 12 - 3), penis and glans, which is a foreign body reaction caused by sarcoptic mite. Intense itching is obvious especially at night. The lesions may appear secondary infection, develop impetigo, furuncle, lymphadenitis or even nephritis. Patients with skin anaesthesia secondary to sensory neuropathy or severe extremity disability can not perceive itch or can not scratch. They develop crusted scabies also called Norwegian scabies easily. It appears as a mass of scales, crust, erythroderma or the warty plaques. There are several millions mites on crusted scabies patients, whose infectiousness is extremely intense.

12. 1. 3   Diagnosis and Differential Diagnosis

Diagnosis is not difficult on the basis of contact transmission history, predilection site, features of skin lesions, intense itching at night.

Absolute confirmation can be made by the discovery of mites in microscopical examination. The lesion should make a differential diagnosis with pruritus of skin, phthiriasis, nodular prurigo and eczema and so on.

12. 1. 4   Prevention and Treatment

Pay attention to good personal cleanliness, and once confirmed patients should be insulated and treated immediately. Close contacts should be treated at the same time. The clothes, bedding of patients should be boiled to disinfect. When the course of treatment is completed, patient should change the disinfectant clothing and bedding. The major clinical management is drug for exterior use antihistamine drug for oral use is helpful to patients with severe itching. In the case with secondary pyogenic infection, anti-infective drug should be used at the same time.

Sulfur ointment 10% (infants and children 5%) is applied from neck to all over the body 1 - 2 times per day after bathing with soap and hot water, continuously 3 - 4 day for a course of treatment. During the medicine applying, don't change clothes and bath to keep the efficacy. 3. 1% r -666 cream frost has a strong acaricidal role, no odor, but toxic. Usually only apply once, do not exceed 30 g in adult, and bath with warm water after 24 hours.

12. 2 Insect Bite Dermatitis

The cutaneous reaction caused by insects biting is called insect bite dermatitis. The frequent types include acaridan dermatitis, mosquito bite, bedbug bite, flea bite, bee sting.

12. 2. 1   Etiology

Acaridans is a kind of tiny insect visible by unaided eye. The biting, secretion, excretion and ecdysis of acaridan can cause allergic response, leading to dermatitis. Tyroglyphidae mite(flour mite) and dermatophagoides mite (dust mite) live on putrefactive organics rather than blood.

Mosquitos include anopheles, culex and aedes, only female mosquito sting and suck blood. All the moisture, temperature, carbon dioxide(CO_2), estrogen and lactic acid secreted from sweat on body surface can attract mosquitos.

The bedbugs hide in bed crevice or mattress, bedclothes, floor crevice during the day, while crawl on the human skin to suck blood at night. Some proteinum included in the saliva can lead to anaphylaxis.

The most frequent biting fleas are ctenocephalides felis (cat flea) and ctenocephalides canis (dog flea) in addition, there are pulex irritans (human flea), rodent flea(common rat flea) and ceratophyllus gallinae (fowl flea).

There are kinds of bees, such as apis mellifera (honey bee), wasp, bumblebee, scoliid, venomous sting after their end stings into the skin causing reaction. Venenum apis contain histamine, hyaluronidase, phospholipase A and macromolecules with active acid phosphatase.

12. 2. 2   Clinical Features

12. 2. 2. 1   Mite dermatitis

The skin lesion was characterized by swollen wheal-like papule, papulovesicle or ecchymosis with blister, occasionally bulla in the center, usually accompany with scratch and scab. General symptoms such as headache, arthralgia, fever, fatigue and nausea were observed in severe cases. Few patients might develop asthma, proteinuria and hypereosinophilia.

12.2.2.2   Mosquito bites

There were petechiae, wheal, papule or ecchymosis in the skin with violent itching after bitten by mosquitoes, and sometimes the skin may have no reaction to the bite. Infants bitten by mosquito may develop angioedema, usually involving the prepuce, dorsal hand, facial region and other exposed body sites. Immediate hypersensitivity, delayed hypersensitivity and even systemic reactions happen in severe cases. Newcomers to the epidemic areas usually develop wheal-like papules lasting for about a week.

12.2.2.3   Cimex bites

Wheal-like papules and itching appeared few hours after cimex bites. There were needle-head-sized hemorrhagic petechiae or blisters in the central of the skin lesion, massive erythema and purpura, accompany with violent itching and pain. Sometimes, linear lesion formed after repeated cimex bites in one night. Pigmentation was usually caused by over scratching.

12.2.2.4   Flea bites

Red maculopapule with petechia was characterized in flea bites skin lesion. Patient allergy to flea saliva might develop blister, erythema multiforme or purpura. The skin lesion usually scattered in groups after being bitten by flea on legs or waist.

12.2.2.5   Bee bites

Significant pain, burning sensation and itching appeared immediately after bee bites. Red swelling of the bitten part was quickly observed, with petechia in the center. Even blisters and bullae are formed sometimes, occasionally tissue necrosis can be found. Massive swellings appear after bee bites in most situations, and few people might develop general symptoms such as nausea, vomit, chill and fever, etc. Swollen erythema, wheal and angioedema are caused by histamine, and in severe cases histamine could initiate allergic shock and patients would quickly die in a few minutes or a few days. Seru-sickness-like delayed hypersensitivity such as fever, urticaria and arthralgia might appear 7 to 14 days after the bee bites.

12.2.3   Diagnosis and Differential Diagnosis

The levels of insects'sting change with the season and the living environment. Before making the final diagnosis, it's very important to enquire the patients the history of exposure to insects depending on the skin injure.

12.2.4   Prevention and Treatment

To prevent the insect sting, ones should to make personal and occupational protection, avoid getting close to pets and fowls, and disinfect the living circumstance using synthetic pyrethroids pesticides.

For those whose injuries have slight inflammation, they can use corticosteroid ointment on it and take antihistamine orally. For those that have serious injured, they can take prednisone orally for a short time.

Draw the anal style instantly after bee bites. Then the lesions should be washed with water, applied with an ice block or cold and wet dressing. If it is a serious injury, patients with obvious symptoms all over the body should be treated in acute, injecting 0.5 ml adrenalin 0.1% into muscle or under the skin. Repeat it if necessary. Injecting into the veil with 500 ml glucose fluid enriched with 200 – 400 mg hydrocortisone. Then continue with 30 – 40 mg/d prednisone, reducing the dose in one to two week.

12.3   Lice

Three varieties of these flattened, wingless insects usually attack humans, although others infest the lower animals or may become temporarily deposited on human hosts.

12.3.1   Etiology and Pathogenesy

Lice belong to arthropod insecta and pertaining to ectoparasite. Each variety of lice has a predilection for certain parts of the body and is highly host-specific. Humans are parasitized by three species of anoplura: the head louse, the clothing or body louse and the pubic or crab louse; that cause pediculosis capillitii, pediculosis corporis and pediculosis inguinalis accordingly. The head louse and the body louse may survive for about 10 days when they depart from the human body, but the pubic or crab louse cannot survive over 24 hours. The head louse and the diameter of hair are almost identical. The body louse's eggs are cemented to clothing fibers and the pubic or crab louse's eggs are cemented to pubisure. Lice attach themselves to the skin and live on the blood they suck. In piercing the skin, the parasites exude an antigenic salivary secretion. This, together with the mechanical puncture, produces pruritic dermatitis. In addition, the louse may be a carrier of disease and through its bite or excretions may transmit an infectious disease-epidemic typhus, relapsing fever, or trench fever.

12. 3. 2   Clinical Features

12. 3. 2. 1   Pediculosis capitis

The head louse is attached to the hair root. Lice are more common on children and the females who are not clean. There is intense pruritus of the scalp, and the lesions are erythema and papule usually. In severe cases, pus and exudate may be produced to make the hair sticking to fasciculation as well as diverging foul smell. Because of the itching, secondary complications with impetigo and furunculosis, eczema are common. The eggs may be seen on the hair attaching to the hair shafts.

12. 3. 2. 2   Pediculosis corporis

The lice live chiefly in the seams of clothing and the collar of underwear and should be sought in the kerchief, bedclothes severely. The body may appear erythema, papule and bolus resulting form the punctures, usually following by parallel linear scratch marks, blood scab. In those who have harbored clothing lice for long periods of time the skin is often hyperpigmented.

12. 3. 2. 3   Pediculosis pubis

There is intense pruritus of the body of crinis pubis. It is generally worst at night. When crab lice (Color Figure 12 - 4) are discovered on the pubic area, other hairy areas of the body should be examined, as these lice may colonize eyebrows, eyelashes, beard, axillae, areolar hair and occasionally scalp hair, particularly the scalp margins. Crab lice are transmitted by close physical contact, usually sexual. The spouse or sexual partner of the patient may occur analogous symptom. The majority patients or their spouse have a history of feculent sexual relations. The gray eggs are found attaching to the pubisure. There is slow-moving crab louse on the skin or the crab louse that half turn to intracutaneous and half expose to outside the skin, following by parallel linear scratch marks, blood scab or lamellar ecchymosis. The underclothes may be spotted with altered blood pigments of infest human.

12. 3. 3   Diagnosis and Differential Diagnosis

The diagnosis usually presents no difficulties. Absolute confirmation can be made by finding the lice or eggs. The lesion should be examined for pruritus of skin, prurigo, and scabies, but pediculosis frequently coexists with these diseases.

12. 3. 4   Treatment

Treatment of phthiriasis aims at destruction of the lice and eggs. The patient of pediculosis capitis should apply the cream after shaving the hair. Combing with a double-edged fine-toothed comb is important to the female. Stemonoe tincture 50% and 25% benzyl benzoate cream form are available. The medicine is then applied twice daily, and shampooing the hair with soap after 72 hours. Laundering the comb, fine-toothed comb, cap, kerchief and bedding are necessary. Boiling the clothing of pediculosis corporis is a most effective means of killing both lice and ova. The patient should bathe with water and soap. To pediculosis pubis, the patients should shave and burn out the pubic hair. 10% sulfur ointment, 0.3% pyrethrins, or 25% benzyl benzoate cream is the standard treatment. In pregnant women and the patients with damaged skin or inflammation, vaseline is perfectly safe and very effective. Although lice and eggs are destructed, pruritus may persist for several days. Symptomatic treatment is available.

▪ Summary

Scabies is a kind of dermatonosis caused by sarcoptic mite. Scabies is usually transmitted by close personal contact. Scabies often involves the tender and thin skin, intense itching at night. The major clinical management is drug for exterior use. Insect bite dermatitis is skin allergy and inflammation reactions to insects stings which may inject poison into human body. The common pathogens are acarians, mosquito, chinch, flea and bee. Diagnosis depends most on the sting injury and the history of exposure to insects. Make protection to avoid insect bite dermatitis. Depending on the symptom, insect bite dermatitis can be treated by topical therapy or systemic therapy. Pediculosis are encountered because of louse parasitize on the human body, which divide into head louse, clothes louse, crab louse.

■ **Questions**

1. Describe the clinical feature of scabies.
2. Make a short description of the treatment to bee bite dermatitis.

3. Describe the clinical feature of all lice patterns.

(**Xiaoqian Zhou** 周晓谦)

Chapter 13

Eczema and Dermatitis

▪ Objectives

To master the knowledge of the causes and clinical features of skin diseases characterized by eczematous lesions.

To have an intimate knowledge of diagnosis and management about contact dermatitis and atopic dermatitis.

▪ Key concepts

Dermatitis is a term for all kinds of inflammation of the skin that presents with erythema alone, erythema and scaling, or erythema, scaling, vesicles and crusts.

Eczema is a descriptive term and not a specific diagnosis. The term of eczema refers to the morphology of erythema, scaling, vesicles, and crusts. Sometimes eczema is used loosely to refer to the infantile form of atopic dermatitis.

Atopic dermatitis is a special form of eczema, characterized by xerosis, relapsing eczematous lesions and extremely pruritus. It is often associated with a family history of atopy and numerous immunologic abnormalities.

Autosensitization dermatitis refers to a phenomenon in which an acute widespread dermatitis develops in response to skin infections or other triggers.

Stasis dermatitis is a common inflammatory skin disease that occurs on the lower extremities as a direct consequence of venous insufficiency.

▪ Introduction

The words "eczema" and "dermatitis" are often used synonymously to describe a group of skin diseases characterized by erythema, papules and vesicles in the acute phase, and by dryness, lichenification and fissure in the chronic phase. Among this group of diseases, atopic dermatitis and contact dermatitis are most common. Diagnosis is mainly based on the clinical features and history. Patch test is helpful to make diagnosis of contact dermatitis and distinguish it from other eczematous lesions. Topical steroid remains the first-line therapy in the management of this kind of diseases.

13.1 Contact Dermatitis

Contact dermatitis is an inflammatory reaction in the skin and occurs when the skin comes in direct contact with an irritating or an allergic substance. It is characterized by lesions localizing to the contact sites.

13.1.1 Etiology

Contact dermatitis can be classified into two types: irritant contact dermatitis and allergic contact dermatitis.

Irritate contact dermatitis is a nonallergic inflammatory reaction of the skin. It is the result of the external agents acting as irritants, which produces direct local cytotoxic effect on the cells of the epidermis, with a subsequent inflammatory response in the dermis. It happens in all people of exposure. Irritant contact dermatitis is common in infants, such as diaper dermatitis is the most common irritant contact dermatitis happening in infants. The most common irritants are alkalis such as soaps and detergents. In occupational settings, other irritants such as oils and coolants, alkalis, acids and solvents may be important. A strong acid or alkalis may cause severe acute irritant contact dermatitis in all exposed individuals. Following contact with strong irritants, the reaction is immediate with blistering and pain, resembling a burn. From application of weak irritants, the reaction develops more slowly, over several days or weeks, with redness, pain or itching, and scaling.

Allergic contact dermatitis is the result of the external agents acting as allergens, where cell-mediated type IV hypersensitivity reaction is involved. The allergen penetrates the epidermis, combing with a protein mediator and then travels to the dermis, where lymphocytes become sensitized. The allergic reaction takes place when people are exposed again to the same allergens. Unlike irritant contact dermatitis, allergic contact dermatitis only occurs in a small number of exposed and sensitized individuals. It is most common during adulthood, but it affects all ages. Common contact allergens are as follows:

(1) Nickel or other metals.
(2) Rubber or latex.
(3) Cosmetics, perfumes and fragrances.
(4) Fabrics and clothing, chromates, dyes.
(5) Adhesives.
(6) Solvents.
(7) Poison ivy, poison oak, poison sumac and other plants.
(8) Medications(antibiotics, topical anesthetics, or others).
(9) Others.

In recent years, allergic contact dermatitis caused by topical steroids is well recognized.

13.1.2 Clinical Features

No matter what the mechanism or cause of the inflammation is, most cases of contact dermatitis have a similar appearance characterized by lesions localizing to the contact sites. Contact dermatitis can be categorized into acute, subacute and chronic phases. Contributing factors include allergen concentration, duration of exposure, and presence of other skin diseases.

Acute contact dermatitis is quick onset and often the result of a single overwhelming exposure or a few brief exposures to strong irritants or caustic agents. The lesions appear in the areas that are exposed and are characterized by well-defined erythema, papules, and vesicles(Color Figure 13 - 1). In severe cases, bullae may appear(Color Figure 13 - 2). Skin becomes exudative and weeps clear fluid if scratched. In acute irritate contact dermatitis, lesions are sharply demarcated and located only in the distribution of the contact sites. In the early stage, irritant contact dermatitis is likely to produce stinging or burning, while allergic contact dermatitis causes itching.

Subacute contact dermatitis is characterized by the formation of papules and dry scales. Edema and vesicles are less seen in this phase.

Chronic contact dermatitis occurs following repetitive exposure to weaker irritants such as detergents, organic solvents, soaps, weak acids and alkalis, and presents with scaling, skin fissuring, and lichenification(Color Figure 13 - 3). Excoriation can be seen in some cases.

Some common cases of contact dermatitis are as followed:

13.1.2.1 Diaper dermatitis

Diaper dermatitis is the most common case of irritant contact dermatitis happened in infants, which is caused by multiple factors, including occlusion, maceration, and friction. Eruptions are located in the diaper areas and present as acute or subacute erythematous lesions.

13. 1. 2. 2　Cosmetic dermatitis

Cosmetic dermatitis remains one of the most common allergic contact dermatitis, caused by deodorants, nail lacquers, lipsticks, and eye make-up. It may be divided into irritant, allergic and photosensitivity reactions and presents as an acute, subacute, or chronic dermatitis depending on the duration of exposure and the concentration of the allergens.

13. 1. 2. 3　Corticosteroid dermatitis

While using topical corticosteroid to treat some skin diseases, corticosteroid dermatitis may occur, characterized by eruptions to become much redder.

13. 1. 2. 4　Nickel dermatitis

Nickel allergy is one of the most common causes of allergic contact dermatitis. Nickel is wildly used in many everyday objects included buttons, earrings, necklaces, bracelets, watches, eyeglass frames and rings, so eczematous lesions caused by nickel can be seen in the area of exposed.

13. 1. 3　*Diagnosis and Differential Diagnosis*

Diagnosis of contact dermatitis is primarily based on the clinical features and a history of exposure to an irritant or an allergen. Location of the dermatitis is helpful in identifying the cause. Patch test is an easy way to identify the allergens. In patients with persistent eczematous eruptions when contact allergy is suspected or cannot be ruled out, patch test is helpful in making the diagnosis.

13. 1. 4　*Treatment*

If the agents causing the dermatitis can be found and successfully avoided, the recovery can be anticipated. But if contact continues, the dermatitis may become chronic. So the primary management consists of thorough washing with lots of water to remove any trace of the offending agent and avoiding further exposure.

Topical steroids and antihistamines are the mainstay of treatment of contact dermatitis and should be used until the inflammation has subsided. In severe cases, systemic corticosteroids may be required and usually tapered gradually over a period of 10 to 14 days to prevent recurrence of the eruptions.

13. 2　Eczema

The term eczema, derived from the Greek word ekzein, meaning to "boil out", refers to a group of skin conditions characterized by erythema, scales, vesicles, and crusts. Some medical staff loosely used the word eczema to refer to infantile form of atopic dermatitis. Eczematous lesions can be seen in many skin conditions such as atopic dermatitis, contact dermatitis, autosensitization dermatitis, seborrheic dermatitis, and scabies. Eczema is a descriptive term and not a specific diagnosis.

13. 2. 1　*Etiology*

The exact cause of eczema remains unknown. There are a lot of internal and external factors which can provoke eczematous lesions. Internal factors include genetic predisposition, stress, chronic infections (such as parasitosis, chronic tonsillitis), disturbance of blood circulation (such as venous insufficiency), endocrine and metabolic changes (such as pregnancy, menstrual disorders). External factors include food allergens (such as cow milk, egg whites, sea foods, soy bean), inhalant allergens (such as house dust mites, pollens, animal danders), environment (air pollution, smoking, hot or dry weather), other daily objects (such as soaps, cosmetics, detergents, synthetic fibers).

13. 2. 2　*Clinical Features*

According to the duration of the lesions and clinical characteristics, eczema can be divided into three phases: acute phase, subacute phase, and chronic phase. Eczema, regardless of cause, manifests similar clinical features characterized by erythema and edema in its acute phase and associated with thickening, lichenification, and scaling in its chronic phase.

In acute phase, lesions are characterized by erythema, edema, papules, and vesicles (Color Figure 13 - 4). In severe cases, bullae, oozing, crusting, or bleeding may appear.

In subacute phase, lesions are characterized by the formation of papules and dry scales. Edema and vesicles are less seen in this phase (Color Figure 13 - 5).

In chronic phase, eruptions present with scaling, skin thickening, fissuring, and lichenification (Color Figure 13 - 6). Excoriation can be seen in some cases.

A type of eczema may be described by location

(hand eczema, eyelid eczema), by specific appearance (eczema craquele or discoid), by possible cause (varicose eczema). Some special types of eczema are as follows:

13. 2. 2. 1   Discoid eczema

Discoid eczema usually begins on the lower legs, but dorsa of the hands and extensor surfaces of the arms can also be involved. Lesions are characterized by coin shaped plaque from 5 to 50 mm in diameter with edema, papules, vesicles and crusting (Color Figure 13 - 7). As new lesions appear, the old lesions expand by tiny papulovesicular satellite lesions presenting at the periphery and fusing with the main plaque. The plaques sometimes ooze and become thickened and scaly. It is usually worse in winter with severe pruritus.

13. 2. 2. 2   Hand eczema

Hand eczema can be caused by contact with an irritant, an allergic reaction to a substance, or an inherited condition. The symptoms of hand eczema can range from a mild, itchy erythema and scaling to severe itching, swelling, and blistering. In severe cases, bacterial skin infections can present.

13. 2. 2. 3   Eczema craquele

Eczema craquele, also known as xerotic eczema, is characterized by the formation of scaling patches with fine crackling, mainly on the lower legs. Favored sites are the anterior shins, extensor arms, and flank. Elderly persons are particularly predisposed, and xerosis appears to be the most common cause of pruritus. It is worse in the dry winter months and is also seen in those who have excessive bathing with hot water and soap.

13. 2. 3   Treatment

During a flare, patients should avoid all kinds of irritant factors such as wet, scratch, spicy foods, alcohol, hot water bathing and excessive using of soap.

13. 2. 3. 1   Topical therapy

Eczema is often treated with topical corticosteroids. They do not cure eczema, but are highly effective in controlling symptoms. Topical steroid should be used until improvement occurs and then withdrawn. The potency of topical corticosteroids should be tailored to the severity of the disease, the sites of lesions and the age of the patient. For mild eczema, a mild-potency steroid, such as hydrocortisone 1 percent, may be effective, whereas for moderate-to-severe cases, a higher-potency steroid may be needed. For children, mild or medium steroids are most-

ly adequate whereas highly potent steroids are not usually required. Do not use potent topical corticosteroids on the face or neck. When the lesions are characterized by edema, weeping and oozing, wet dressing may help to settle the acute flare.

13. 2. 3. 2   Systemic therapy

Antihistamine, especially sedating antihistamine, can be useful in controlling pruritus. In severe cases, short-term using of oral steroids such as prednisolone may also be prescribed.

13.3   Atopic Dermatitis

Atopic dermatitis (AD), which was first reported by Robert Willan in 1808, is a pruritic, chronically relapsing inflammatory skin disease often associated with a family history of atopy (asthma, hay fever, and AD). In 1892, Besnier described it as prurigo diasthetique. In 1923, Coca and Cooke used the term atopy to describe a hypersensitive state in human characterized by an enhanced capacity to form reagins in response to a variety of antigens. "Atopy" has the meaning of "without place or a strange thing". The term atopic dermatitis was used by Wise and Sulzherger in 1935 and now is accepted universally. This disorder, primarily occurring in infants and children, is commonly seen in pediatric dermatology clinics.

The prevalence of AD displays both geographical and ethnic variations. The exact incidence is difficult to establish, as many of the mild cases are not noted. The prevalence of AD has been increased significantly worldwide over the past few decades, especially in developed countries. It has been reported that the incidence rate of AD was 10% to 20% in America, Japan, Hong Kong and European countries, but it is rather lower in China.

13. 3. 1   Etiology

Although it is a common disease, the exactly pathogenesis of AD is still obscure. AD is more likely to result form the interaction between genetic and environmental factors.

Around 60% of AD patients have a family history of atopy. If one of the parents is suffering from an atopic disease, there is a 60 percent chance of the child to be atopic, and the rate reaches to 80% if both parents are affected. The mode of inheritance is not entirely clear, but appears to be polygenic.

AD patients are known to have numerous immunologic abnormalities. Most patients have elevated numbers of circulating eosinophils and serum IgE levels. IgE is raised in approximately 60% of patients with AD. The elevated IgE responses and eosinophilia reflects an increased expression of Th2 cytokines such as IL-4, IL-5, and IL-13. Some studies also show that patients with AD have an expanded subset of activated CLA＋T cells in their circulation. CLA＋T cell in AD expressing either CD4 or CD8 spontaneously secrete IL-5 or IL-13, functionally prolong eosinophil survival, and induce IgE synthesis. AD patients are more susceptible to viral infections with herpes simplex, associated with diminished cell-mediated immunity.

Provoking factors for AD exacerbations include the following:

(1) Microbial colonization(*Staphylococcus aureus*).

(2) Defects in skin barrier function.

(3) Exposure to aeroallergens(pets, house-dust mites, pollen).

(4) Sensitization to food allergens(cow's milk, hen's egg, wheat, soy beans and peanut).

(5) Sweating.

(6) Sensory irritant(wool).

(7) Stress.

13. 3. 2   Clinical Features

AD is divided into three phases, in which both the sites and the morphology of the lesions vary with age.

Infantile phase(up to 2 years of age): The onset of AD occurs during the first year of life in 60% and before the age of 5 in 85% of affected individuals. The eruption starts on the cheeks(Color Figure 13 - 8), forehead or scalp, and often affects the lateral aspects of the extensors of the extremities. Trunk may also be involved but the diaper area is often spared. The lesions, which are extremely pruritic, are characterized by poorly defined erythema with edema, papules and vesicles(Color Figure 13 - 1). Crusting and oozing can be present if scratched. Generalized xerosis is quite seen(Color Figure 13 - 9).

Childhood phase(from age 2 to puberty): In this phase, the typical sites of predilection are the flexural areas(Color Figure 13 - 10). Children are more likely to present the lichenified papules and plaques showing the more chronic disease and involving the hands, feet, wrists, ankles, and antecubital and popliteal regions(Color Figure 13 - 11).

Adult phase(from puberty onward): Predomi-

nant areas of involvement in adult phase include the flexural folds, the face and neck, the arms and back, the hands and feet. The lesions are characterized by dry, scaling erythematous papules and large lichenified plaques.

13. 3. 3   Diagnosis and Differential Diagnosis

Diagnosis of AD is based on the clinical features. In 1980, Harnifin and Rajka established standardized criteria for the diagnosis of AD, which is accepted worldwide.

13. 3. 3. 1   Basic features (must have three or more)

(1) Pruritus.

(2) Typical morphology and distribution.

Flexural lichenification or linearity in adults.

Facial and extensor involvement in infants and children.

(3) Tendency toward chronic or chronically relapsing dermatitis.

(4) Personal or family history of atopy(asthma, allergic rhinitis, AD).

13. 3. 3. 2   Plus three or more of the following

(1) Xerosis.

(2) Ichthyosis/palmar hyperlinearity/keratosis pilaris.

(3) Immediate(type I)skin test reactivity.

(4) Elevated serum IgE.

(5) Early age of onset.

(6) Tendency toward cutaneous infections(esp. *Staphylococcus aureus*)and herpes simplex/impaired cell-mediated immunity.

(7) Tendency toward nonspecific hand or foot dermatitis.

(8) Nipple eczema.

(9) Cheilitis.

(10) Recurrent conjunctivitis.

(11) Dennie-Morgan infraorbital fold.

(12) Keratoconus.

(13) Anterior subcapsular cataracts.

(14) Orbital darkening.

(15) Facial pallor/facial erythema.

(16) Pityriasis alba.

(17) Anterior neck folds.

(18) Itch when sweating.

(19) Intolerance to wool and lipid solvents.

(20) Perifollicular accentuation.

(21) Food intolerance.

(22) Course influenced by environmental/emotional factors.

(23) White dermographism/delayed blanch.

Harnifin's criteria has been very useful but some of the features do not occur in young children and some of the minor features may be present in normal population.

In 1994, Williams, with the UK Working Group, proposed criteria for the diagnosis of AD, which was mainly used in epidemiological studies. These criteria have a sensitivity of 80% and a specificity of 97% in children and are easy to use in daily work. The diagnosis requires evidence of itchy skin(or parental report of scratching or rubbing)plus three or more of the following:

(1) History of flexural involvement(folds of the elbows, behind the knees, front of ankles, around the neck, and the cheeks in children under 10 years of age).

(2) Personal history of hay fever or asthma(or a history of atopy in a relative of a child under 10 years of age).

(3) A history of generalized day skin in the last year.

(4) Visible flexural eczema(or eczema involving he cheeks/ forehead and outer limbs in children under 4 years).

(5) Onset under the age of 2 years(this is not used if the child is under 4 years of age).

The differential diagnosis of AD includes scabies, seborrheic dermatitis, contact dermatitis and psoriasis. Scabies may produce nonspecific eczematous changes on the entire body. Burrows and pustules on palms, soles, genitalia and between fingers help to establish diagnosis. Both Seborrheic dermatitis and AD can affect scalp and sometimes are difficult to distinguish but in AD the scale is dry and excoriations are frequent whereas in seborrheic dermatitis the scale is yellow and greasy. The infant with seborrheic dermatitis appears comfortable whereas children with AD often feel extremely itching. Contact dermatitis is not common in children and patch test may help to make a diagnosis. In young children, psoriasis is mostly seen in the diaper area and scalp but may be seen anywhere. It is characterized by scaly erythematous, well-demarcated small plaques, typical silver scale. In some cases, skin biopsy can help distinguish psoriasis from AD.

13. 3. 4   Treatment

Although there is no cure for AD, It can be treated effectively through a combination of prevention and drug therapy.

13. 3. 4. 1   Basic therapy

Basic treatment of AD should comprise education patients or parents about the nature of the disease, addressing the skin barrier defect with regular use of emollients and skin hydration, along with identifications and avoidance of trigger factors.

13. 3. 4. 2   Topical therapy

(1) Emollients

A key feature of AD is intense dryness of the skin caused by a dysfunction of the skin barrier with increased transepidermal water loss, so the regular use of emollients is important for handling this problem. Emollients should be used continuously, even if no actual inflammatory skin lesions are obvious.

(2) Topical steroids

Topical steroids still remain the mainstay of management for AD and should be used until improvement occurs and then withdrawn. Consider the age of the patient and the sites of the lesions while using topical steroids. Potent steroids should never be used on thin skin areas such as face, neck, axillae, and groin, where 1% hydrocortisone ointment is effective. For children, mild or medium steroids are mostly adequate whereas potent steroids are not usually required.

(3) Wet dressing

Wet dressing is an effective adjunct to topical steroids to settle an acute flare, especially when the lesions are characterized by edema, weeping and oozing.

(4) Topical calcineurin inhibitors

Topical tacrolimus and pimecrolimus have both been shown to be effective in the treatment of AD and can be used when topical steroids have failed or cannot be tolerated. Don't use topical Calcineurin Inhibitors as first-line treatment for atopic dermatitis of any severity. Consider topical Calcineurin Inhibitors for facial atopic dermatitis in children requiring long-term or frequent use of mild topical corticosteroids. 0. 03% tacrolimus ointment and 1% pimecrolimus cream can be safely applied in children older than 2 years of age whereas 0. 1% tacrolimus ointment can only be used in adults. Mild burning sensations are the most common side effects of these two preparations.

13. 3. 4. 3   Systemic therapy

(1) Antihistamine

Short-term using of sedating antihistamine can be useful in promoting sleep and controlling severe pruritus during a flare.

(2) Antibiotic

Systemic antibiotic is considered when there is a sign of widespread bacterial secondary infection(primarily S aureus).

(3) Corticosteroids

In severe cases, patients might benefit from a short course of systemic steroids therapy, but long-term use should be avoided.

(4) Immunosuppressive agents

Cyclosporin A and azathioprine can be used in severe AD patients but should evaluate the benefits and risk before using.

(5) Phototherapy

UVA, narrow-band UVB and PUVA may be help to improve AD lesions in some cases. Overexposure to ultraviolet light carries its own risks, particularly potential skin cancer from exposure.

13. 4 Autosensitization Dermatitis (Autoeczematization)

Autosensitization dermatitis refers to a phenomenon which an acute widespread dermatitis develops at cutaneous sites distant from an inflammatory focus, and where the secondary acute dermatitis is not explained by the inciting cause of the primary inflammation.

13. 4. 1 Etiology

Autosensitization dermatitis is a skin reaction involving the development of a variety of skin lesions in response to infections(virus, bacteria, fungus, and parasite), inflammatory skin conditions or other triggers.

13. 4. 2 Clinical Features

The skin reaction may have considerable change in appearance from itchy red skin to the development of blisters and may involve variable portions of the body.

Clinically, autosensitization dermatitis occurs after 1 week to several weeks of a localized dermatitis, usually lower leg dermatitis. Often somewhat suddenly widespread, symmetrical, pruritic erythematous, 1 – 2 mm papulovesicular lesions appear. The palms may be affected in a pattern resembling pompholyx. The eruption may spread to confluence, and some areas may become weepy and crusted. The eruption usually persists until the triggering focus is improved. Histologically, the lesions show spongiotic

dermatitis.

Infectious eczematoid dermatitis is a special kind of autosensitization dermatitis and appears around the ulcer, sinus, chronic purulent otitis media or fistula on the abdomen with overabundant discharges.

13. 4. 3 Diagnosis and Differential Diagnosis

Autosensitization dermatitis should be considered when the acute dermatitis appears distant from an inflammatory focus. And infectious eczematoid dermatitis should be considered when the patient has ulcer, sinus or chronic purulent otitis media.

13. 4. 4 Treatment

Autosensitization dermatitis is treated by identifying the original inciting dermatitis and eliminating it. Systemic corticosteroid therapy will clear the eruption, but unless the triggering dermatitis is appropriately managed, the widespread dermatitis is likely to recur. Systemic corticosteroids are often required, but in mild cases topical steroids, soaks, and antipruritics may be adequate. Coexistent infection either secondary or in the original triggering focus (e. g. an infected leg ulcer) should be aggressively treated with oral antibiotics.

13. 5 Stasis Dermatitis

Stasis dermatitis is a common inflammatory skin disease that occurs on the lower extremities in patients with chronic venous insufficiency with venous hypertension.

13. 5. 1 Etiology

Stasis dermatitis occurs as a direct consequence of venous insufficiency. Disturbed function of the one-way valvular system in the deep venous plexus of the legs results in backflow of blood from the deep venous system to the superficial venous system, accompanying with venous hypertension. The pooled venous blood in the legs compromises the endothelial integrity in the microvasculature, resulting in fibrin leakage, local inflammation, and local cell necrosis.

13. 5. 2 Clinical Features

Stasis dermatitis typically affects middle-aged and elderly patients. It rarely occurs before the fifth decade of life, except in patients with acquired venous insufficiency due to surgery, trauma, or thrombosis. Stasis dermatitis is usually the earliest cutaneous sequela of venous insufficiency, and it may be a precursor to more problematic conditions, such as venous leg ulceration and lipodermatosclerosis.

Initially, hyperpigmentation and red-brown discoloration from RBC extravasation appear. Later, eczematous changes develop and manifest as erythema, scaling, weeping, and crusting, all of which can be made worse by bacterial superinfection or by contact dermatitis caused by many topical treatments often applied. When chronic venous insufficiency and stasis dermatitis are both inadequately treated, stasis dermatitis may progress to frank skin ulceration, chronic edema, thickened fibrotic skin, or lipodermatosclerosis(a painful induration resulting from panniculitis, which, if severe, gives the lower leg an inverted "coke-bottle" shape with enlargement of the calf and narrowing at the ankle).

13.5.3 Diagnosis and Differential Diagnosis
Stasis dermatitis is easily diagnosed according to the typical skin lesions and the varicosity on the lower leg. But this disease should be differentiated with contact dermatitis, autosensitization dermatitis and progressive pigmentary purpuric dermatosis, and the ulceration should be differentiated with other conditions with ulcer on the lower leg.

13.5.4 Treatment
The overall mainstay of treatment has always been aimed at lessening the clinical impact of the underlying venous insufficiency, which is typically accomplished with compression therapy.

Topical treatment of stasis dermatitis has much in common with the treatment of other forms of acute eczematous dermatitis. Open excoriations and erosions should be treated with a topical antibiotic, such as bacitracin or polysporin. Obvious superficial impetiginization should be treated with topical mupirocin or a systemic antibiotic with activity against Staphylococcus and Streptococcus species (e.g. dicloxacillin, cephalexin, cefadroxil, levofloxacin). Patients with chronic, refractory stasis dermatitis can be treated with ligation of the vessels.

■ Summary

Eczema refers to a group of skin diseases and its etiology remains unknown. According to the duration of the lesions and clinical characteristics, eczema can be divided into three phases: acute phase, subacute phase, and chronic phase. It is characterized by erythema, papules and vesicles in the acute phase and by dryness, lichenification and fissure in the chronic phase.

Contact dermatitis is an inflammatory reaction in the skin resulting from exposure to external agents. It can be classified into two types: irritant contact dermatitis which happens in all people of exposed and allergic contact dermatitis which only occurs in a small number of exposed and sensitized individuals. Contact dermatitis is characterized by lesions localizing to the area of contact and well-defined. Patch test is helpful to make the diagnosis and distinguish it from other eczematous lesions.

Atopic dermatitis often occurs in infants and children and is characterized by xerosis, relapsing eczematous lesions and extremely pruritus. It is often associated with a family history of atopy and numerous immunologic abnormalities. In young children, the eruption often affects face, scalp and the lateral aspects of the extensors of the extremities. In old children and adults, the typical sites of predilection are the flexural areas, especially antecubital and popliteal regions.

Topical steroids still remain the mainstay of management for eczema, contact dermatitis and atopic dermatitis. Wet dressing is an effective adjunct to topical steroids to settle an acute flare, especially when the lesions are characterized by edema, weeping and oozing. Short-term using of sedating antihistamine can be useful in controlling severe pruritus. In severe cases, patients might benefit from a short course of systemic steroids therapy, but long-term use should be avoided.

Autosensitization dermatitis refers to a phenomenon in which an acute widespread dermatitis develops in response to skin infections or other triggers. It should be treated by identifying the original inciting dermatitis and eliminating it.

Stasis dermatitis is a direct consequence of venous insufficiency. The mainstay of treatment has always been aimed at lessening the clinical impact of the underlying venous insufficiency.

▪ Questions

1. What is the clinical feature of contact dermatitis and how to diagnose and treat it?

2. What is the clinical feature of atopic dermatitis and how to manage it?

3. What is the cause of autosensitization dermatitis and how to treat it?

4. What is the cause of stasis dermatitis and how to treat it?

（**Huan Xing** 邢嬛）

Chapter 14

Drug Eruption

- **Objectives**

To master the knowledge of the clinical features of drug eruption.

To have an intimate knowledge of diagnosis and management of the disease.

- **Key concepts**

Drug eruption is the inflammatory lesions caused by medication.

Cross-allergy phenomena are that patients, under the condition of hypersensitivity, are allergic to the drugs that have similar chemical groups to allergenic drugs.

Polyvalent allergy is more deathful than cross allergy because drugs different from allergenic drugs can cause drug eruptions when the patient is under the hypersensitivity.

Drug eruption, also called dermatitis medicamentosa, is the inflammatory eruption in the skin and mucosal that can be caused by oral drugs, externally applied medicines, injection medicines, enema medicines, suppository medicines. Multi-systems can be involved during the most serious drug eruption. The non-treatmental reactions of medications are usually defined as adverse reactions to medications. Drug eruption is only one of the manifestations.

14.1.1 Etiology

14.1.1.1 Individual factors

The sensitivity of different individuals to the same medicine is different. The same person could even react differently to the same medicine. Genetic factors, allergic constitutions, enzyme defect, pathological or physiological conditions contribute to causing these differences.

14.1.1.2 Drug factors

There are many different drugs that can cause drug eruptions. The common medicines include:

(1) Antipyretic and analgesic drugs

Aspirin, aminopyrine, paracetamol, phenylbuta-zone.

(2) Antibiotics

β-lactam penicillin is the most common drug to induce drug eruption, including semi-synthetic penicillin(ampicillin and amoxycillin), sulfonamides such as azole compound sulfamethoxazole, streptomycin, furazolidone, tetracycline, chloromycetin, and so on.

(3) Sedative hypnotics and antiepileptic drugs

Such as phenobarbital, phenytoin, meprobamate, and carbamazepine. Among which phenobarbital is the most common drug to cause drug eruption.

(4) Heterogeneous serum preparations and vaccines

Tetanus antitoxin, rabies vaccine, venom serum and so on.

(5) All kinds of biological agents.

(6) Some Chinese medicines have been also found to induce drug eruptions.

14.1.2 Pathogenesis

The pathogenesis of drug eruption involves two types of mechanisms: immune mechanism and non-immune mechanism.

14.1.2.1 Immune mechanism

It is an allergic reaction. Most drug eruptions are attributed to this mechanism. Drugs are various and can be classified by protein and small molecule compounds. The latter is the common. Macromolecules, such as serum products, biological agents, vaccines, can directly induce immune response. However, small molecules must be combined with macromolecules(for example protein, polysaccharide, and polypeptide)in the body to become the complete antigen that will cause immune reactions. Semi-complete antigens include drugs, degradation products or metabolites of drugs, excipients and impurities. A few drugs such as sulfonamides, quinolones, tetracycline, contraceptives can be transformed to antigens after illumination and then cause light allergy.

There are four kinds of allergic reactions:

(1) IgE-dependent allergic reaction(type Ⅰ)

It can cause urticaria, angioedema or anaphylactic shock.

(2) Cytotoxic type hypersensitivity(type Ⅱ)

The pathogenesis of thrombocytopenic purpura, hemolytic anemia or neutropenia is this type of reaction.

(3) Immune complex-type reaction(type Ⅲ)

It includes vasculitis, urticaria, serum sickness, and serum sickness-like syndrome that are always accompanied by joint and kidney disorders.

(4) Delayed type hypersensitivity(type Ⅳ)

Eczematous drug reactions, measles-like drug eruptions, exfoliative dermatitis. The pathogenesis of drug reactions is very complicated because every type of reactions can act alone or act together during the course of the disease.

Characteristics of drug reactions induced by immune mechanism are explained as followed:

(1) Occurring only in a small part of population.

(2) The degree of seriousness of the skin rash does not correlate with the pharmacological and toxicological effects of the drug, or the dosage of the drug.

(3) They have latency. The latency period is about 4 to 20 days(mostly 7 to 8days)after the first drug administration and is about several minutes to 24 hours after the second drug administration.

(4) They have various clinical manifestations that are not specific. The same person can show different kinds of drug eruptions even he or she has the same drugs.

(5) Cross-allergy and polyvalent allergy phenomena: under the condition of hypersensitivity, patients can be allergic to the drugs that have the similar chemical groups to ever allergic drugs. Polyvalent allergy is more serious than cross allergy because drugs different from allergenic drugs can cause drug eruptions when the patient is under the hypersensitivity.

(6) Treatment with glucocorticoid is effective. The disease will vanish if the patients stop using the allergic drugs.

14.1.2.2 Non-immune reaction

This type of drug reactions is rare. The possible mechanisms include:

(1) Drugs induce the release of inflammatory mediators, for example radiological contrast agents, aspirin, polymyxin-B, opiates. These drugs can induce degranulation of mast cells and basophils, release histamine that causes urticaria and angioedema. Some drugs such as non-steroidal anti-inflammatory drugs can increase the formation of leukotriene through inhibition of cyclo-oxygenase and then induce the drug reactions.

(2) Over-dosage reactions: They always occur

in elder people or patients with liver and kidney dysfunction. Ammonia neopterin and methotrexate frequently induce this type of drug reactions.

(3) Accumulative function: Some drugs have a slow excretion rate or they have been administered for a long time. These drugs cause eruptions in patients with liver and kidney dysfunction. Lodide and bromide can cause acne-like rash. Arsenic can cause pigmentation, hyperkeratosis, or even squamous cell carcinoma.

(4) Enzyme defect or enzyme inhibition led by genetic factors influence the normal metabolic pathways of certain drugs; then the drug reactions may occur.

(5) Phototoxic reactions: Some drugs can be transformed into toxic products after ultraviolet irradiation.

14.1.3 Clinical Features

Adverse drug reactions will be discussed by their morphologic patterns. The most common patterns are as followed:

14.1.3.1 Fixed drug eruption

Many antipyretic and analgesic drugs, sulfonamides, phenobarbital drugs are responsible for the majorities of fixed drug eruptions. They may present anywhere, but often occur on the perioral location, glans, and some skin-mucosa junctions. They present as edematous erythema with diameter of 1 to 4 cm and a clear boundary which is round or oval (Color Figure 14 – 1). There is usually only one patch, but occasionally several patches can occur. Patients can feel mild itching without any systemic symptoms. More serious eruptions are blisters or bullous on the patches. Exudative erosion may occur on the mucosa. If the condition is worse, painful ulcers will form with secondary infection. The eruptions will enlarge and increase in numbers when recurring on ingestion of the offending drug. Plaques will resolve 1 week after stopping using the drug and maybe leave a long-lasting characteristic hyperpigmentation.

14.1.3.2 Urticarial drug eruption

Serum products, penicillin and sulfonamides, β-lactam antibiotics, aspirin and nonsteroidal anti-inflammatory drugs (NSAIDs) are the most common causes of urticarial reactions. Medications may induce urticaria by immunologic and non-immunologic mechanisms. Clinically the lesions are pruritic wheals, edematous erythema that are similar to urticaria (Color Figure 14 – 2), but the lesions last longer and are frequently accompanied with serum sickness-like symptoms such as joint pain, fever, adenopathy, angioedema, even proteinuria and so on. The most serious manifestation is the anaphylactic shock. If the drug has a slow metabolism rate, or the patient frequently contacts the allergic drug during normal life, chronic urticaria will occur.

14.1.3.3 Morbilliform drug eruption and scarlatiniform drug eruption

They are exanthema types and the most common types in the clinical manifestations. Penicillin, antipyretic and analgesic drugs, sulfonamides, barbitone are responsible for these eruptions, especially semi-synthetic penicillin. The lesions occur suddenly 1 week after the medication and are always accompanied by systemic symptoms such as fever.

Lesions of morbilliform drug eruption are red pinhead sized or rice sized patches and rashes that are scattered or dense, symmetrically distributed and generalized all over the body, especially the trunk. In some serious cases, there are some purpuras on the skin that resemble measles, but the lesions are better than measles (Color Figure 14 – 3).

Scarlatiniform drug eruption begins with small pieces of erythema on the face, neck, upper limb, trunk and then extends to the other sites of the body. The lesions can spread all over the body in 1 – 4 days and can fuse together, especially on the fold sites and flexor folds of the side parts and limbs. The clinical manifestations resemble scarlet fever, but it has the better prognosis. The patients have obvious itching feelings.

These two types drug eruptions don't have the characteristic symptoms besides the similar lesions with measles and scarlet fever. After 1 – 2 weeks, the lesions will fade with bran-like desquamation and the fever will disappear. If the drug eruptions are ignored, they might deteriorate to the heavy drug eruption.

14.1.3.4 Eczematous drug eruption

Contact dermatitis will occur after first using or contacting penicillin, streptomycin, or sulfonamides. Then, when the same medicines or similar medicines (with the same chemical structures) are used again, the eczematous drug eruption will occur. The lesions are characterized by different-sized erythema, papules, papulovesicles and vesicles that tend to generalize and confluent. Secondary leakage, erosion, scaling can be seen on the top of the lesions. Pruritus varies in different people. Long time medication will lead to dry skin, invasive hypertrophy. The drug reactions have a long course about over 1 month. Systemic symptoms are rare.

14.1.3.5 Purpuric drug eruption

Barbiturates, antibiotics, diuretics or quinine are responsible for this type of drug reaction that is caused by type Ⅱ allergic reaction or type Ⅲ reaction. The former induces thrombocytopenic purpura and the latter induces vasculitis that shows purpura. Both lower limbs are the most common involved sites. Mild cases are characterized by red petechia or ecchymosis, scattered or dense, slight uplifted. Serious cases are characterized by wheal, vesicles or blood blisters. Some other systemic symptoms include bellyache, joint swelling and pain, hematuria, blood in stool, mucosal bleeding, anemia and so on.

14.1.3.6 Erythema multiforme drug eruption

This type of drug reaction is caused by antipyretic and analgesic drugs, sulfonamides and barbiturates. The lesions are characterized by round or oval edema erythema with clear boundary. The lesions are dusky in the center. Bullae are seen in the center and become the typical iris-like lesions. The mild skin lesions appear on the proximal extremities. Pruritus is common. The serious skin lesions can scatter all over the body. Bullae, erosion and exudation can form on the base of the erythema, papules and vesicles, especially on the eyes, oral mucosa, anus and genitals. Pain is very severe. WBC may be elevated in the blood. Patients may suffer from liver and kidney dysfunction and secondary infection. This type of drug reaction is one of the serious drug eruptions that can cause death.

14.1.3.7 Drug-induced bullae epidermolysis

It is the most serious drug eruption. Antipyretic and analgesic drugs, sulfonamides, barbiturates, and antibiotics are the common causes. This drug reaction occurs suddenly and rapidly. Some patients present with diffuse dark red or purple patches resembling erythema multiforme drug eruption, scarlatiniform drug eruption, or morbilliform drug eruption. Rapidly, the patches spread over the body. Then different sized relaxed vesicles or bullae appear on the base of red patches. The lesions cause a positive Nikolsky sign (Color Figure 14 – 4). External force can make the lesions form erosion surface and can form large sized epidermal necrolysis followed by erosion and leakage resembling scald. The patient can feel severe tenderness. Oral mucosa, conjunctival mucosa, respiratory or gastrointestinal mucosa can be involved. The symptoms of systemic poisoning are very severe. Patient can also suffer from high fever, vomiting, fatigue, nausea, diarrhea and some other symptoms. Secondary infection, electrolyte imbalance, liver and kidney dysfunction, visceral bleeding, proteinuria, or azotemia that the patients suffer from can lead to death.

14.1.3.8 Drug-induced exfoliative dermatitis

It is one of the severe drug reactions. The antibiotics, antipyretic and analgesic drugs, barbiturates, sulfonamides, antiepileptic drugs (carbamazepine) are the common causes. This type of drug eruption always occurs after a long time of medication. Latency of the first occurrence is about 20 days. Continuing medication or improper treatment to scarlatiniform drug eruption, morbilliform drug eruption, or eczematous drug eruption can also cause exfoliative dermatitis. The lesions fuse to be diffuse flushing erythema, swelling. Hands, feet and face are the most common involved locations (Color Figure 14 – 5). Sometimes there are some blisters, erosion, and leakage on the base. 2 – 3 weeks later, the erythema fades gradually and is followed by some scaly or leaf-like scaling. There are characteristic manifestations on the hands and feet: gloves-like and sock-like scaling. It is difficult to swallow because of the blisters, painful erosion in the oral mucosa. Conjunctival hyperemia, swelling, photophobia, increased secretion, even more serious corneal ulcer can be seen in some patients. The hair, finger nails and toe may shed sometimes, but they can come out again. The systemic symptoms are very severe, including high fever, chills, adenopathy, bronchial pneumonia, drug-induced hepatitis, increase or decrease in peripheral blood leukocytes, even agranulocytosis. This type of drug eruption has a long duration. Without the rapid diagnosis and correct treatment, the disease may lead to death due to secondary infection and systemic failure.

14.1.3.9 Acneiform drug eruption

This type of drug reaction is caused by a long time of using iodine, bromine agent, contraceptives, glucocorticoid, or isoniazid. It has a long latency period. Face, chest and back are the most commonly involved sites. Follicular papules, papulopustules resembling acne are the most typical manifestations. Systemic symptoms are rare. The disease progresses slowly. Long-term use of bromine agent can lead to granuloma-like lesions.

14.1.3.10 Photosensitive drug eruption

This kind of drug reactions occur when patient

receives sunlight irradiation or ultraviolet irradiation after using sulfonamides, tetracycline, psoralen, quinolones, phenothiazine, chlorpromazine, griseofulv-in or contraceptives. It is classified into two types:

(1) Photo toxic erythema

Anybody can get the disease after the first-time administration of the drugs. The pathogenesis is non-immune mechanism. It is correlated to the dosage of medication and the level of exposure to sunlight. The lesions are found 7 – 8 hours after sunlight exposure. Lesions resemble sunburn and can disappear rapidly after stopping the medication.

(2) Photo allergic eruption

Only a minority of people can get the disease that has a latency period. Eczematous eruptions are found not only on the exposure sites, but also the non-exposure sites. It has a long duration.

14. 1. 3. 11　Drug hypersensitivity syndrome

It is accompanied by the increase in eosinophils and systemic involvement. Antiepileptic drugs, sulfonamides are responsible for the drug eruption. It always occurs in people who have epoxide hydrolase defect. The drug eruption begins within 2 – 6 weeks after medication. It is a sudden disease that is characterized by morbilliform lesions on face, upper trunk and limb. The lesions tend to become exfoliative dermatitis. Infiltration of the lesions occurs because of edema of the hair follicle. Swelling of face is characteristic. Sometimes sterile pustules and purpura are also present. Systemic symptoms include fever, adenopathy and hematological abnormalities. Death rate is about 10%.

Clinically, drug-induced bullae epidermolysis, erythema multiforme drug eruption and drug-induced exfoliative dermatitis are called serious drug reactions.

Besides those above drug reaction, there is other drug eruption such as skin pigmentation, systemic lupus erythematosus-like reaction, lichenoid lesions, pemphigus-like rash, pseudo-lymphoma syndrome and so on.

14. 1. 4　Laboratory Examination

There are two methods of detecting allergic medicines: tests in vivo and in vitro.

14. 1. 4. 1　Tests in vivo

(1) Skin test

The most common used methods are: ① prick test, ② intradermal test, ③ cut test, ④ Patch test, ⑤ Skin window test. Among them, intradermal test, prick test and patch test are the more common used tests. The result of intradermal test is very specific. Intradermal test is used for detecting rapid onset of skin allergy that may be allergic reactions from penicillin, antiserum or procaine. However, a negative result can not exclude the possibility of occurrence of allergic reaction completely. Then it is prohibited to be used on the most hypersensitive individuals. Epinephrine, oxygen equipment and other first aid measures should be prepared before the test in order to prevent the occurrence of anaphylactic shock. Eczematous drug eruption can be diagnosed by patch test auxiliarily and safely.

(2) Drug provocation test

Half a month after the disappearance of drug reaction, we can give the patient experimental dosage of the drug(1/8 to 1/4 or less than the treating dosage)in order to find the allergic drugs. The test can be used under the condition that the patient need the medications(for example: anti-TB drugs or antiepileptic drugs) very much and the drug eruption is mild. Because the test is dangerous for the patients, the patients who have rapid onset of skin allergy and serious drug reactions should not be tested.

14. 1. 4. 2　tests in vitro

They are safer than test in vivo. Basophil degranulation test, lymphocyte transformation test in vitro, allergen assay radiation test and agar diffusion test are included. The results are not stable.

14. 1. 5　Diagnosis and Differential Diagnosis

14. 1. 5. 1　Diagnosis

Diagnosis of drug reactions is based on several factors as followed:

(1) Definite medication history;

(2) A certain degree of latency;

(3) Symmetrical distribution of lesions that are fresh red;

(4) Obvious itching.

Excluding the diseases resembling drug eruption and the contagious eruptive diseases. It is difficult to find the allergic drug if the patient are taking more than two medications. Then, we should try to get the correct diagnosis based on medication history, drug reaction history and the relationship between the incidence and medications.

14. 1. 5. 2　Differential diagnosis

(1) Morbilliform drug eruption should be differentiated with measles and scarlatiniform drug eruption should be distinguished from scarlet fe-

ver. The lesions caused by drug reactions are lighter red than infectious eruptive diseases. The pruritus is more severe in drug eruption and the systemic symptoms are milder. Manifestations of drug reactions are lack of characteristic symptoms and signs that are special to measles and scarlet fever.

(2) Drug-induced bullae epidermolysis should be differentiated with staphylococcal scalded skin syndrome.

(3) When fixed drug eruption occurs on genital area, it should be distinguished from chancre and genital herpes.

14.1.6 Treatment

Stop using all potential allergic drugs and accelerate metabolites excretion.

14.1.6.1 Rescue measures and treatment of anaphylactic shock

Anaphylactic shock is the most serious drug reaction. Penicillin injection is the most common cause. It occurs suddenly within several minutes to half an hour after injection or intradermal test. The patient will suffer from face flushing, chest tightness, gasp, dizziness, palpitations and limb numbness at the beginning, and then pallor or cyanosis, cold sweat, cold limbs, weak pulse, hypotension, unconsciousness, even coma. It can be accompanied by urticaria, angioedema and other drug eruptions.

Rescue measurement and treatment:

(1) We must rescue the patient immediately after the diagnosis has been made.

(2) 0.1% epinephrine(0.5 - 1 ml) should be injected intramuscularly or added to 40 ml 50% glucose solution for intravenous use in order to relieve airway mucosal edema, smooth muscle spasm and hypotension.

(3) Intramuscular or bolus injection of 5 - 10 mg dexamethasone firstly, then adding 200 - 400 mg hydrocortisone into 500 or 1 000 ml 5% - 10% glucose solution for intravenous use.

(4) After these steps above, if the systolic blood pressure is still lower than 80 mmHg, we can give the patient vasopressor .

(5) We should give the patient 0.25 g aminophylline for intravenous use in order to reduce severe bronchospasm. When the laryngeal edema causes respiratory obstruction, tracheotomy is necessary.

(6) CPR must be done when cardiopulmonary arrest occurs.

14.1.6.2 Mild drug eruptions

The lesions often disappear quickly after stopping allergic medications. Vitamin C, antihistamine are always used for treatment. Moderate doses of prednisone(30 - 60 mg/d) can be given to patient with severe lesions and tapered down according to the degree of the lesions. Local treatment: calamine lotion or corticosteroid cream can be used for erythema or papules. 3% boric acid solution or 0.1% chlorhexidine solution should be used by wet compress on the erosion or leakage lesions. After wet compress, zinc oxide oil or corticosteroid cream may be used on lesions.

14.1.6.3 Severe drug reactions

We must rescue patients immediately and prevent complications and sequelae. We should enhance the care, shorten the course of disease and reduce mortality.

(1) Early use of corticosteroids in sufficient quantities

It is the premise to reduce mortality. Hydrocortisone 300 - 400 mg/d intravenous infusion or dexamethasone 10 - 20 mg/d intravenous infusion is the usual treatment. Increasing the amount of glucocorticoid is better for severe drug-induced bullae epidermolysis. We should balance drug delivery within 24 hours. If the amount of glucocorticoid is sufficient, the condition should be controlled in 3 - 5 days. Otherwise, we should increase the amount of glucocorticoid(1/3 - 1/2 of the original dose). When the old eruptions become light and there are no new eruptions appearing, we will reduce the doses of the drug gradually.

(2) Prevent infection and complications

It is the key factor to reduce mortality. When choosing antibiotics, we should pay attention to the cross allergy and polyvalent allergy. We should avoid using allergic drugs. Before the bacteriological test results come out, broad-spectrum antibiotics that is not prone to drug allergy should be considered first. After the bacteriological test results come out, we should choose antibiotics on the basis of bacteria strains and antimicrobial susceptibility test results. The possibility of fungal infection should be considered if the antibiotic drug doesn't work. Please pay attention to the side effects of high-dose glucocorticoid.

(3) Supportive treatment

We should promptly correct the water and electrolyte disturbances and hypoproteinemia that are induced by difficult eating, high fever, erosion and skin stripping. Please note the intake of protein. Sometimes it is necessary to infuse blood or plasma albumin in order to maintain the colloid osmotic pressure that can reduce the leakage. If there are signs of liver damage, liver therapy should be given.

(4) Strengthen the care and topical treatment

It can shorten the course and guarantee the successful treatment. It should be noted to prepare warm, sterilized and isolated ward for the patient that have a wide area of skin lesions, severe erosion and exudation. Oozing skin lesions should be treated by 3% boric acid solution or saline wet dressing. Lesions of drug-induced bullae epidermolysis should be treated by wet dressing and exposure to the dry environment alternatively. We should pay attention to eye care such as regular washing to prevent infection and adhesion between the sclera and conjunctiva. The patients having difficulty in closing the eyes should be covered by gauze on the eyes in order to prevent corneal damage from long-term exposure.

14.1.7 Precaution

Drug eruption is a iatrogenic disease. Therefore, precaution is very important. We should pay attention to the following factors:

(1) Before any treatment, we should ask the history of drug allergy and the symptoms in detail. Then we can avoid using the known allergic drugs and similar drugs that have similar structures to the allergic drugs.

(2) When using penicillin, streptomycin, serum products, procaine or other drugs, we should take the intradermal test as required. Before the test, emergency medicines should be prepared. The patient with positive test result can not use the drug.

(3) Avoid misusing drugs, take the correct route of administration, choose the less allergic drugs for allergic people, especially pay attention to the known allergic drugs in the compound.

(4) Note the early symptoms of drug eruption, for example: sudden pruritus, fever, erythema and other reactions. If these symptoms appear, please stop using the suspicious drugs and give it a close observation and timely treatment.

(5) If the diagnosis of drug reactions is made, the allergic drug should be recorded in medical record page. We should tell the patient to keep the allergic drug in mind so patient can tell other doctors not to use the drug.

▪ Summary

Drug eruption, also called dermatitis medicamentosa, is the inflammatory eruption in the skin and mucosal that can be caused by medication. Several systems can be involved. It is classified to 11 types of drug eruptions. After excluding other diseases, the diagnosis can be made according to drug using history and characteristic clinical features. Systemic and topical treatments are necessary to cure the disease.

▪ Questions

Describe the clinical features of all kinds of drug eruptions.

(Shaoxia Zi 訾绍霞, Haiping Zhang 张海萍)

Urticarial Dermatoses

Chapter
15

▪ Objectives

To master the knowledge of the causes, clinical features and treatment of urticaria and acquired angioedema.

To have an intimate knowledge of special types of urticaria.

▪ Key concepts

Urticaria is characterized by transient swelling of the skin and mucosa due to vasodilation and increased capillary permeability.

Angioedema is an acute, evanescent, localized edema in the loose part of hypodermis and mucous membrane.

15. 1 Urticaria

Urticaria is a common disease, characterized by transient swelling of the skin and mucosa due to vasodilation and plasma leakage. Up to 25% of the population will experience at least one episode of urticaria in their lifetime.

15. 1. 1 Etiology

The causes of urticaria are complex, and there are no definitive causes in the most patients. Common factors are as follow:

15. 1. 1. 1 Food and food additives

Foods are a frequent cause of acute urticaria. The most common allergenic foods are fish, nuts, chocolate, shellfish, tomatoes, eggs, berries, milk, and spices. Eggs and milk are associated with urticaria in children. Many food additives can aggravate chronic urticaria. Allergen can induce immunological mast cell activation, or directly result in mast cell degranulation.

15. 1. 1. 2 Drugs

Some drugs can cause immunological reaction, such as penicillin and related antibiotics, serum products, bacterin, furazolidone and sulfonamides. Aspirin, salicylates, NSAIDs, opiates, codeine, quinine, hydralazine, atropine, pilocarpine, papaverine and polymyxin b can cause urticaria by inducing release of histamine.

15.1.1.3　Infections

Viral infections(viral upper-respiratory tract infections, hepatitis, infectious mononucleosis syndrome and coxsackievirus infection), bacterial infections(staphylococcus aureus septicemia and streptosepticemia, tonsillitis, chronic otitis media, sinusitis), fungal infections(superficial and deep fungal infections)and parasitic infestations, may cause urticaria.

15.1.1.4　Insect and plant factors

Insect bites and stings or some inhalants including pollens, animal dander, feathers, dust and spore have been known to cause urticaria.

15.1.1.5　Physical factors

Physical stimulus including cold, heat, solar, friction, vibration and pressure may cause urticaria.

15.1.1.6　Psychological factors

Psychological stress as a cause of chronic urticaria can increase release of acetylcholine.

15.1.1.7　Systemic diseases and other factors

Urticaria has been known to be associated with rheumatism, thyroid autoimmunity, systemic lupus erythematosus and cancers. Chronic urticaria may occur in the menses, menopause or gestation.

The pathogenesis of urticaria involves mast cells activation through immune-mediated and non-immune-mediated mechanisms. Immune-mediated urticaria can be caused by 3 of 4 types of immune response. The type I allergic IgE response, as the main immunologic type, is initiated by a given antigen binding to an antigen-specific IgE on the surface of a mast cell. As a result, the mast cell degranulates, releasing histamine and vasoactive mediators. Type II response usually occurs in the transfusion reaction. Type III response can cause urticarial vasculitis. Non-immune-mediated urticaria occurs through direct mast cell degranulation, induced by agents including some foods, drugs, curare and physical factors.

15.1.2　Clinical Features

Urticaria can be divided into acute urticaria or chronic urticaria depending on the duration. Acute urticaria is defined as the presence of wheals lasting less than 6 weeks, whereas chronic urticaria lasts longer. There are several special types in addition.

15.1.2.1　Acute urticaria

The eruption of itching erythemas or wheals of-ten occurs in variable shapes including rounded, annular, serpiginous and bizarre patterns. When plasma leakage is intense, wheals may present pale with a tangerine skin-like surface(Color Figure 15 – 1). After several hours, wheals may be transformed into erythemas, and resolve with no residuals, usually lasting less than 24 hours. But while some lesions resolve, others may appear.

In serious patients with allergic shock, palpitation, dysphoria, nausea, vomiting, or hypotension may occur. Angioedema may target the gastrointestinal system resulting in nausea, vomiting, abdominal pain, or diarrhea. The emergency is respiratory tracts problems with wheezing, dyspnea or anaphylaxis. The patients with urticaria caused by infections may suffer from systemic toxic symptoms, such as chill, high fever, rapid pulse.

15.1.2.2　Chronic urticaria

Daily episodes of urticaria lasting more than 6 weeks is designated chronic urticaria, in which systemic symptoms are less than acute urticaria. Repeated episodes of wheals last usually more than several months or years.

15.1.2.3　Special types

(1) Dermatographism

Also known as factitious urticaria, a localized itching edema or wheal may arise from stroking of the skin with a surrounding erythematous flare within seconds to minutes(Color Figure 15 – 2). Dermatographism may occur in some patients with urticaria.

(2) Cold urticaria

Exposure to cold may result in edema and whealing on the exposed areas, usually the face and hands. Cold urticaria is classified into familial cold urticaria and acquired cold urticaria. Familial cold urticaria has an autosomal dominant inheritance pattern, and occurs after born or primary with onset all life. The severe ones may be accompanied by fever, chills, headache, arthralgia, myalgia, and abdominal pain. The mouth and pharynx may swell after drinking cold liquid. The ice cube test is negative. Acquired cold contact urticaria is classified into primary and secondary cold urticaria. In the primary, it is usually ice cube test positive. The secondary is associated with an underlying systemic disease, such as cryoglobulinemia and paroxysmal nocturnal hemoglobinuria.

(3) Cholinergic urticaria

Cholinergic urticaria usually occurs in young

adults after sweating during physical exercise, taking a bath, raising the body temperature, and emotional stress, which can cause the action of acetylcholine on the mast cell by increasing in core temperature. This disorder is characterized by pinpoint sized, highly pruritic, an eruption of small red macules and papules(2 to 5 mm) surrounded by areas of erythema, appearing within 30 – 60 minutes. Cholinergic urticaria may be associated with systemic syndromes (salivate, headache, slow pulse, miosis, abdominal spastic pain and diarrhea) by increase acetylcholine. In patients with this disorder, injection of acetylcholine(1 ∶ 5 000)into normal-appearing skin produces a wheal and flare reaction, often surrounded by smaller satellite lesions.

(4) Solar urticaria

Edema or wheals with itching appear soon after unshielded skin is exposed to visible, long-or short-wave ultraviolet radiation, especially 300 wave ultraviolet. The lesions may erupt in very sensitive patients following sun exposure through glasses. In severe ones, systemic symptoms may occur including headache, nausea, wheezing, dizziness, syncope, and, rarely, anaphylactic shock.

(5) Pressure urticaria

The pathogenesis of pressure urticaria is unknown, but it is closely related to dermatographism. The development of swelling with pain often occurs on the feet or buttocks after local sustained pressure, usually lasting 8 to 24 hours. The severity may be accompanied by systemic symptoms of malaise, arthralgias, fever, chills, and leukocytosis.

15. 1. 3 Diagnosis and Differential Diagnosis
The diagnosis of urticaria is usually made on clinical features. However, it is frequently difficult to determine the cause. The differential diagnosis includes popular urticaria and urticarial vasculitis, in which the lesions usually last longer. The case with abdominal pain or diarrhea may be accompanied by acute abdominal disease or gastro-enteritis.

15. 1. 4 Treatment
The mainstay of treatment of urticaria is administration of antihistamines, reduce the plasma leakage of the skin vascular and avoiding the possible factors.

15. 1. 4. 1 System treatment

(1) Acute urticaria

The first-generation and second-generation H_1 antihistamines are the mainstay of treatment, and vitamin C or calcium can decrease capillary permeability. The case with bellyache should be prescribed to take probanthine, 654 – 2, atropine. The case with severe infections should be treated with antibiotics.

In severe case with shock or angioedema involving the upper airway, the patient should be treated with a 0. 5 – 1 ml dose of 0. 1% epinephrine every 10 – 20 minutes, a nebulized 5% solution of metaproterenol and oxygen therapy. Second-line therapy includes intramuscular antihistamines(25 – 50 mg of promethazine), systemic steroidal medication(200 – 300 mg hydrocortisone), and 200 mg aminophylline for bronchus convulsion.

(2) Chronic urticaria

The main treatment of chronic urticaria also is administration of antihistamines. Prescribe drugs time should be adjusted according eruption of hives, and after suppresses the hives, the medications should be continued for a periods with gradually reducing dose. If a kind of antihistamine is ineffective, 2 and 3 kinds may be taken or alternatively. In stubborn cases, the combination of H1 and H2 antihistamines(hydroxyzine, cimetidine or ranitidine) may be more effective. There are other medications that may be added, such as reserpine, euphyllin, chloroquine and tripterygium wilfordii.

(3) Special urticarias

The combination of medicines should be used according to different special types in addition to antihistamines. Patients with dermatographism may take ketotifen. Patients with cold urticaria may take ketotifen, vimicon and reserpine. Patients with cholinergic urticaria may take ketotifen, probanthine, and atropine. Patients with solar urticaria may take chloroquine. Patients with pressure urticaria may take hydroxyzine.

15. 1. 4. 2 Topical treatment

In summer, calamine lotion may be used, whereas, emulsion should be used in winter.

15. 2 Angioedema

Angioedema's synonym is giant urticaria. Angioedema is an acute, evanescent, localized edema in the loose part of hypodermis and mucous membrane. Angioedema is divided to two types, hereditary angioedema and acquired angioedema.

15. 2. 1 Etiology
Hereditary angioedema, inherited in an autosomal

dominant fashion, is characterized by low antigenic and dysfunctional plasma levels of a normal C1-esterase inhibitor(C1-INH). The causes of acquired angioedema are similar to those of urticaria, such as food, drugs, inhalants or physiological stimulus.

15.2.2   Clinical Features

15.2.2.1   Acquired angioedema

The swelling often occurs in the loose subcutaneous tissue(eyelids, lips, lobes of the ears and external genitals), or the mucous membranes of the mouth, tongue, or larynx. The lesions with obscure boundary may be salmon pink, skin color or slightly pale(Color Figure 15 - 3). Lasting for a few hours, or occasionally 2 - 3 days, the edema may disappear without trace. It is often in combination with urticaria. In a case with laryngeal edema, the patient may be accompanied with respiratory complaints of shortness of breath, dyspnea or asphyxiation. Gastrointestinal edema is manifested by nausea, vomiting, severe colic and diarrhea.

15.2.2.2   Hereditary angioedema

Hereditary angioedema commonly occurs in primarily childhood throughout life, lasting for 2 to 5 days. Local swelling in subcutaneous tissues(faces, hands, arms, legs, genitals, and buttocks)may appear after trauma, surgery or infections. Swelling is typically solitary and may be painful, and urticaria or itching does not occur. It may occur in a bdominal organs(stomach, intestines, bladder)mimicking surgical emergencies, and the upper airway(larynx)that can be life threatening.

15.2.3   Diagnosis and Differential Diagnosis

The diagnosis of angioedema is usually made on clinical features. The patient should be diagnosed with hereditary angioedema if angioedema occurs primarily, and half-apart members in family are associated. The low levels of plasma C1NH is help to diagnosis.

15.2.4   Treatment

Antihistamines are effective to acquire angioedema, however, the response of hereditary angioedema to treatment is generally poor. Replacement therapy with fresh frozen plasma is effective to complement C1 inhibitor on acute onset. A prophylactic treatment is to using androgens.

■ Summary

Urticaria is a common disease characterized by transient swelling of the skin and mucosa due to vasodilation and increased capillary permeability. Clinical presentations are itching erythemas or wheals in clear size. It can be divided into acute urticaria and clinical urticaria depending on the duration. There are 5 special types of urticaria. The diagnosis of urticaria is usually made on clinical features. The mainstay of treatment of urticaria is administration of antihistamines, reduce the plasma leakage of the skin vascular and avoiding the possible causes.

Angioedema is an acute, evanescent, localized edema in the loose part of hypodermis and mucous membrane. The diagnosis of angioedema is usually made on clinical features. Antihistamines are effective to acquire angioedema. On acute hereditary angioedema onset, fresh frozen plasma should be used to complement C1 inhibitor.

■ Questions

Describe the clinical features and treatment of urticaria.

Describe the treatment of significant angioedema involving the upper airway.

(Yu Wang 王瑜, Shi Lian 连石)

Chapter 16

Disorders due to Physical Agents

▪ Objectives

To master the knowledge of definition and clinical feature of sunburn, specific clinical presents of polymorphic light eruption, definition of estival dermatitis, definition and grouping of miliaria, definition and clinical presents of perniosis.

To have an intimate knowledge of treatment of polymorphic light eruption, clinical presents of estival dermatitis, treatment of perniosis.

▪ Key concepts

Sunburn is the acute local cutaneous inflammation of intensive exposure to sunlight in short duration.

Polymorphic light eruption is a common sunlight-induced disease. It may have several different morphologies and appear severe in spring and summer.

Estival dermatitis is an inflammatory dermatosis which caused by high temperature and sweater in summer.

Miliaria occurs in the environment of high temperature and will recover after departure.

Perniosis occurs in cold seasons and will recover after departure.

▪ Introduction

Physical dermatoses are a group of diseases which caused by physical factors in environment. In this chapter we will cover photodermatoses, estival dermatitis, miliaria and perniosis.

16. 1　Photodermatoses

16. 1. 1　Sunburn

Sunburn, also named solar dermatitis, is an acute local cutaneous reaction of the intensive exposure to sunlight. The condition can occur in all races and ages, while the reaction may be different.

16.1.1.1 Etiology

Sunburn is the reaction to sunlight, mostly UVB in excess of tolerance dose.

16.1.1.2 Clinical features

The eruptions onset 4 to 6 hours after the sun exposure and peak at 12 to 24 hours after that. Diffused erythema with pain and burning sensation may appear (Color Figure 16 - 1). In severe cases, vesicles, blisters and edema may occur. General symptoms, such as fever, headache and collapse, may be present when lesions confluens and spread widely. The lesions release 1 to 2 days later, leaving with pigmentation. But in severe cases, that secondary infections may occur, will recover in 1 to 2 weeks.

16.1.1.3 Diagnosis and differential diagnosis

Diagnosis depends on the history of definitive sun exposure and classical clinical feature. The differential diagnosis includes contact dermatitis. Contact dermatitis, without sun exposure, has definitive contact with stimulator and the lesions localized at the contact area, may occur in any season.

16.1.1.4 Treatment

Sunburn is best prevented by avoiding sun exposure and using protective medicines.

(1) Topical therapy

In slight cases, topical methods of dephlogistication, analgesia and soothing, may be effective.

(2) System therapy

Oral antihistamine and NSAIDS (non-steroidal anti-inflammatory drugs) should be required. Systemic corticosteroids may help those with severe conditions.

16.1.2 *Polymorphic Light Eruption*

Polymorphic light eruption, which can affect all races and skin types, is a common sunlight-induced disease. The eruption may have several different morphologies. It may recur but appears severe in spring and summer.

16.1.2.1 Etiology

The etiology is unknown. The immunological reaction of T cell mediation, evoked by the sunlight is considered recently.

16.1.2.2 Clinical features

Eruption appeared several days after exposure to sunlight, accompanied with itching. The involved areas include the face, the neck, the V area of the chest and the arms. In some severe conditions, sever-

al unexposure areas may be affected. The eruption may have many different morphologies, such as erythemas, papules, papulovesicles, wheals or plaques. But usually in the individual patient, the morphology is constant. The eruption appears severely in the spring and summer, and may release without exposure to sunlight in autumn and winter. But the condition may recur or aggravate after exposure again.

16.1.2.3 Diagnosis and differential diagnosis

Diagnosis depends on the clinical features, which the eruptions usually appear on the exposure area due to the sunlight, and occur in springtime and summertime.

Eczema should be considered to complete the differential diagnosis, while it has nothing to do with sunlight, and eruptions may have several morphologies simultaneously.

16.1.2.4 Treatment

Patients need restriction of sunlight exposure, using protective methods.

(1) Topical therapy

The use of topical medicines depends on the morphologies and location of the eruptions. Using topical steroids is effective.

(2) System therapy

Systemic chloroquine and hydroxychloroquine are effective, and antihistamine should be used for itching conditions. For patients with severe disease, oral corticosteroids and azathioprine is necessary.

16.2 Estival Dermatitis

Estival dermatitis is an abnormal inflammatory response to hot conditions in summer.

16.2.1 *Etiology*

Estival dermatitis produces an eruption that is common in hot, humid climates such as the tropics and the hot summer months in temperate climates. It appears in persons who often work in a hot environment for a long time (temperature $>30°C$).

16.2.2 *Clinical Features*

Estival dermatitis occurs mostly in adult women. It often exclusively involves anterior shins, extensor arms, and trunk. The eruption is usually symmetrical. It usually begins as erythematous macules or papules. Lesions evolve into papulovesicles. Pruritus is a constant feature, and leads to scratching. The scratching may cause excoriation, crust, thickening of the skin, or hyperpigmented. Complete remission of estival dermatitis in cool seasons is the rule.

16. 2. 3　Diagnosis and Differential Diagnosis

Typical estival dermatitis is not difficult to diagnose. Dermatosis resembling estival dermatitis may be miliaria or pruritus aestivalis.

16. 2. 4　Treatment

Place the patient in a cool environment is the most effective treatment. The use of circulating air fans to cool the skin is next best.

Topical calamine lotion or corticosteroid creams may be effective. Antihistaminics may be used to aid in the relief of the severe pruritus.

16. 3　Miliaria

Although sweat retention can occur as a secondary phenomenon in a variety of skin conditions, it also represents the primary pathologic process in a group of disorders listed under the generic designation "miliaria".

16. 3. 1　Etiology

Miliaria, the retention of sweat as a result of occlusion of eccrine sweat ducts and pores, produces an eruption that is common in hot, humid climates and during the hot summer months in temperate climates. The essential fundamental steps in the development of miliaria can be simply stated as keratinous obstruction of the eccrine ducts followed by their rupture and the formation of a sweat retention vesicle. Adherent parakeratotic plug of the sweat duct, most commonly as a result of maceration and requiring bacteria, is the initial essential major event.

16. 3. 2　Clinical Features

Three types of miliaria, each reflecting reactive keratinous obstruction of sweat ducts at different levels, from the stratum corneum to the dermo-epidermal junction, are known:

(1) Miliaria crystallina

Miliaria crystallina appears in bedridden patient in whom fever produces increased perspiration or in situations in which fever produces increased perspiration or in situations in which clothing prevents dissipation of heat and moisture. It is characterized by small, clear, and very superficial vesicles with no inflammatory reaction. The lesions are asymptomatic and their duration is short lived because they tend to rupture at the slightest trauma.

(2) Miliaria rubra

The most common and clinically important form of miliaria is miliaria rubra, which is characterized by small erythematous macules surmounted by a punctate vesicle. The site of injury and sweat escape is in the prickle cell layer, where spongiosis is produced. The site most frequently affected are the antecubital and popliteal fossae, the trunk, the inframammary areas (especially under pendulous breasts), the abdomen (especially at the waistline), and the inguinal region. The lesions of miliaria rubra appear as discrete, extremely pruritic, erythematous papulovesicles accompanied by a sensation of prickling, burning or tingling. They later may become confluent on a bed of erythema.

(3) Miliaria pustulosa

Miliaria pustulosa is always preceded by some other dermatitis that has produced injury, destruction, or blocking of the sweat duct. The pruritic pustules occur most frequently on the intertriginous areas, on the flexure surfaces of the extremities, on the scrotum, and on the back of bedridden patients.

(4) Miliaria profunda

This form is observed only in the tropics and usually follows a severe bout of miliaria rubra. The occlusion is in the upper dermis. Miliaria profunda typically occurs on the trunk and proximal extremities. When large numbers of sweat glands are occluded and essentially deactivated, these individuals are at risk for significant thermoregulatory problems. Nonpruritic, flesh-colored, deep-seated, whitish papules characterize this form of miliaria. A compensatory hyperhidrosis of the face is rather routinely observed and can be searched for in the screening of large groups suspected of having this dangerous and potentially disabling clinical problem. Under conditions of heat stress, patients can develop weakness, dyspnea, tachycardia, fever and ultimately collapse because of their inability to cool themselves properly.

16. 3. 3　Diagnosis and Differential Diagnosis

Each type of miliaria presents such a classic clinical picture that its diagnosis is usually readily apparent to the knowledgeable physician. In infants with miliaria rubra, other eruptions must be excluded, especially erythema toxicum neonatorum, contact dermatitis and folliculitis. Close inspection of miliaria lesions to confirm their extra-follicular location and when necessary a biopsy, should clarify the diagnosis. Amyloidosis, papular mucinosis and papular sarcoidosis may have to be excluded in some patients with miliaria profunda, although the temporal correlation of such lesions with sweating and their tendency to regress or disappear with its cessation essentially clinch the diagnosis.

16.3.4 Treatment
Management of all types of miliaria requires placement of the patient in a cool environment, in which sweating stops, for several days to 2 to 3 weeks. Mild cases may respond to dusting powders, such as cornstarch or baby talcum powder. An oily "shake" lotion such as calamine lotion, with 1% or 2% phenol, may be effective. Oral retinoids and ascorbic acid have been advocated therapeutically, but their efficacy awaits substantiation.

16.4 Perniosis

Perniosis is an abnormal inflammatory response to cold, damp, nonfreezing conditions. It is most common in areas without central heating.

16.4.1 Etiology
Exposure to cold, wet conditions is the major risk factor for perniosis. This condition is common in those whose homes lack central heating. The precise pathogenesis of perniosis is unknown, but the condition is thought to have a vascular origin. In children, it may be associated with cryoglobulins or cold agglutinins.

16.4.2 Clinical Features
Perniosis occurs repeatedly during cold weather and disappears during warm weather. Lesions are often symmetrically distributed on the distal toes and fingers, and less often on the heels, nose and ears (Color Figure 16 – 2). Deep perniosis may be seen on the thighs, calves and buttocks as blue-erythrocyanotic plaques. Perniosis presents with single or multiple erythematous to blue-violet macules, papules or nodules. In severe cases, blistering and ulceration may be seen. Patients describe itching, burning or pain. Lesions often resolve in 1 to 3 weeks, except among elderly patients with venous insufficiency in whom lesions can become chronic.

16.4.3 Diagnosis and Differential Diagnosis
Idiopathic perniosis needs to be distinguished from several other cold-induced syndromes, including chilblains lupus erythematous and cold-sensitive blood dyscrasias.

16.4.4 Treatment
Adequate clothing and avoidance of cold, damp conditions are important preventive measures as are keeping feet dry and avoidance of smoking. Vasodilators, such as nifedipine, are used to improve circulation. Other anecdotal remedies include nicotinamide, phenoxybenzamine, sympathectomy and erythemogenic ultraviolet B phototherapy.

■ Summary

Physical dermatoses are a group diseases which caused by physical factors in environment. Sunburn is the acute local cutaneous inflammation of intensive exposure to sunlight in short duration. Polymorphic light eruption is a common sunlight-induced disease. It may have several different morphologies and appear severe in spring and summer. Estival dermatitis is an inflammatory dermatosis which caused by high temperature and swelter in summer. Miliaria occurs in high temperature environment and will recover after departure. Perniosis occurs in cold seasons and will recover after departure.

■ Questions

Describe the clinical feature of each physical dermatoses.

(**Xiaoyang Wang** 王晓阳, **Xiaoling Chu** 褚晓玲, **Junying Zhao** 赵俊英)

Chapter 17

Pruritus

▪ Objectives

To master the knowledge of the clinical features of pruritus, lichen simplex chronicus and prurigo.

To have an intimate knowledge of how to diagnose and treat pruritus, lichen simplex chronicus and prurigo.

▪ Key concepts

Pruritus is a disorder manifested by itching exclusive to the skin, without primary cutaneous lesions. Clear diagnosis can be made based on systemic or local itching with secondary rather than primary skin lesions. This disease should be treated promptly after excluding systemic disorders. Generally, local irritation, scratching, hot-water bath, inappropriate treatment and spicy food should be avoided.

Lichen simplex chronicus, also known as neurodermatitis, is a common skin disorder with chronic cutaneous neurological dysfunction. Diagnosis is fairly easy for this disorder based on disease history, typical skin lesions and clinical features. Treatment of lichen simplex chronicus needs both systemic and topical medications.

Prurigo is a pruritic inflammatory dermatosis, characterized by urticarial wheals, nodules and irresistibly severe itching. It includes three types: acute prurigo, chronic prurigo and symptomatic prurigo. Treatment of prurigo needs both topical remedies and drug medications.

▪ Introduction

Pruritus is a sensation associated with skin or mucous membrane that causes scratching desire. Although histamine, serotonin, protease, prostaglandin E, neuropeptide and related chemical substances can cause pruritus, the specific mechanisms are still to be determined. Pruritic skin diseases are highlighted by itching and common vicious cycle of itching-scratching-itching with seemingly complex etiology and unknown pathogenesis. In this chapter, we will introduce three main diseases of pruritic: pruritus, lichen simplex chronicus and prurigo.

17.1   Pruritus

Pruritus refers to skin diseases collectively with itching exclusive to the skin, without primary lesions. It's caused by various intrinsic and extrinsic factors.

17.1.1   Etiology
Etiology of this disease is complex.

17.1.1.1   Generalized pruritus

The most common cause is xerosis cutis such as asteatotic eczema. Neuropsychiatric factors include depression, parasitophobia, emotional stress, anxiety, fear, agitation and melancholia can induce this disease frequently. Systemic diseases such as uremia, biliary cirrhosis, hyperthy roidism or hypothyroidism, diabetes mellitus, lymphoma, leukemia and other malignancies can also cause this disease. Pregnancy, drugs or food, temperature, humidity, environment, living habits (e. g. soaps, cleansing skin care cosmetics and clothing in direct contact with skin) can also cause systemic pruritus.

17.1.1.2   Local pruritus

Etiology is sometimes identical to that of systemic pruritus. Infection (e. g. fungus, trichomonas, and pubic lice), clothing and drug irritation can cause vulvar and scrotal pruritus; hemorrhoids, anal fissure and pinworm infection can cause perianal pruritus.

17.1.2   Clinical Features
Usually without primary lesions, itching is as the characteristic symptom of this disease, maybe accompanying with the sensation of burning and ant-creeping.

17.1.2.1   Generalized pruritus

Generalized pruritus is usually characterized by unfixed itching sites and wide variations of itching degrees. It's usually paroxysmal and apt to be most severe at night. Scratching can cause scratches, blood scab, pigmentation or hypopigmentation and other secondary lesions. Eczema-like change or lichenification may occur with time. In addition, the secondary infections of skin may also occur, such as folliculitis, furuncle and lymphadenitis.

Special types of generalized pruritus including:

(1) Pruritus senilis

It usually appears in trunk and frequently results from dysfunction of secretion of sebaceous glands, cutaneous xerosis and atrophy.

(2) Pruritus hiemalis

It is usually induced by cold, accompanying with skin xerosis and can be aggravated at the time of undressing for bed.

(3) Pruritus aestivalis

It is often induced by high-heat and moisture and aggravated by sweating.

(4) Pruritus gestationis

It frequently occurs in late trimester of pregnancy and also in early trimester of pregnancy sometimes. Some of them are accompanied by jaundice. Spontaneous alleviation or healing after labor has been observed for most cases. This disease can lead to premature birth, fetal distress or even stillbirth.

17.1.2.2   Local pruritus

Local pruritus manifests as local paroxysmal severe itching. It usually occurs in areas such as vulva, scrotum, perianal area, legs and scalp.

17.1.3   Diagnosis and Differential Diagnosis
It's necessary to search for primary diseases actively. This often requires comprehensive investigations including X-ray chest film, blood, urine and stool routine tests, liver and kidney function tests, blood glucose test.

Once secondary skin lesions occur, systemic pruritus needs to be differentiated from scabies, insect bite dermatitis, prurigo and lichen simplex chronicus; local pruritus needs to be differentiated from local fungus, trichomonas infection, contact dermatitis and eczema.

17.1.4   Treatment
17.1.4.1   Topical therapy

Calamine lotion, peppermint tincture, camphor tincture, lidocaine, prilocaine or procaine preparations can be selected; Vitamin E cream and other emollients can be used for dry skin; Short-term application of corticosteroid preparations can be used to relieve symptoms of severe itching.

17.1.4.2   Systemic therapy

Anti-histamine drugs, sedative hypnotics and tricyclic antidepressants can be administered orally; Intravenous injection of calcium preparation and vitamin C can also be used; intravenous procaine blocking is an option for severe cases.

Consume less spicy food and eat high-fiber diet. Avoid excessive cleansing, hot water bath or irritative hygiene products.

17.2   Lichen Simplex Chronicus

Lichen simplex chronicus, refers to skin diseases characterized by pruritus and lichenification caused by a variety of factors, also known as neurodermatitis.

17.2.1   Etiology
Etiology of this disease is unknown and may be related to irascible temperament, excessive contemplation, tension, depression, fatigue and insomnia; in addition to gastrointestinal dysfunction, endocrine disturbances, drinking alcohol, eating spicy food, fish and shrimp, wearing rigid collar and woolen fabrics, chemical substances, infectious lesions, sweat soaking and other local irritations. Scratching and chronic friction may induce or exacerbate this disease, while the vicious cycle of repetitive itching-scratching-itching may be the major factors responsible for onset or gradual aggravation of the disease.

17.2.2   Clinical Features
This disease involves middle-aged and young adults frequently. The disease is mostly seen on one side or symmetrical distribution on both sides in the neck and upper eyelids, also usually in both sides of elbow extensors, lumbosacral region, calves, vulva, scrotum and perianal area and other areas susceptible to scratching. Patients often feel paroxysmal itching that often aggravates during local irritation or anxiety, especially at night. Basic skin lesions are usually polygonal flat papules from needle tip to grain size with pink, light brown or normal skin color and fairly firm shinning textures. There may be small amount of furfuraceous scales on the surface. The skin lesions may merge and expand gradually with time to form lichenification. The central lesions are larger and more obvious with flat papules readily visible scattering by the clear borderlines (Color Figure 17 - 1). Some patients may have widely distributed lesions. Lesions and their surroundings usually have scratching marks or blood scabs. This disease is characterized by its chronic course, persistent unhealed lesion or recurrent attacks.

17.2.3   Diagnosis and Differential Diagnosis
Diagnosis of this disease is fairly easy based on the typical clinical manifestations.

Necessarily, it should also be differentiated from chronic eczema, atopic dermatitis, lichen planus and local cutaneous amyloidosis.

17.2.4   Treatment
17.2.4.1   External medication
Drugs (e.g. antipruritics, tars or glucocorticoids) and dosage forms should be selected rationally based on lesion types, locations and seasons of onset. Medicated bath, spa bath and ultraviolet therapy are options for patients with generalized skin lesions.

17.2.4.2   Internal medication
Anti-histamine drugs can be administered orally with supplementary application of oryzanol and complex vitamin B. Diazepam or doxepin and other sedative hypnotics can be used after dinner or before bedtime for uncontrollable pruritus. Intravenous procaine blocking is an option for severe cases.

Scratching, friction and other irritations should be avoided with supportive psychotherapy to break the vicious cycle of itching-scratching-itching.

17.3   Prurigo

Prurigo is an acute or chronic inflammatory dermatosis, characterized by pruritic urticarial wheals, nodules, severe unbearable itching and local skin erosion: skin hypertrophy, lichenification, pigmentation, etc. In clinical it includes three types: acute prurigo, chronic prurigo and symptomatic prurigo.

17.3.1   Etiology
The cause of prurigo is unknown. Most scholars believe that allergic reaction is probably relative. Other multiple factors may contribute, including insect bites, food or drug allergy, gastrointestinal disorder, focal infection, neuropsychiatric disorders and genetic irritable physique.

17.3.2   Clinical Features
17.3.2.1   Acute prurigo
Acute prurigo is also called papular urticaria. Insect bites, intestinal parasites and allergies of certain foods may relate to acute prurigo. It usually affects children or adolescents, primarily occurring in the spring and fall. The waist, back, abdomen, buttocks, calves are the most frequent sites affected. Lesions are red urticarial wheals, 1 - 2 cm in di-

ameter, spindle-shaped or round-shaped, usually with papulovesicles, or blisters or bullae in central, mostly in clusters but less integration. Patients feel itching consciously and if they scratch repeatedly, it will lead secondary infection (Color Figure 17 - 2). Usually rashes subside 1 week later. It will be recurrent if the cause is not removed.

17.3.2.2　Chronic prurigo

(1) Prurigo adultorm

It usually affects the young and middle-aged adults, mostly occurring in women. The trunk and the extensor surfaces of the extremities are the most frequent sites affected. Sometimes the scalp and face are involved too. Basic lesions are multiple firm papules, the color of which is light red or skin colored, the size of which is millet to mung bean. Prurigo adultorm is with severe itching. There are wheal-like plaques and papulovesicles after scratching, sometimes with small blisters and crusts. Recurrent rash and scratching may thicken the skin and make it rough, sometimes with lichenification and pigmentation. The course of the disease is chronic and the lesions evolve slowly.

(2) Prurigo infantilis

Prurigo infantilis also called prurigo of early onset or Hebra prurigo. It occurs chiefly in children before 3 years old, especially around 1 years old. Extensor extremities are the most frequent sites affected. Basic lesions are urticarial wheals of mung bean size. Gradually the lesions turn into firm pimples of skin color. Children with prurigo infantilis are often with severe itching. After scratching there are often scratches and blood scabs. After a long time the skin may appear the lichenification, eczema-like change, purulent infection with inguinal lymphadenectasis. The course of the disease is chronic and persistent.

(3) Prurigo nodularis

Nodules are situated chiefly on extremities, especially on the anterior surfaces of the legs. The lesions at the beginning are firm papules which are red and edematous. Gradually the lesions grow into hemispherical nodules with soy sized or larger. When fully developed they become verrucous, obviously at the top, and rough on the surface, the color of which turn brownish (Color Figure 17 - 3). The lesions are often scattered or occasionally in dense clusters. Itching is severe and paroxysmal, often unbearable. The lesions can be self-limited and leave pigmentations or scars. Also scratching the nodules to re-

lieve the itch may often induce blood crusts, scratches and lichenifications.

17.3.2.3　Symptomatic prurigo

Symptomatic prurigo often occurs in pregnant women (called as gestational prurigo) or patients with tumors (such as lymphoma or leukemia). It may be related to the endogenous metabolic productions or allergic factors. The occurrence rate of gestational prurigo is about 2%. It mainly affects women who are pregnant more than twice. Generally the symptoms go away in the third or fourth week of the postpartum period. It usually occurs in the upper trunk and proximal extremities. Essential lesions are urticarial wheals with sever itching, and sometimes are papulovesicles. After scratching there are scratches, blood scabs and pigmentations and other changes of skin.

17.3.3　Diagnosis and Differential Diagnosis

First, according to characteristics of lesions and severe itch it can be diagnosed as prurigo. Then according to medical history, age, course of disease and accompanying diseases, the different types of disease can be identified.

Acute prurigo should distinguish from urticaria and varicella; Prurigo adultorm should be identified among atopic dermatitis, chronic eczema, scabies, etc; Prurigo nodularis should differentiate from verruca vulgaris, verrucous lichen planus and primary cutaneous amyloidosis.

17.3.4　Treatments

Remove various pathogenic factors (such as insect bites, local stimulation, associated diseases, etc.).

17.3.4.1　Topical treatment

It is mainly to relieve itching and diminish inflammation. Also glucocorticoid and horny stripping agent can be used, especially with closed packet to enhance the efficacy. Lesions injection of corticosteroids can also be taken.

17.3.4.2　Drug treatment

Oral antihistamines or procaine intravenous closure can be used. In patients with neuropsychiatric disorders, sedative hypnotic drugs may be appropriate to apply; Short-term systematic low-dose corticosteroids (such as prednisone 30 - 40 mg/d orally) can be taken by patients with extensive nodules and unbearable severe itching; UVB phototherapy or PUVA treatment to intractable skin lesions are often effective.

▪ Summary

Pruritus refers to skin diseases collectively with mere skin itching caused by various intrinsic and extrinsic factors without primary skin lesions. The main etiologic factors responsible for pruritus include neuropsychiatric factors, systemic diseases and endocrine abnormalities such as pregnancy, environment and clothing. This disease can be divided into systemic pruritus and local pruritus per scope of illness. Diagnosis of pruritus can be confirmed based on typical clinical manifestations and lack of primary skin lesions. Therapeutic principle requires a combination of systemic treatment, local drug application and emphasis of protection.

Lichen simplex chronicus, refers to skin diseases characterized by pruritus and lichenification caused by a variety of factors, also known as neurodermatitis. Scratching and chronic friction play an important role in the disease. Apart from those, stress, depression, fatigue, gastrointestinal dysfunction, endocrine disturbances and certain kinds of chemical substances are also contributed. According to its typical lesion and symptom, it's easy to make a diagnosis. Internal medicine and external medicine should be used at the same time.

Prurigo is a pruritic inflammatory dermatosis, characterized by urticarial wheals, nodules and severe unbearable itching. According to characteristics of lesions and severe itch it can be diagnosed. In clinical it includes three types: acute prurigo, chronic prurigo and symptomatic prurigo. The treatment includes topical treatment and drug treatment.

▪ Questions

1. Describe the etiological factors of generalized pruritus.

2. Describe the clinical features of Lichen simplex chronicus.

3. Describe the classification of prurigo and its clinical features.

(**Cang Zhang** 张苍, **Li Jin** 金力)

Chapter 18

Skin Disorders with Erythema and Scaling

▪ Objectives

To master the clinical feature, differential diagnosis and the treatment of the main skin disorders with erythema and scaling.

To have an intimate knowledge of the pathogenesis of the main skin disorders with erythema and scaling.

▪ Key concepts

Erythema multiforme is an acute recurrent inflammatory mucocutaneous disease. Its typical clinical characteristic is the "target lesion" or "iris lesion".

Psoriasis is a chronic, autoimmune, systemic skin disease hard to be radical cured and characterized by red maculopapule with silvery white scale, Auspitz's sign and Koebner phenomenon.

Pityriasis rosea is an acute, self-limited disease. Its typical lesions locate along the lines of cleavage of the trunk and often begin with a single oval scaly plaque called "mother patch". The course of pityriasis rosea is about 6 – 8 weeks.

Lichen planus is a recurrent rash characterized by purple, flat-topped, polygonal papules with Wickham stria.

▪ Introduction

Skin disorders with erythema and scaling include a group of skin diseases with different etiology and pathogenesis. Despite the clinical features of these diseases are quite different from each other, they all display erythema and the formation and shedding of keratin scale during the course of diseases. Among this group of diseases, erythema multiforme, psoriasis, pityriasis rosea and lichen planus are most common and will be discussed in this chapter. Diagnoses of those skin disorders are based on the typical clinical lesions and histopathology. Symptomatic treatments are effective and enough for most mild cases, but for serious cases, systemic and supportive treatments are quite important.

18. 1　Erythema Multiforme

Erythema multiforme (EM) is an acute recurrent inflammatory mucocutaneous disease with immunological basis. Its typical clinical characteristic is the target-shaped plaques lesions called "target lesion" or "iris lesion". The serious cases of EM need optimal management to reduce the risk of death.

18. 1. 1　Etiology

The etiology of EM is complex and still unclear. Chronic infection (Herpes virus, bacteria, fungi, M. pneumoniae etc.), drugs, vaccine, foods and physical factors such as cold, sunlight and radiation are considered to be the causes of EM. Many systemic diseases such as rheumatic fever, connective tissue diseases and malignant tumors also can display the same lesions as EM.

18. 1. 2　Pathogenesis

EM appears to have an immunological basis. Cell-mediated immunoreactions play important roles in the genesis of EM as showed in literature. Active T cells have been found in the lesions: $CD4^+$ lymphocytes in the dermis while $CD8^+$ cells in the epidermis.

Most cases of EM are related to infections especially HSV. The presence of HSV DNA in EM lesions has been reported in numerous studies using the PCR assay. Monocytes, macrophages and Langerhans cells can pick up HSV DNA and transport fragments to distant skin sites leading to recruitment of HSV-specific T cells, including cytotoxic cells, and then initiate the inflammatory cascade.

18. 1. 3　Clinical Features

EM can occur at any age, but often involves children and young women. It often attacks at spring and autumn with self-limited course of disease. Prodromal symptoms are usually mild, including fever, headache, rhinitis, malaise, myalgia and arthralgia. Lesions have multiform appearances such as macule, maculopapule, papule, blister, bulla, wheal, purpura and so on, but often have a major lesion type in individual cases. Depends on the appearance of lesions, EM is divided into three types: macule-papule form, blister-bulla form and Steven-Johnson syndrome form.

18. 1. 3. 1　Macule-papule form

The most common type of EM with or without mild constitutional symptoms. Lesions including macule, papule and the "Target Lesion" or "iris lesion" with a diameter of 0. 5 – 2cm are distributed on face, neck and the distal extremities (Color Figure 18 – 1). Oral, ocular and genital mucous membranes also can be involved. Patients can feel itching, mild pain or burning. The lesions can last 2 – 4 weeks before disappearance.

18. 1. 3. 2　Blister-bulla form

This type of EM often aggravates from the macule-papule form with constitutional symptoms such as myalgia, arthralgia, fever, hematuria, albuminuria, increased ESR, etc. Besides the distal extremities, lesions can expand to the whole body. Blisters, bullae, even blood bullae with an outer ring of erythema is the major appearance of lesions. Nikolsky sign of the bulla is negative. Mucous membranes symptoms are much worse than the macule-papule form, including erosion, ulcer and effusion (Color Figure 18 – 2).

18. 1. 3. 3　Steven-Johnson Syndrome (SJS)

Form The most serious type of EM. It is an acute life-threatening mucocutaneous reaction characterized by extensive necrosis and detachment of the epidermis with marked constitutional symptoms of high fever, malaise, myalgia, arthralgia and even respiratory failure. The skin lesions are multiform, including maculopapule, bullae, petechiae, and even pustule. Nikolsky sign of the bulla is positive. Lesions can sudden onset distributing on the whole body surface. Mucous membrane involvement is observed in approximately 90 percent of cases. It begins with erythema followed by painful erosions of the buccal, ocular, and genital mucosa. Visceral involvement is also possible, particularly with pulmonary and digestive complications. Abnormalities of liver function, acute hemorrhagic necrotizing pancreatitis, haematuria or even renal tubular necrosis may be present. Untreated, the mortality can be up to 5% – 15% from infection, toxemia or renal damage. The course of SJS can last for 3 – 6 weeks or even longer.

18. 1. 4　Pathology

The pathologic changes depend on the type of EM. The basic changes include keratinocyte necrosis, liquefaction degeneration of basal cells, blister under epidermis, vasodilatation of upper dermis blood vessels, erythrocyte extravasation, lymphocytes and eosinocyte infiltration around blood vessels.

18.1.5 Diagnosis and Differential Diagnosis

Diagnosis can be made based on the clinical features. The typical "target lesion" is helpful for diagnosis. Classification can be made based on the number of blisters, bullae, and the extent of mucous membranes reaction.

Differential diagnoses include lupus erythematosus, chilblain, bullous pemphigoid, pemphigus, syphilis, pityriasis rosea, etc.

18.1.6 Treatment

Try to find the causes of disease onset. Stop taking any drugs doubted to be associated with the genesis of EM. Mild cases with self-limited course just need symptomatic treatments, but serious cases with high mortality require optimal management.

18.1.6.1 Topical treatment

The effusion and erosion lesions should be covered by gauze with 3% boric acid or physiological saline. As for lesions without effusion or erosion, corticosteroids creams are suitable. Antibiotic salve can be used to prevent skin infection. Intensive nursing is needed to prevent ablepsia and secondary infection.

18.1.6.2 Systemic treatment

Anti-histamine drugs are effective for mild cases. But for serious cases, corticosteroids should be used enough and as quickly as possible. Antibiotic should be used if necessary. Fluid replacement must be started as soon as possible and adjusted daily to maintain the water and electrolyte balance in serious cases. Other supportive treatments to protect liver, kidney and digestive tract function should be taken into account.

18.2 Psoriasis

Psoriasis is a chronic, autoimmune, recurrent systemic skin disease characterized by pink to red plaques covered with silvery white scales. It is universal in occurrence and involves all races and both sexes. The incidence of psoriasis is 1%–3% in the US, as for china, the rate is about 0.123%. Although psoriasis can involve people of any age, from babies to seniors, it is most likely to begin between the ages of 15 to 30 years. About 75% patients develop psoriasis before 40. Another common age of onset for psoria-

sis is between the 50 to 60 years.

18.2.1 Etiology and Pathogenesis

The causes of psoriasis are still not fully understood. However, it is recognized that genetics and immune system play major roles in its development.

18.2.1.1 Genetic factors

Psoriasis has a large hereditary component and nearly one third of the cases have family history. It is recognized as a polygenic disease. Psoriasis susceptibility 1 through 9 (PSORS1 through PSORS9) are associated with psoriasis based on the literatures.

18.2.1.2 Immunological factors

The immune system is somehow mistakenly triggered, which causes a series of events, such as acceleration of skin cell growth. T cells become active, migrate to the dermis and trigger the release of cytokines (TNFα in particular) which cause inflammation and the rapid production of keratinocytes. Normal keratinocytes maturing and falling off the body need 28 to 30 days, while in psoriasis patients they just take 3 to 4 days to mature, and instead of falling off, the cells pile up on the surface of the skin, forming psoriasis lesions.

18.2.1.3 Environmental factors

Various environmental factors have been suggested as aggravating factors to psoriasis, including stress, trauma, streptococcal infection, drugs, sunlight, withdrawal of systemic corticosteroid, excessive alcohol consumption and smoking. But few have been shown statistical significance.

18.2.2 Clinical Features

Psoriasis has many different appearances. Based on the symptoms, it is divided into four types: psoriasis vulgaris, psoriatic arthritis, pustular psoriasis and erythrodermic psoriasis.

18.2.2.1 Psoriasis vulgaris

Psoriasis vulgaris is the most prevalent form of the disease characterized by raised, inflamed, red lesions covered by a silvery white scale (Color Figure 18 – 3). Lesions are distributed on elbows, knees, scalp and lower back. The typical lesions have multilayer silver scales, Auspitz's sign (removal of the thinned suprapillary epidermis, by gentle scraping, reveals vascular bleeding points) and Koebner phenomenon (occurrence of new psoriatic lesions at the site of skin injury, also known as the isomorphic response). Nails can also be involved, showing nail pitting and onychodystrophy. The major complaint is pruritus. According to disease activity, psoriasis vulgaris can be divided into progressive stage, resting stage, and regression stage.

Guttate psoriasis is a special form of psoriasis vulgaris that often involves children or young adult. It is associated with streptococcal infection, typically streptococcal pharyngitis. The typical lesions of this form are small, red, individual spots distributed on the trunk and limbs.

18. 2. 2. 2   Pustular psoriasis

Pustular psoriasis is primarily seen in adults, characterized by white blisters of noninfectious pus (consisting of white blood cells) surrounded by ring of erythema. It begins with the reddening of the skin followed by formation of pustules and scaling. Depends on the distributing of lesions, it is conveniently divided into two subtypes: localized pustular psoriasis and generalized pustular psoriasis. Localized pustular psoriasis is the mild type, lesions of which are confined to hands and feet and tends to be chronic. It consists of palmoplantar pustulosis and acrodermatitis continua. Generalized pustular psoriasis is much more serious often caused by sudden withdrawal of systemic corticosteroid. It can involve the whole body, and the course of which may be subacute, acute or even fulminating and life-threatening.

18. 2. 2. 3   Psoriatic arthritis

Psoriatic arthritis is autoimmune inflammation arthritis of the musculoskeletal system that occurs in patients with psoriasis or with a strong family history of psoriasis. About 10 – 15 percent of psoriasis patients will suffer from psoriatic arthritis during the course of disease. In about one-half of these patients, psoriasis appears an average of a decade earlier than the arthritis, while in the other half arthritis is roughly contemporaneous or even precedes the skin disease. According to the Moll and Wright classification, psoriatic arthritis can be divided into five clinical groups: predominantly peripheral mono-or asymmetrical oligoarthritis, predominantly distal interphalangeal arthritis, predominantly symmetrical polyarthritis, arthritis mutilans and predominantly axial arthritis. Nail matrix is always affected. Serological test for rheumatoid factor is always negative and nearly no rheumatoid nodules occur in the disease.

18. 2. 2. 4   Erythrodermic psoriasis

Erythrodermic psoriasis is characterized by periodic, widespread, fiery redness of the skin and the shedding of scales in sheets, rather than smaller flakes (Color Figure 18 – 4). Two forms exist. In the first, chronic plaque psoriasis may worsen to involve most or all of the skin surface, but patients remain relative responsive to therapy and the prognosis is good. In the second form, lesions may present suddenly and unexpectedly, or result from intolerance to local applications, UV therapy, and of loss of control over the disease. The reddening and shedding of the skin are often accompanied by severe itching and pain, heart rate increase, and fluctuating body temperature. Lower extremity edema, high-output cardiac failure and impaired hepatic and renal function may also occur.

18. 2. 3   Pathology

The typical changes of psoriasis include hyperkeratosis, parakeratosis, thin or loss of the granular cell layer, acanthosis (uniform elongation of the rete ridges), vasodilatation and the formation of spongiform pustules and parakeratotic microabscesses. Spongiform pustules of Kogoj refers to neutrophils aggregation in the Malpighian layer, while Munro microabscess refers to neutrophils accumulation in the parakeratotic layer. The latter is characteristic of psoriasis vulgaris, and the former is usually seen in pustular psoriasis (Color Figure 18 – 5).

18. 2. 4   Diagnosis and Differential Diagnosis

Diagnosis of psoriasis can be made based on the appearance of lesions. In atypical cases, skin biopsy or scraping may be needed to rule out other disorders and to confirm the diagnosis.

Differential diagnoses include pityriasis rosea, eczema, lichen planus, seborrheic dermatitis, drug eruption and secondary syphilis.

Fibromyalgia, seronegative or seropositive rheumatoid arthritis, intercurrent arthritides and repetitive motion-induced musculoskeletal syndromes should be excluded before the diagnosis of psoriatic arthritis.

18. 2. 5   Treatment

Psoriasis is a lifelong condition. There is currently no cure, but various treatments can help to control the symptoms.

18. 2. 5. 1   Topical treatment

Topical medications include topical corticosteroids, vitamin D analogue creams, topical retinoids, moisturizers, topical immunomodulators, coal tar, anthralin, and others.

18.2.5.2 Systemic treatment

The three main traditional systemic treatments are methotrexate, cyclosporine and retinoids. Methotrexate and cyclosporine are immunosuppressant drugs; retinoids are synthetic forms of vitamin A. Antihistamine drugs, NSAID and biologics are also used in the treatment of psoriasis.

18.2.5.3 Phototherapy and photochemotherapy

The UVB narrowband lamp, psoralen and ultraviolet A phototherapy (PUVA) are widely used.

18.3 Pityriasis Rosea

Pityriasis rose is an inflammatory self-limited cutaneous disease. Its typical clinical characteristic is a "herald" or "mother" patch and oval, scaly, pink patches distributed on the chest, back, arms, and legs. The lesions always last for 6 – 8 weeks before disappearance.

18.3.1 Etiology

The etiology is still unclear. Epidemiological and clinical features suggest that it is associated with infection. The pathogens include bacteria, fungi, and most notably, viruses. Two herpes viruses, HHV-6 and HHV-7, are considered as causes for the eruption. Cell immunity reaction may also play a role in the occurrence of this disease.

18.3.2 Clinical Features

Pityriasis rosea can involve people of all age, but most commonly attacks between the ages of 10 and 35. It often attacks at spring and autumn with self-limited course of disease. Lesions usually begin with a large, scaly, pink patch on the chest or back, which is called a "herald" or "mother" patch. Within a week or two, more oval faint pink to deep red patches spread over trunk and extremities (Color Figure 18 – 6). Patches may also occur on the neck, but rarely on the face. Typical lesion has a dry surface and an inner circlet of scaling with or without itch. The itching is often non-specific, and worsens if scratched. Rashes usually fade and disappear within 6 to 8 weeks, but sometimes can last much longer. Recurrence is very rare.

18.3.3 Diagnosis and Differential Diagnosis

Diagnosis can be made based on the typical clinical features. If the diagnosis is in doubt, tests may be performed to differentiate similar conditions such as tinea versicolor, guttate psoriasis, nummular or discoid eczema, drug eruptions, other viral exanthems, and especially secondary syphilis.

18.3.4 Treatment

Pityriasis rosea usually requires no special treatment due to its self-limited course. However, topical or systemic treatment should be taken into account in itching conditions and for the purpose to reduce the rash. Oral antihistamines or topical steroids may be prescribed to decrease itching. Soothing medicated lotions and lubricants may be helpful for over-dryness management. Ultraviolet light treatments are also effective.

18.4 Lichen Planus

Lichen planus (LP) is a recurrent inflammatory cutaneous disease with immunological basis. Its typical clinical characteristic is purple polygonal papules with Wickham stria. Topical steroids treatment is effective for mild cases, while more intensive therapy is needed for severe cases.

18.4.1 Etiology

The etiology of LP is still unclear. Some drugs, such as those containing arsenic, bismuth, or gold can cause a reaction. Exposure to certain chemicals can also produce a similar rash. Other unusual causes of lichen planus include liver disease, viral infection, etc. Some of the latest studies have shown a co-association of LP with a rare variety of Hepatitis-C. It also has been suggested that LP lesions may present on the mucosa or skin during times of stress. Furthermore, LP may be influenced by genetic predisposition.

18.4.2 Clinical Features

The typical rash of LP is characterized by well-defined pruritic, planar, purple, polygonal papules varying in size from 1 mm to greater than 1 cm in diameter. They can be discrete or arranged in groups of lines or circles (Color Figure 18 – 7). Characteristic fine white lines, called Wickham stria often can be found on the papules. Besides the typical lesions, many morphological varieties of the rash may occur: actinic, annular, atrophic, erosive, follicular, hypertrophic, linear, pigmented, and vesicular/bullous. Wrist and the ankle are the commonly affected. The rash tends to heal with prominent blue-black or brownish discoloration that persists for a long time. Pruritus is common but varies in severity depending on the type of lesion and the extent of involvement.

In addition to the cutaneous eruption, LP can involve the mucous membranes, the genitalia, the nails, and the scalp. About half of the people affected with LP have the rash inside of their mouths (oral mucosa). The oral rash often occurs prior to any skin involvement. Oral lesions tend to last far longer than cutaneous lesions. In more than 50% of patients with cutaneous disease, the lesions resolve within 6 months, and 85% of cases subside within 18 months.

18. 4. 3 Pathology

The typical pathologic appearances of LP include: hyperkeratosis, thickening of the granular cell layer, degeneration of the basal cell layer, infiltration of lymphocytic inflammatory cells into the subepithelial layer and Civatte or colloid body formation (Color Figure 18 - 8).

18. 4. 4 Diagnosis and Differential Diagnosis

Diagnosis can be made based on the typical clinical features. Sometimes the LP eruptions, especially in early states, may resemble to some other diseases like atopic dermatitis, psoriasis, candidiasis (in mouth), leukoplakia (mouth), aphthous ulcers (mouth). Also, LP of nails alone could resemble psoriatic nails and fungus infection. If necessary, a skin biopsy should be done to help confirm the diagnosis.

18. 4. 5 Treatment

LP is hard to be cured. Topical and systemic treatments are available to reduce the effects of the inflammation.

18. 4. 5. 1 Topical treatment

Topical treatment especially topical corticosteroid as the first line therapy is effective for mild cases to deal with the lesions and itch. For localized, itchy, thick lesions, injections of corticosteroids may be given.

18. 4. 5. 2 Systemic treatment

For severe cases, especially those with scalp, nail, and mucous membrane involvement, intensive therapy should be taken into account. Antihistamines and low-dose oral corticosteroids may be helpful to reduce itch, though it may return after the drug has been discontinued. Ultraviolet light (PUVA, narrowband or broadband UV-B) treatment may be useful

in condition of widespread LP. For painful lesions within the mouth, special mouthwashes containing a painkiller (such as lidocaine) may provide some relief.

■ Summary

This chapter has introduced four main skin disorders with erythema and scaling: erythema multiforme, psoriasis, pityriasis rosea and lichen planus. The pathogeneses of those diseases are still unclear and clinical features are quite different from each other.

Erythema multiforme (EM) is an acute recurrent inflammatory mucocutaneous disease with immunological basis. Its typical clinical characteristic is the "target lesion" or "iris lesion". Depends on the appearance of lesions, EM is divided into three types: macule-papule form, blister-bulla form and Steven-Johnson syndrome form. SJS is the most serious type of EM with high mortality. The diagnosis of EM is mainly based on the clinical typical features. For serious cases, optimal management is important to reduce the mortality.

Psoriasis is a chronic, autoimmune, systemic skin disease. Immune system and genetics play major roles in its development. It is characterized by pink to red plaques that are covered with silver-white scales. It is classified by symptoms into four types: psoriasis vulgaris, psoriatic arthritis, pustular psoriasis and erythrodermic psoriasis. Auspitz's sign and Koebner phenomenon are the characteristic features of the psoriasis. The typical pathological changes include hyperkeratosis, parakeratosis, thin or loss of the granular cell layer, acanthosis, vasodilatation and the formation of spongiform pustules and parakeratotic microabscesses. There are various treatments can help to control the symptoms: topical medications, systemic treatment and PUVA.

Pityriasis rosea is an inflammatory, self-limited cutaneous disease characterized by a "herald" or "mother" patch and oval, scaly, pink patches on the trunk and extremities. Itching is often non-specific. Oral antihistamines, topical steroids and ultraviolet light may be effective.

Lichen planus (LP) is a recurrent inflammatory cutaneous disease with immunological basis. The rash is characterized by purple, flat-topped, many-sided (polygonal) papules and Wickham stria. Itch is the major symptom. The typical pathologic appearances are distinctive. Topical steroids, antihistamines, oral corticosteroids and ultraviolet light should be taken into account to control the symptoms.

▪ Questions

1. Try to describe the classification and clinical feature of erythema multiforme.

2. Try to describe the clinical feature of four types of psoriasis.

3. What are Auspitz's sign and Koebner phenomenon?

4. What is the typical lesion of pityriasis rosea?

5. What are the typical pathologic appearances of lichen planus?

(**Shiguang Peng** 彭世光，**Yanling He** 何焱玲)

Chapter 19

Connective Tissue Diseases

▪ Objectives

To master the knowledge of the causes and clinical features of skin diseases characterized by discoid lupus erythematosus, subacute cutaneous lupus erythematosus, and systemic lupus erythematosus lesions. To have an intimate knowledge of diagnosis and management discoid lupus erythematosus.

To handle the knowledge of the clinical feature of dermatomyositis. To familiar with diagnosis and treatment of dermatomyositis.

To master the knowledge of clinical features, diagnosis and treatment of scleroderma. To have an intimate knowledge of two patterns of scleroderma (localized scleroderma and systemic sclerosis).

▪ Key concepts

Lupus erythematosus is a category for a collection of diseases with similar underlying problems with immunity. Symptoms of these diseases can affect many different body systems, including joints, skin, kidneys, blood cells, heart, and lungs.

Dermatomyositis is a muscle disease characterized by inflammation and a skin rash. It is an ongoing, long-term inflammation of many muscles throughout the body. These can include the muscles of the lungs, esophagus, and throat. It is linked in some cases to specific types of cancer, such as lung cancer.

Scleroderma is an autoimmune disease of the connective tissue featuring skin thickening, spontaneous scarring, blood vessel disease, varying degrees of inflammation, associated with an overactive immune system. It is classified into localized scleroderma and systemic sclerosis. Patients with scleroderma can have specific antibodies in their blood which suggest autoimmunity. Treatment of scleroderma is directed toward the individual's symptoms that are most debilitating.

▪ Introduction

Connective tissue diseases are a group of multi-system illnesses of unknown etiology, which include systemic lupus erythematosus, dermatomyositis, scleroderma, polymyositis, rheumatoid arthritis, Sjögren's syndrome, and et al. Connective tissue diseases are grouped among the autoimmune diseases therefore the autoantibodies present in the sera of some patients with these diseases. Therapy with topical corticosteroids, and antimalarial agents is usually effective.

19.1   Lupus Erythematosus

Lupus erythematosus (LE) is a multisystem disease of unknown origin characterized by the production of numerous diverse types of autoantibodies that, through immune mechanisms in various tissues, cause several combinations of clinical signs, symptoms, and laboratory abnormalities. Symptoms of these diseases can affect many different body systems, including joints, skin, kidneys, blood cells, heart, and lungs. LE is usually divided into two main types: discoid lupus erythematosus (DLE), and systemic lupus erythematosus (SLE). Subacute cutaneous lupus erythematosus (SCLE) is described as a subset intermediate between DLE and SLE. And the other special types of lupus erythematosus: lupus erythematosus profundus (LEP), drug-induced lupus erythematosus (DIL) and neonatal lupus erythematosus (NLE). The risk of a patient with DLE developing over SLE varies from 1.3% to about 6.5%. The risk is higher in patients with disseminated DLE (22%) than in DLE confined to the head and neck (1.2%). And discoid lupus erythematosus may occur in patients with systemic lupus erythematosus (SLE).

Etiology

(1) Genetic factors

An important role for a genetic contribution to lupus susceptibility in humans is suggested by the high concordance of disease in identical twins (65%). Of all cases, 4% are familial, with marked concordance of disease expression between parents and offspring. Positive associations with HLA-B7, -B8, -Cw7, -DR2, -DR3 and-DQw1 are reported.

(2) Hormonal factors

As markedly more females than males are af-fected in early adult life, it has been suggested that endocrine factors may be involved. Pregnancy may initiate and exacerbate lesions.

(3) Environmental factors and others

Ultraviolet light exposure is a well-described trigger of lupus flares. Photosensitivity is present in 50% of patients with discoid lupus erythematosus. Skin lesions clinically and histologically compatible with lupus erythematosus (LE) were induced by UVB and UVA radiation in 42% of patients with DLE, 64% of patients with SCLE and 25% of patients with SLE. Streptococcus and Epstein-Barr virus infections may initiate and exacerbate lesions. Drug-induced lupus erythematosus (DIL) may be induced by a variety of drugs, most notably hydralazine, procainamide, isoniazid, methyldopa, chlorpromazine, and quinidine.

Mechanism

Lupus is thought to be a dysregulation of T cells causing the activation of B cells, producing a variety of autoantibodies directed against cellular antigens such as DNA, RNA, and RNA-protein complexes. Tissue and organ damage in LE is mediated by the deposition or in situ formation of immune complexes and subsequent complement activation and inflammation. Tissues targeted by immune system activity in lupus include the skin, where immune complexes and complement are deposited in a linear pattern, the glomeruli, and heart valves.

19.1.1   *Discoid Lupus Erythematosus (DLE)*

Patients with DLE have a low incidence of systemic disease. The disease is more common in females, and it has a peak incidence in the fourth decade. Trauma and ultraviolet light exposure (UVB) may initiate and exacerbate lesions.

19.1.1.1   Clinical features

The face and scalp are the most commonly affected areas, but lesions may occur on any body surface. Lesions are usually asymmetrically distributed and begin as asymptomatic, well-defined, elevated, erythematous, 1 – 2 cm, flat-topped plaques with firmly adherent scale. Follicular plugs are prominent, peeling the scale reveals an undersurface that looks like a carpet penetrated by several carpet tacks; it is called "tin-tack" sign.

Epidermal atrophy gives the surface either a smooth white or a wrinkled appearance in the central or inactive area. These lesions endure for months and either resolve spontaneously or progress with further atrophy, ultimately forming smooth white or hyperpigmented depressed scars with telangiectasia and scarring alopecia. Scalp disease begins with erythema, scaling, and follicular plugging. Hair follicles are destroyed, resulting in irreversible, scarring alopecia. Hair loss is haphazard in distribution. Most patients have disease limited to the head and neck (localized DLE), but a few have much more extensive disease, potentially affecting any area of the skin (disseminated DLE).

19. 1. 1. 2 Laboratory findings

The laboratory abnormalities of some patients with DLE manifest leucopenia, raised serum globulin, raised erythrocyte sedimentation rate, false-positive syphilis serology, positive rheumatoid factor and positive anticardiolipin antibodies (mainly IgM).

Some (approximately 20%) manifest a positive antinuclear antibody (ANA) when tested with human substrates. Anti-Ro (SS-A) autoantibodies are present in approximately 1%–3% of patients. Antinative DNA (double-stranded or nDNA) or anti-Sm antibodies usually reflect SLE, and they may occur in some patients (<5%).

19. 1. 1. 3 Histopathology and immunopathology

The characteristic histopathologic alterations observed in discoid lupus erythematosus include vacuolar alteration of the basal cell layer, thickening of the basement membrane, follicular plugging, hyperkeratosis, atrophy of the epidermis, incontinence of pigment, and inflammatory cell infiltrate (usually lymphocytic) in a perivascular, periappendiceal, and subepidermal location.

Approximately 80% of patients with discoid lupus erythematosus manifest a positive direct immunofluorescence (DIF) test which is called lupus band test (LBT) on lesional skin. Immunohistology shows the presence of immunoglobulins IgG, IgA, IgM and complement at the dermal-epidermal junction, in skin lesions present for 6 weeks or more, but rarely present in uninvolved skin.

19. 1. 1. 4 Diagnosis and differential

Diagnosis depends on the typical symptoms, laboratory findings, histopathologic and immunopathology.

DLE must be differentiated from SLE, lichen planus, psoriasis vulgaris, actinic keratosis, tinea corporis/capitis, and subacute cutaneous lupus erythematosus.

19. 1. 1. 5 Treatment

A sunscreen cream or lotion should be prescribed, and a preparation with a UVB protection factor of at least 15 is required; UVA protection is at least as important.

(1) Topical steriod can frequently control and sometimes clear lesions without systemic treatment. Intralesional corticosteroid injections are helpful in resistant cases, even on lips, mouth and ears.

(2) Oral therapy

1) Antimalarials: There is little doubt that in most cases first-line oral treatment should be with one of the antimalarials. Most would start therapy with hydroxychloroquine, initially at 200 mg twice daily, reducing to 200 mg/d once a response is achieved. Chloroquine sulphate is equally effective, usually at a dosage of 200 mg twice daily, but hydroxychloroquine is used first by most prescribers because side effects, particularly eye toxicity, are less likely provided that the dosage limitations of 6. 5 mg/kg lean body weight are adhered to.

2) Thalidomide: For cases not responding to topical steroids, antimalarials and sunscreens, oral thalidomide has proved remarkably effective in suppressing lesions, and also in the treatment of chilblain LE. The originally employed dosage of 100 mg/d seems to be equally effective.

3) Corticosteroid: For patients with severe, extensive or scarring disease, particularly affection the scalp, oral prednisolone is often the most helpful initial treatment. A dosage of 0. 5 mg/kg, rapidly tapered over 6 weeks, is quickly effective, minimizes scarring, and allows the slower acting agents such as antimalarials to work.

19. 1. 2 Subacute Cutaneous Lupus Erythematosus (SCLE)

Subacute cutaneous lupus erythematosus (SCLE) is a specific 'subset' of lupus first described by Sontheimer et al. in1979, which comprises approximately 10% of patients with LE. It is most common in white, young to middle-aged women. Antibodies to the Ro/SS-A antigen are closely associated with this subgroup. SCLE may be induced by a variety of drugs, most notably hydrochlorothiazide and calcium channel blockers. Patients exhibit mainly cutaneous disease and usually have a good prognosis.

19. 1. 2. 1 Clinical features

Two morphologic varieties are a non-scarring papulosquamous pattern (2/3) and an annular polycyclic pattern (1/3). Both most often occur above the waist and particularly around the neck, on the trunk and on the outer aspects of the arms. A subtle grey-white hypopigmentation and telangiectasia are frequently seen in the center of annular lesions, bordered by erythema and a superficial scale. Follicular plugging, adherent hyperkeratosis, scarring, and dermal atrophy are characteristic of DLE but not prominent features of SCLE. Other dermatologic manifestations are photosensitivity (85% to 52%), periungual telangiectasia (51% to 22%), discoid LE (35% to 19%), and vasculitis (12%). Systemic manifestations [arthritis/arthralgia (74% to 43%), renal disease (19% to 11%), serositis (12%), and central nervous system symptoms (19% to 6%)] are not severe and follow a benign course.

19. 1. 2. 2　Laboratory findings

The antinuclear antibody titer is elevated in 50%–72% of cases. Using human cell lines as substrates, homogeneous antinuclear antibodies are found in approximately 60% and anti-Ro/SS-A antibodies in approximately 80% of patients, rising to higher levels in females. Anticardiolipin antibodies occur in 16%. Anti-La/SS-B coexists with anti-Ro/SS-A and is usually not present as a unique antibody. Leucopenia is present in 25%–50% of patients with SCLE.

19. 1. 2. 3　Histopathologic and immunopathology

SCLE can be differentiated from DLE by the presence of more epidermal atrophy and less hyperkeratosis, basement-membrane thickening, follicular plugging and inflammatory infiltration. Colloid bodies and epidermal necrosis are present in more than 50%, especially in those with Ro/SS-A antibodies. Dust-like particles of inter-and intracellular IgG in the basement layers of the epidermis may be a specific feature. Subepidermal immunoglobulin is found in approximately 60% of lesions, and is more frequent in papulosquamous (88%) than annular lesions (29%), and 30% of uninvolved skin.

19. 1. 2. 4　Diagnosis and differential

The diagnosis of SCLE is confirmed by clinical-pathologic correlation. Skin biopsy reveals similar features to those observed in DLE, but there is less prominent follicular plugging and less frequent epidermal atrophy. Although patients frequently have antibodies to Ro/SS-A, their presence is not diagnostic and their absence is not exclusionary. Immunofluorescence microscopy is useful only in selected pa-

tients and the findings must be interpreted within the context of the clinical findings.

SCLE must be differentiated from drug eruptions (especially thiazides), dermatomyositis, secondary syphilis, psoriasis, cutaneous T cell lymphoma, seborrheic dermatitis, and tinea corporis.

19. 1. 2. 5　Treatment

The condition in most patients is controlled by sunscreens, topical or intralesional corticosteroids or the macrolides, pimecrolimus and tacrolimus. In those not responding to these agents, antimalarial drugs are often helpful. These can be used as either hydroxychloroquine or chloroquine base, although the former is safer from the ophthalmological point of view and requires less ophthalmological monitoring. The antimalarial mepacrine (quinacrine) does not have ocular side effects but does induce yellow discoloration of the skin. There is evidence that a combination of antimalarials may be more effective than either alone and that they are less effective in smokers. Patients not responding to antimalarials may respond to oral corticosteroids, methylprednisolone, etretinate, acitretin, isotretinoin, and dapsone; or oral, intravenous and subcutaneous methotrexate and thalidomide, UVA, IFN-α, long-term cefuroxime axetil, mycophenolate mofetil, intravenous immunoglobulin, etanercept and efalizumab.

19. 1. 3　Systemic Lupus Erythematosus (SLE)

Systemic lupus erythematosus (SLE) is a multiorgan system autoimmune disease that results from immune system-mediated tissue damage. It is characterized by an autoantibody response to nuclear and cytoplasmic antigens. Manifestations of SLE can involve the skin, joints, kidney, central nervous system, cardiovascular system, serosal membranes, the hematologic, and immune systems. The female-to-male ratio is approximately 8 : 1 to 9 : 1 in adults, and most cases are diagnosed between the ages of 15 and 44 years.

19. 1. 3. 1　Clinical features

The main clinical features include fever, rashes and arthritis, but renal, pulmonary, cardiac and neurological involvement may occur, with increased mortality.

(1) Musculoskeletal system

Involvement of the joints occurs at some time in approximately 90% of patients, arthralgia being more common than arthritis. A rheumatoid-like deformity is present in approximately 25% of cases, with marked soft-tissue swelling, especially of the dorsa of the fingers, hands and wrists, although joint erosions on X-ray are not a feature. Fibromyalgia, characterized by painful trigger points at characteristic locations, commonly accompanies SLE and can contribute to fatigue and depression. Numerous cases of patients with SLE and concomitant avascular bone necrosis have been reported; the disease itself or systemic corticosteroids may cause the necrosis.

(2) Skin

Approximately 80% of cases have a rash at some stage. ① The erythematous facial rash with a butterfly distribution across the malar and nasal prominences and sparing of the nasolabial folds is the classic rash of SLE. The butterfly rash is often triggered by sun exposure(Color Figure 19–1). ②Telangiectasia occurs on the palms and fingers in association with palmar erythema; it resembles that observed in liver disease and pregnancy. ③Lesions resembling chronic discoid lesions are initial manifestations in approximately 10% of patients and occur in the course of the disease in approximately 33%; they may be more common in men. ④ The hair is usually coarse, dry and fragile, especially on the frontal margin. This leads to an unruly appearance with short, broken-off hair, the so-called "lupus hair". ⑤Lupus should be considered in all patients who experience painless or painful oral or vaginal ulcers.

(3) Hematologic system

Anemia, leucopenia (particularly lymphopenia), thrombocytopenia are observed.

(4) Renal system

Kidney involvement in SLE is common, with 74% of patients being affected at some time in the course of disease, and is a poor prognostic indicator. The renal system can be affected leading to renal failure. Specific signs and symptoms of renal disease may not be apparent until advanced nephrotic syndrome or renal failure is present; therefore, obtaining a urine analysis, serum BUN and creatinine levels on a regular basis is important.

(5) Cardiovascular system

Cardiac disease in lupus erythematosus may appear as pericarditis, myocarditis, or cardiomegaly and possibly lead to heart failure. Pericarditis has been estimated to occur in 25% of cases. It is usually associated with small effusions, but it may involve larger effusions when uremia is concomitant. Myocarditis can cause heart failure, arrhythmias, and sudden death.

(6) Pulmonary system

Transient pleurisy is the most common feature. Involvement of the lungs is shown mainly as transient infiltration, sometimes with mottling and reticulation. Tachypnea, cough, and fever are common manifestations of lupus pneumonitis.

(7) Gastrointestinal system

Gastrointestinal findings include vague abdominal discomfort, nausea, and diarrhea. Acute crampy abdominal pain, vomiting, and diarrhea may signify vasculitis of the intestine.

(8) Neuropsychiatric involvement

The most common manifestations that are probably attributable to SLE cerebritis include cognitive dysfunction, present in 17% to 66% of SLE patients; psychosis or mood disorder, the former reported in up to 8% of patients; cerebrovascular disease in 5% to 18% of patients; and seizures, present in 6% to 51% of patients. Headaches are also common.

19. 1. 3. 2　Histopathologic and immunopathology

The primary lesions of SLE are fibrinoid necrosis, collagen sclerosis, necrosis and basophilic body formation, and vascular endothelial thickening. The basophilic (haematoxylin) bodies are aggregates of homogeneous material staining blue with haematoxylin and staining positively for DNA by the Feulgen technique.

Immunoglobulins, predominantly IgG, but less frequently IgM and IgA, together with complement (C1, C3) can be demonstrated at the dermal-epidermal junction by immunofluorescence techniques. They occur in more than 80% of skin lesions of DLE and SLE.

19. 1. 3. 3　Diagnosis and differential

The American College of Rheumatology classification criteria for systemic lupus erythematosus (SLE) were updated in 1997 (www. rheumatology. org)(Table 19–1). The presence of four or more of the 11 parameters, serially or simultaneously, is believed to be compatible with the diagnosis of LE.

19. 1. 3. 4　Treatment

(1) Corticosteroids

Oral prednisone in doses ranging from 5 to 30 mg daily is effective in treating constitutional symptoms, arthralgias, pericarditis and pleuritis, and skin disease. Topical corticosteroids are sometimes applied to cutaneous lesions. For more serious disease, particularly active nephritis, central nervous system disease, or systemic vasculitis, prednisone at

60 mg daily or 1 g of intravenous methylprednisolone administered daily for 3 days can often gain control of disease activity.

(2) Immunosuppressive agents

Cyclophosphamide is a cytotoxic agent that has been one of the more reliable and studied treatments for severe organ system manifestations of lupus, particularly lupus nephritis and central nervous system involvement. Azathioprine has been used for the treatment of lupus nephritis and as a steroid-sparing agent in SLE for many years.

(3) Others

Clinical manifestations of lupus that do not involve major organ systems can often be managed with nonsteroidal anti-inflammatory drugs, low-dose corticosteroids, and antimalarials.

Table 19 - 1　American College of Rheumatology: The 1997 revised criteria for classification of systemic lupus erythematosus

Definition	Criterion
1. Malar rash	Fixed erythema, flat or raised, over the malar eminences, tending to spare the nasolabial folds
2. Discoid rash	Erythematous raised patches with adherent keratotic scaling and follicular plugging; atrophic scarring may occur in older lesions
3. Photosensitivity	Skin rash as a result of unusual reaction to sunlight, by patient history or physician observation
4. Oral ulcers	Oral or nasopharyngeal ulceration, usually painless, observed by physician
5. Arthritis	Nonerosive arthritis involving 2 or more peripheral joints, characterized by tenderness, swelling, or effusion
6. Serositis	a) Pleuritis - convincing history of pleuritic pain or rubbing heard by a physician or evidence of pleural effusion OR b) Pericarditis-documented by ECG or rub or evidence of pericardial effusion
7. Renal disorder	a) Persistent proteinuria greater than 0.5 mg per day or greater than 3+ if quantitation not performed OR b) Cellular casts-may be red cell, hemoglobin, granular, tubular or mixed
8. Neurologic disorder	a) Seizures-in the absence of offending drugs or known metabolic derangements; e. g. uremia, ketoacidosis, or electrolyte imbalance OR b) Psychosis-in the absence of offending drugs or known metabolic derangements; e. g. uremia, ketoacidosis, or electrolyte imbalance
9. Hematologic disorder	a) Hemolytic anemia-with reticulocytosis OR b) Leukopenia-less than 4×10^9/L total on 2 or more occasions OR c) Lymphopenia-less than 1.5×10^9/L on 2 or more occasions OR d) Thrombocytopenia-less than 100×10^9/L in the absence of offending drugs
10. Immunologic disorder	a) Anti-DNA: antibody to native DNA in abnormal titer OR b) Anti-Sm: presence of antibody to Sm nuclear antigen OR c) Positive finding of antiphospholipid antibodies based on ① an abnormal serum level of IgG or IgM anticardiolipin antibodies; ② a positive test result for lupus anticoagulant using a standard method; or ③ a false-positive serologic test for syphilis known to be positive for at least 6 months and confirmed by *Treponema pallidum* immobilization or fluorescent treponemal antibody absorption test. Standard methods should be used in testing for the presence of antiphospholipid
11. Antinuclear antibody	An abnormal titer of antinuclear antibody by immunofluorescence or an equivalent assay at any point in time and in the absence of drugs known to be associated with "drug-induced lupus" syndrome

Hochberg MC. Arthritis Rheum, 1997, 40: 1725.

The proposed classification is based on 11 criteria. For the purpose of identifying patients in clinical studies, a person shall be said to have systemic lupus erythematosus if any four or more of the 11 criteria are present, serially or simultaneously, during any interval of observation.

19.1.4 Other Special Types of Lupus Erythematosus

19.1.4.1 Lupus erythematosus profundas (LEP)

Lupus erythematosus profundas (LEP) is a rare disease. It is characterized clinically by deep subcutaneous nodules or plaques, with central erythematous and atrophic features, distributed on the face, scalp, proximal extremities, trunk or lower back. Hydroxychloroquine is the agents of first choice for LEP.

19.1.4.2 Drug-induced lupus erythematosus (DILE)

Many drugs have been reported to cause a syndrome similar to systemic lupus erythematosus. Procainamide, hydralazine are the most common cause of drug related lupus. DILE is characterized by arthralgia and/or arthritis, myalgia, serositis, fever, hepatomegaly, splenomegaly, and skin manifestation. ANA is an important marker for DILE. Anti-nuclear antibodies in DILE are fairly specific and mainly directed against histones or single-stranded DNA (ssDNA). DILE resolves in weeks and rarely in years after drug withdrawal. It does not usually require treatment.

19.1.4.3 Neonatal lupus erythematosus (NLE)

NLE is a rare disorder caused by transplacental autoantibodies from the mother to the fetus, which is caused by the transplacental passage of maternal IgG anti-Ro/SS-A and/or anti-La/SS-B or anti-U$_1$ RNP. This syndrome is characterized by one or more of the following findings: subacute cutaneous lupus-like annular and polycyclic lesions, congenital heart block, cardiomyopathy, cholestatic hepatitis, and thrombocytopenia. The lesions heal without scarring or atrophy within 6 months. The congenital heart block is a permanent defect. Patients with heart block may be asymptomatic or require pacemakers.

19.2 Dermatomyositis

Dermatomyositis is a type of inflammatory myopathy. It is a rare but treatable disorder which, in some cases, can result in serious complications, such as difficulty breathing, difficulty swallowing, pneumonia, gastrointestinal ulcerations, lung cancer, and complications of pregnancy.

The incidence of dermatomyositis (DM) has been estimated at 5.5 – 8.0 cases per million. However, it appears that the incidence is increasing. It occurs in all ages but is most common in middle-age adults and school-age children. Women are affected twice as often as men.

19.2.1 Etiology

The cause of dermatomyositis is unknown but is believed to have relationship with autoimmune reaction in which the body immune system attacks muscle cells mistaken for dangerous substances. Increasing evidences indicate that the cause of dermatomyositis is related to genetic factors, immunological abnormalities and infection. It is also linked in some cases to specific types of cancer, such as lung cancer.

19.2.2 Clinical Features

There are six dermatologic features of dermatomyositis:

(1) Heliotrope erythema of eyelids

Periorbital edema and violet discoloration may be either the earliest cutaneous sign or a residual finding as diffuse erythema fades (Color Figure 19 - 2).

(2) Gottron'papules

Gottron'papules, a pathognomonic sign of dermatomyositis, are round, 0.2 to 1.0 cm, smooth, violaceous-to-red, flat-topped papules that occur over the knuckles, along knees and elbows.

(3) Violaceous scaling patches

A characteristic violet erythema with or without scaling occurs in a localized or diffuse distribution. Dermatomyositis typically involves the knuckles and spares the skin over the phalanges.

(4) Periungual erythema and telangiectasia

The telangiectasia is most prominent on the proximal nailfold and appears as irregular, red, linear streaks. The cuticles are thick, rough, hyperkeratotic, and irregular.

(5) Poikiloderma

Poikiloderma is a descriptive term for the pattern that consists of finely mottled white areas and brown pigmentation, telangiectasia, and atrophy. It may occur in the same sun-exposed areas.

(6) Scaly red scalp

Scalp scaly may be a sign of dermatomyositis. Erythematous, scaly, atrophic scalp lesions initially diagnosed as psoriasis, seborrheic dermatitis, or lupus erythematosus were reported in a series of patients with dermatomyositis.

This process results in the typical symptoms of dermatomyositis which include muscle weakness. Symptoms can occur suddenly or they can develop slowly over a period of months. Symptoms of dermatomyositis can also include muscle pain and joint pain. Symptoms can lead to difficulties performing the activities of daily living, such as dressing, walking, bathing, and eating.

19.2.3 Diagnosis and Differential Diagnosis

Diagnosing dermatomyositis and its root cause begins with taking a thorough personal and family medical history, including symptoms, and completing a physical examination, including a neurological examination. A neurological exam evaluates the muscles, nerves and nervous system and such functions as reflexes, sensation, movement, balance, coordination, vision, and hearing. Making a diagnosis of dermatomyositis may require the collaborative effort of a variety of specialists. These include a neurologist, a specialist in neurological diseases and disorders, and a rheumatologist, a specialist in disorders and diseases of the joints, muscles, and connective tissue. Diagnostic tests may include a muscle biopsy. In a muscle biopsy a small sample of muscle tissue is removed and examined under a microscope. Other tests may include blood tests that measure the levels of certain antibodies that made in dermatomyositis. Diagnostic tests may also include an electromyography (EMG) which tests the nerve and electrical activity of muscles. A nerve conduction test may also be performed to test how fast the nerves transmit impulses to the muscles.

Dermatomyositis must be differentiated from lupus erythematosus and scleroderma.

19.2.4 Treatment

Oral corticosteroids are the treatment of first choice for most adults who have skin and muscle symptoms. Adjuvant immunosuppressive drugs are used if muscle symptoms do not respond to oral steroids. Physical therapy is essential to prevent joint contractures and muscle atrophy. Shin disease is treated with topical steroids and sunscreen.

(1) Corticosteroids

Corticosteroids suppress immune system, limiting the production of antibodies and reducing skin and muscle inflammation, as well as improving muscle strength and function. Corticosteroids, especially prednisone, are usually the first choice in treating inflammatory myopathies such as dermatomyositis. It may start with a very high dose, and then decrease it as the signs and symptoms of dermatomyositis

improved. Improvement generally takes about two to four weeks, but therapy is often needed for years. Doctors may also prescribe topical corticosteroids for the patient.

Oral prednisone(0.5 to 1.5 mg/g) is given in single daily dose(not every-other-day dosing) until serum cytokine (CK) is normal. Most patients begin to improve after the first month. Muscle strength improvement usually lags behind decreasing CK values. The dosage is lowered over a 12 to 24 month period as disease activity improves, as indicated by improving clinical signs and decreasing levels of muscle enzymes. Another regimen involves oral prednisone in a divided daily dose of 40 to 60mg/day (1 – 2mg/kg in children) until the CK has normalized; consolidation of the prednisone into a single daily dose, which is then reduced by one fourth every 3 to 4 weeks only if the CK value is still normal; and continuation of the prednisone until a maintenance dose of 5 to 10 mg/d is reached, at which time this dosage is continued for 1 year.

(2) Immunosuppressants

Methotrexate: Start oral methotrexate at 7.5 to 10 mg per week, increased by 2.5 mg per week to total of 25 mg per week. Intravenous dosage is 10 mg per week, increased by 2.5 mg per week to total of 0.5 to 0.8 mg per kg. Azathioprine: Start oral medication with 2 to 3 mg/kg per day tapered to 1 mg/kg per day once steroid is tapered to 15 mg per day. Reduce dosage monthly by 25 mg intervals. Maintenance dosage is 50 mg per day. Cyclophosphamide: The drug is less effective than azathioprine. Start oral medication at 1 to 3 mg/kg per day, with prednisone.

(3) Antimalarial medications

Antimalarials are sometimes effective in treating the cutaneous lesions of dermatomyositis. Hydroxychloroquine sulfate(200 to 400 mg/d) is prescribed.

(4) Antibody therapy

Intravenous immunoglobulin (IVIg). Immunoglobulin contains healthy antibodies from blood donors. High doses can block the damaging antibodies that attack muscle and skin in dermatomyositis.

(5) Immunosuppressive therapies

In addition to corticosteroids and immunosuppressive drugs, other treatments to suppress the immune system include: tacrolimus (Prograf). This transplant-rejection drug may work to inhibit the immune system. Tacrolimus is often used topically to treat dermatomyositis and other skin problems.

When taken orally, it may be helpful if you have dermatomyositis complicated by interstitial lung disease.

(6) Physical therapy

Bed rest is essential for patients with active muscle disease. Physical therapy is very important in the management of dermatomyositis to prevent atrophy and contractures. Prednisone and immunosuppressive agents treat inflammation, but they do not make muscles strong. An aggressive-passive physical therapy program should be started, and, as muscle pain decreases, an active exercise program should be adopted.

19.3 Scleroderma

Scleroderma is a disease characterized by sclerosis of the skin and visceral organs, vasculopathy (Raynaud's syndrome), and autoantibodies. The spectrum of disease is wide, with systemic and localized forms.

19.3.1 Etiology

Scleroderma is caused by the immune system attacking the body's own tissues mistakenly. The immune system attack causes inflammation and an overproduction of collagen. Too much collagen causes the skin, and sometimes the internal organs, to become hard and tight. The main histological feature in the early stage of scleroderma is infiltrates of inflammatory cells in the dermis. Inflammatory cells are a key source of released cytokines, which in turn produce growth factors such as transforming growth factor-beta and connective tissue growth factor and initiate the sequential events of fibrosis. Various cytokines produced by immune-activated cells modulate the synthesis of extracellular matrix (ECM) by fibroblasts. Over-deposition of ECM results in tissue fibrosis in scleroderma. Both genetics and environment may play a role.

19.3.2 Clinical Features

Scleroderma can be classified in terms of the degree and location of the skin involvement. Accordingly, it has been categorized into two major groups, localized and systemic.

19.3.2.1 The localized scleroderma

Tends to have far less skin involvement with skin thickening confined to the skin of the fingers and face. The skin changes and other features of disease tend to occur more slowly than in the systemic form. The localized scleroderma have at least two variants: morphea, linear scleroderma.

Morphea: Morphea is more common in females, it can occur at any age, but is more common after 30 (Color Figure 19 – 3).

Linear scleroderma: Lesions of linear scleroderma have bands of sclerotic skin that often cross joint lines and lead to mild but occasionally severe and disabling joint contractures. Unlike oval plaque morphea, the inflammatory and fibrotic process may involve the underlying subcutaneous tissue and muscles, causing the fibrotic band to be more firmly anchored(Color Figure 19 – 4).

19.3.2.2 The systemic sclerosis

The usual initial symptom of systemic sclerosis is swelling, then thickening and tightening of the skin at the ends of the fingers. Raynaud's syndrome, in which the fingers suddenly and temporarily become very pale and tingle or become numb, painful, or both in responses to cold or emotional upset is also common. Fingers may become bluish. Heartburn, difficulty in swallowing, and shortness of breath are occasionally the first symptoms of systemic sclerosis. Aches and pains in several joints often accompany early symptoms. Sometimes inflammation of the muscles (polymyositis), with its accompanying muscle pain and weakness develops. Organ disease can occur early on and be serious. Organs affected including esophagus, bowels, and lungs with scarring (fibrosis), heart, and kidneys. High blood pressure can be a troublesome side effect.

(1) Skin changes

Systemic sclerosis can damage from large areas of skin or only the fingers. Sometimes systemic sclerosis tends to stay restricted to the skin of the hands. Other times, the disorder progresses. The skin becomes more widely taut, shiny, and darker than usual. The skin on the face tightens, sometimes resulting in an inability to change facial expressions. Sometimes dilated blood vessels (telangiectasia often referred to as spider veins) can appear on the fingers, chest, face, lips, and tongue, and bumps composed of calcium can develop on the fingers, on other bony areas, or at the joints. Sores can develop on the fingertips and knuckles.

(2) Joint changes

Sometimes, a grating sound can be felt or heard as inflamed tissues move over each other, particularly at and below the knees and at the elbows and wrists. The fingers, wrists, and elbows may become stuck (forming a contracture) in flexed positions because of scarring in the skin.

(3) Gastrointestinal system changes

Scarring commonly damages the lower end of the esophagus. The damaged esophagus can no longer propel food to the stomach efficiently. Swallowing difficulties and heartburn eventually develop in many people who have systemic sclerosis. Abnormal cell growth in the esophagus occurs in about 33% of the people, increasing their risk of esophageal blockage due to a fibrous band or their risk of esophageal cancer.

(4) Lung and heart changes

Systemic sclerosis can cause scar tissue to accumulate in the lungs, resulting in abnormal shortness of breath during exercise. The blood vessels that supply the lungs can be affected, so they cannot carry as much blood. Therefore blood pressure within the arteries that supply the lungs can increase. Systemic sclerosis can also cause several life-threatening heart abnormalities, including heart failure and abnormal rhythms.

(5) Kidney changes

Severe kidney disease can result from systemic sclerosis. The first symptom of kidney damage may be an abrupt, progressive rise in blood pressure. High blood pressure is an ominous sign, although treatment usually controls it.

(6) CREST syndrome

CREST syndrome, also called limited cutaneous systemic sclerosis is usually a less severe form of the disorder that is less likely to cause serious internal organ damage. It is named for its symptoms: calcium deposits in the skin and throughout the body, Raynaud's syndrome, esophageal dysfunction, sclerodactyly (skin damage on the fingers), and telangiectasia (dilated blood vessels or spider veins). Skin damage is limited to the fingers. People who have CREST syndrome can develop pulmonary hypertension, which can cause heart and lung failure. The drainage system from the liver may become blocked by scar tissue (biliary cirrhosis), resulting in liver damage and jaundice.

Systemic sclerosis is divided into 2 major clinical variants: diffuse cutaneous systemic sclerosis (dcSSc) and limited cutaneous systemic sclerosis (lcSSc). They are distinguished from one another primarily based on the degree and extent of skin involvement. In most cases, the initial complaint of lcSSc is Raynaud's phenomenon, whereas patients with dcSSc often initially present with generalized swelling of the hands, skin thickening, or arthralgias with or without Raynaud's.

19.3.3 Diagnosis and Differential Diagnosis

The diagnosis of the scleroderma is based on the finding of the clinical features of the illnesses. A skin biopsy is not usually important for confirmation of the diagnosis although it is sometimes performed to help differentiate scleroderma from other syndromes. Early lesions are characterized by a dense inflammatory infiltrate composed of lymphocytes, macrophages, plasma cells, and occasionally, eosinophils and mast cells. The fibrotic phase follows the inflammatory stage, characterized by thickened, hyalinized collagen bundles extending from the deep reticular dermis to more superficial structures.

In addition, nearly all patients with scleroderma have blood tests that suggest autoimmunity, because antinuclear antibodies (ANAs) are usually detectable. Ninety-five percent of patients with scleroderma have a positive antinuclear staining pattern; A particular antibody, the anticentromere antibody, is found almost exclusively in the limited, or CREST, form of scleroderma. Anti-Scl 70 antibody (antitopoisomerase I antibody) is most often seen in patients with the diffuse form of scleroderma. Anti-RNA polymerase I and III are found in patients with SSc especially associated with skin and renal involvement, whereas anti-RNA polymerase II is found in patients with either SSc or systemic lupus erythematosus.

Other tests are used to evaluate the presence or extent of any internal disease. These may include upper and lower gastrointestinal tests to evaluate the bowels, chest X-rays, lung-function testing (pulmonary function test), and CAT scanning to examine the lungs, EKG and echocardiograms, and sometimes heart catheterization to evaluate the pressure in the arteries of the heart and lungs.

Other autoimmune and connective tissue disorders: Several other autoimmune conditions that affect connective tissue can strongly resemble, or occur together with scleroderma. They include the following: rheumatoid arthritis, systemic lupus erythematosus, polymyositis, symptoms of such diseases may also include fever, arthritis, muscle aches, rash, and lung and heart problems.

Eosinophilic fasciitis: Eosinophilic fasciitis is a muscle disorder that is known to occur after intense hard work. It can cause symptoms similar to scleroderma, including pain, swelling, and tenderness in the hands and feet, as well as skin thickening. The disorder can be ruled out with blood tests.

19. 3. 4 Treatment

Currently, there is no cure for scleroderma.

(1) The treatment options that are currently available for the management and treatment of localized scleroderma, including:

In the early age patient can be given intravenous drip penicillamine. External use glucocorticoid, and psoralen photochemotherapy (PUVA), a daily physical therapy program emphasizing full range of motion of all large joints is important.

(2) The medications that are prescribed for the management and treatment of systemic sclerosis, including:

Systemic therapy: Penicillamine, methotrexate, photopheresis, relaxin, interferons, and cyclosporine have all been studied in controlled trails with variable outcomes. Many other case reports for other drugs exist. Penicillamine (500 to 1 500 mg/d) is often the treatment of choice for progressive systemic sclerosis. The clinical response to this agent is variable. There is no advantage to using penicillamine in doses higher than 125 mg every other day.

Management of cutaneous disease: Cutaneous ulcers are protected with an occlusive dressing such as DouDerm. Ischemic digital-tip ulcers may be protected with a small plastic "cage". Infection is signaled by abrupt erythema, swelling, and increased pain and is usually due to staphylococcus. Adequate skin lubrication is difficult to maintain. Patients should bathe less and use moisturizers. Pruritus tends to occur early in the course of diffuse disease, especially over the forearms, and disappears after months or several years. Antipruritic moisturizers such as Sarna lotion may help. No satisfactory medical approaches to calcinosis have yet been developed. A daily physical therapy program emphasizing full range of motion of all large joints is important.

A detailed overview of new treatments that are currently under investigation for the treatment of systemic sclerosis, including: interferons, tumor necrosis factor alpha blockers, halofuginone, plasmapheresis, autologous stem cell transplantation, etc. Although we now have some moderately effective therapies for many aspects of scleroderma, the basic process of fibrosis awaits proven effective therapy.

■ Summary

Lupus erythematosus is a category for a collection of diseases with similar underlying problems with immunity. Symptoms of these diseases can affect many different body systems, including joints, skin, kidneys, blood cells, heart, and lungs. This disease requires close cooperation between the treating physician and the pathologist. Patients may be treated with corticosteroids and immunosuppressive agents. However, these patients are immunocompromised and infections are common. Death is usually secondary to infectious complications, renal failure, or central nervous system disease. There are several well-established variants, such as Discoid Lupus Erythematosus (DLE), that involve selected organ systems and present with different ANA patterns.

Dermatomyositis is a medical condition that most often affects the skin and muscles, resulting in weakness and rashes. It is more common in women than in men, and typically affects people who are either 5 – 15 or 40 – 65 years old. The cause of dermatomyositis is unclear, although it might be connected to issues with the immune system. Its most common symptoms include muscle weakness, inflammation, shortness of breath, stiffness, difficulty swallowing, discolored upper eyelids, and a widespread red or purple rash. The muscle weakness can either develop gradually or occur very abruptly. So far, no cure for dermatomyositis has been found. The most frequent treatment is a corticosteroid such as prednisone, which can help to control the symptoms. In many cases, physical therapy is recommended so that the muscles remain strong and have less risk of atrophying. Treatment is beneficial to most patients, and it is possible for the dermatomyositis to go into remission.

Scleroderma is a disease characterized by sclerosis of the skin and visceral organs, vasculopathy (Raynaud's syndrome), and autoantibodies. The spectrum of disease is wide, with systemic and localized forms. Typical scleroderma is classically defined as symmetrical skin thickening, with about 90% of cases also presenting with Raynaud's phenomenon, nail-fold capillary changes, and anti-nuclear antibodies. Patients may or may not experience systemic organ involvement. Atypical scleroderma may show any variation of these changes without skin changes or with finger swelling only. Additional symptoms of scleroderma typically present themselves within two years of Raynaud's phenomenon. There is no direct cure for scleroderma. Because the exact cause is unknown, any treatment is patient-specific and aimed at ameliorating symptoms of the disease. For example, patients who experience Raynaud's phenomenon may be treated with agents to increase blood flow to the fingers, including nifedipine, amlodipine, diltiazem, felodipine, or nicardipine.

▪ Questions

1. What are the clinical features, diagnosis and treatment of DLE, SCLE, and SLE?

2. What patterns of lupus erythematosus can be divided, and the difference between this patterns?

3. What are the clinical feature of dermatomyositis and how to diagnose and treat it?

4. What are the clinical features, diagnosis and treatment of scleroderma?

5. What patterns of scleroderma can be divided, and the difference between the two patterns?

(Gaoyun Yang 杨高云)

Chapter 20

Bullous Dermatosis

▪ Objectives

Master the causes and clinical features of bullous dermatosis.

Understand how to diagnose and treat pemphigus and bullous pemphigoid.

▪ Key concepts

Pemphigus is a chronic immunobullous disease, characterized by intraepithelial blister formation. Patients develop cutaneous and mucosal lesions with flaccid blisters. Erosions are common to see when blisters ruptured. The Nikolsky sign is positive. Histopathology shows the blisters within epidermal. Anti-desmogleins are detected in epidermal cells and the serum as well. Pemphigus is divided into four major types, according to typical symptoms, histopathology and immunopathology. Corticosteroids are the preferred treatment for pemphigus.

Bullous pemphigoid (BP) is a kind of immunobullous disease which is characterized by thick-walled, tense, subepidermal bullae. Histopathology shows subepidermal blisters. Immunopathology demonstrates deposits of IgG and/or C3 along the basement membrane zone. Antibody to the basement membrane zone can be found in the blood. Treatment aims to control the primary lesions, lessen the severity of itchiness and prevent secondary lesion. Medications include glucocorticoid hormone and other immunosuppressive agents.

Dermatitis herpetiformis (DH) is a chronic and recurrent bullous dermatosis. The cause is still unclear. Most patients are associated with gluten-sensitive enteropathy. Diagnosis depends on the typical symptoms and characteristic histology and immunology. A strict gluten-free diet, diaminodiphenyl sulphone(DDS) oral and topical drugs are the main treatment methods.

▪ Introduction

Bullous dermatosis is relatively rare but important, for it may be the first sign of a severe and potentially fatal problem. In adults the main group of blistering problem is associated with autoantibody formation, while in children, the rare but important group of genodermatosis is associated mainly with mechanical defects in and around the basement membrane zone.

Blisters may arise for two reasons. One is the disruption of the desmosome between keratinocytes in the epidermis, causing an intraepidermal blister; another is the defect in the basement membrane zone between the epidermis and dermis, leading to a subepidermal blister.

The clinical picture may be suggestive. However, definitive diagnosis of blistering dermatoses requires a biopsy of a small, newly formed lesion and also a piece of perilesional skin frozen for immunopathological studies. In some cases, electron microscopy is also needed.

According to etiopathogenesis, bullous dermatosis can be classified as autoimmune bullous disease and non-autoimmune bullous disease (also called as hereditary bullous dermatosis). According to histopathology, bullous dermatosis can be classified as intraepidermal and subepidermal blistering disease (Table 20 - 1). In this chapter, some primary autoimmune bullous dermatoses, including pemphigus, bullous pemphigoid and dermatitis herpetiformis will be introduced.

Table 20 - 1　The classification of bullous dermatoses

	Autoimmune	Non-autoimmune (hereditary)
Intraepidermal	Pemphigus	Epidermolysis bullosa simplex (EBS) Familial benign chronic pemphigus
Subepidermal	Bullous pemphigoid (BP) Cicatricial pemphigoid Dermatitis herpetiformis (DH) Linear IgA bullous dermatosis (LAD) Epidermolysis bullosa acquisita (EBA) Pemphigoid gestationis (PG)	Junctional epidermolysis bullosa Dystrophic epidermolysis bullosa

20. 1　Pemphigus

Pemphigus is a chronic immunobullous disease, characterized by intraepithelial blister formation. Patients develop cutaneous and mucosal lesions with flaccid blisters. Erosions are common to see when the blisters got ruptured. The Nikolsky's sign is positive. Histopathology shows blisters within epidermal. Antidesmoglein are detected in epidermal cells and also in the serum.

20. 1. 1　Etiology
The etiology of pemphigus is largely unknown. The molecular basis for blister formation is the loss of adhesion between keratinocytes caused by circulating autoantibodies (auto-Ab) directed against intercellular adhesion structures.

20. 1. 2　Clinical Features
It usually affects male and occurs in middle-age. Pemphigus vulgaris is the most common form of

pemphigus. Other forms include pemphigus vegetans, pemphigus foliaceus, pemphigus erythematosus, paraneoplastic pemphigus, drug-induced pemphigus, intercellular IgA dermatosis, and pemphigus herpetiformis.

20. 1. 2. 1　Pemphigus vulgaris (PV)

This type is the most common and serious disease, occurring in middle-aged people, which rarely involves children. It mainly affects the oral mucosa, scalp, face, chest, back and widespreadly in severe case. Almost all patients develop oral mucosal lesion, which is the only symptom in some patients. Flaccid blisters arise on normal skin or erythematous base. The Nikolsky's sign is positive. The blisters are easy to rupture and produce erosions and crusts(Color Figure 20 - 1). Prognosis of PV is bad in pemphigus. Before the application of corticosteroids, 75% of patients died. However, the mortality is still 21.4% when corticosteroids are used. The most common cause of death is the infection resulted from applying high-doses and long-time cortico steroids.

20.1.2.2 Pemphigus vegetans

It is a subtype of pemphigus vulgaris, rarely, which is characterized by vegetating erosions. The vegetations often occur in armpit, groin, vulva, four limbs and so on. Oral mucosal lesion occurs later and less seriously. Flaccid blisters present firstly and the Nikolsky's sign is positive. Then there is papillary proliferation of granulation on the erosion surface after blisters rupture(Color Figure 20 - 2). Prognosis is better than pemphigus vulgaris.

20.1.2.3 Pemphigus foliaceus (PF)

This form affects chiefly in middle-aged adults. Lesions involve the scalp, face, chest and upper back. It rarely affects oral mucosa. Blisters arise on erythematous bases. The Nikolsky's sign is positive. Bliter wall is thinner and easier to rupture. There are greasy scales and crusts on the erosion surface (Color Figure 20 - 3). PF is less severe than PV.

20.1.2.4 Pemphigus erythematosus

It is a subtype of PF. The form affects "seborrheic" areas: the scalp, face, chest, upper back and upper limbs. Lower limbs and mucosa are rarely involved. Erythematous scaly lesions with hyperkeratosis, butterfly distribution over the nose and cheeks, similar lesions as seborrheic dermatitis on trunk are common to see in pemphigus erythematosus(Color Figure 20 - 4). Antinuclear antibodies (ANA) and rheumatoid factors (RF) can be found in serum. Immune globulins are deposited in the basement membrane. So it needs to be carefully differentiated from erythematous lupus. Prognosis of pemphigus erythematosus is mostly good in addition to few may become PF.

20.1.2.5 Special types of pemphigus

(1) Paraneoplastic pemphigus (PNP)

This form is most commonly associated with underlying lymphatic system tumor. Patients have severe mucosal erosions and polymorphous cutaneous signs including blisters, bullae, erythema multiforme-like and lichen planus-like lesions. PNP is generally refractory to the treatment of corticosteroids.

(2) Drug-induced pemphigus

It usually occurs when taking some medicine for many months or even more than one year, which usually contains sulfhydryl groups such as D-penicillamine, captopril, piroxicam and rifampicin. Mucosal involvement is few and mild. It has similar features as PF and can be self healing after quitting the drug.

(3) IgA pemphigus

This form chiefly affects middle-aged women. The fold area is the most frequent site affected. Lesions are flaccid vesicles or pustules arising on erythematous, associated with pruritus. Nikolsky's sign is usually negative. Immune globulins deposited in spinous cells and antibodies found in peripheral blood are both IgA.

(4) Herpetiform pemphigus

This form chiefly affects the middle-aged adults. The lesions spread symmetrically on the trunk and proximal extremities. Widespread clusters of pruritic vesicles and papules develop on erythematous background. Mucosal lesions are uncommon. Nikolsky's sign is negative. Itching is obvious.

20.1.3 Histopathology and Immunopathology

The basic pathologic changes of pemphigus are acantholysis, intraepidermal slits and blisters. The sites of acantholysis are different in forms of pemphigus. Direct immunofluorescence (DIF) shows deposites of IgG and C3 in prickle cells in a network distribution. IgM or IgA can also be found. Indirect immunofluorescence (IIF) shows the antibodies of pemphigus exist in serum of 80%-90% of patients (Color Figure 20 - 5).

20.1.4 Diagnosis and Differential Diagnosis

Diagnosis depends on the typical symptoms, histopathology and immunopathology. Pemphigus needs to be differented from bullous pemphigoid, epidermolysis bullosa, and erythema multiforme major.

20.1.5 Treatment

The purpose of treatment is to control the occurrence of new lesions and prevent secondary infection. The key of treatment is correct application of corticosteroid and immunosuppressants and to prevent the complications.

20.1.5.1 General therapy

Note the equilibration of water and electrolyte and supporting treatment. Give the nutritive and digestible diet. Supplement the plasma or albumin in time to patients with severe mucosal lesions and much extravasate.

20.1.5.2 Topical therapy

Nursing of cutaneous and mucosal lesions and prevention of opportunistic infection are important to reduce mortality and relieve symptoms. Potassium permanganate and typical antiseptics can help to reduce the risk of cutaneous infection.

20. 1. 5. 3 Systemic therapy

(1) Corticosteroids

Corticosteroids are the preferred treatment for pemphigus. The dosage is decided by different types and lesion areas. Patients of Pemphigus vulgaris need the higher doses. Prednisone 0. 5 – 2. 0 mg/(kg · d) is sufficient to control disease in many patients. Intravenous (IV) pulse therapy of either methylprednisolone or dexamethasone is recommended for severe pemphigus. When new blisters fail to present for one week, reduction of corticosteroids should be taken into consideration, gradually. In the opposite situation, higher dose or immunosuppressive agents as adjuncts is necessary. Low-dose prednisone (≤7. 5 mg/d) as maintenance dose is recommended when most lesions subsided.

(2) Immunosuppressive agents

A number of immunosuppressive agents are recommended as adjuncts to oral corticosteroids. The combination of steroids and cyclophosphamide (CTX) 1 – 3 mg/(kg · d) is more effective than corticosteroids alone. Monthly IV pulses of cyclophosphamide 600 – 1000 mg combined with corticosteroids are also effective. Azathioprine is used in a dose of 2. 5 mg/(kg · d). And methotrexate 10 – 17. 5 mg/week is permitted withdrawal of prednisolone in steroid-dependent patients. Ciclosporin and mycophenolate mofetil can also be used as adjuvant therapy for pemphigus.

(3) Anti-infectives

Opportunistic infection is the major cause of death in patients with widespread blistering. Timely select suitable anti-infective agents.

20. 2　Bullous Pemphigoid

Bullous pemphigoid (BP) is a kind of immunobullous disease which is characterized by thick-walled, tense, subepidermal bullae. BP occurs most frequently in the middle-aged and elderly. Histopathology shows subepidermal blisters. Immunopathology shows IgG and/or C3 deposit at basement membrane zone. There are autoantibodies to components for the basement membrane zone in serum.

20. 2. 1　Etiology

The cause is unknown. There is autoantibody to components for the basement membrane zone in serum of most patients. Immune electron microscopy revealed that the antibody binds in the lamina lucida of the basement membrane zone. Thus it is also organ-specific autoimmune disease.

Target antigens of BP circulating antibodies are localized to the BP antigen 1 (BPAg1, also known as BP230) and BP antigen 2 (BPAg2, also known as BP180) on the hemidesmosomes. BP230 is intracytoplasmic protein. BP230 has reaction with serum in 80% to 90% of patients, but the serum passive transfer test of its antibody can not cause BP. BP180 is transmembrane protein, with its intracellular portion (N-terminal) localized in hemidesmosomal plaque and the extracellular portion (C-terminal) localized in basement membrane zone. Injecting the antibodies of anti-BP180 N-terminal into BALB/C mice can clone BP animal models similar to human's BP. Thus anti-BP180 antibodies are the pathogenic antibodies of BP. It has been confirmed that there are auto-reactive T lymphocytes against BP180 in pemphigoid patients, which can spontaneously identify BP180. In blister formation it could be attributed to the antigen-antibody reaction in the lamina lucida of the basement membrane zone, with the participation of complements to leukocyte chemotaxis and enzyme releasing.

20. 2. 2　Clinical Features

BP occurs most frequently in the elderly over 50 years of age, with a predilection for the thorax, abdomen and proximal extremities. The tense blisters or bullae may arise on normal skin or erythematous patches. The blisters are thick-walled and dome shaped, obtaining a diameter of less than 1 centimeter to several centimeters. Their contents are usually clear serous exudates, occasionally it is bloodstained. Blisters are tough and may remain intact for several days. After the bullae rupture, large denuded areas are seen, often covered with crusts or blood scabs, and also may show a tendency to heal spontaneously. Nikolsky sign shows negative (the absence of acantholysis) (Color Figure 20 – 6). In small number of patients there are oral mucosal lesions, which are less severe and itching in various degrees. Note that atypical presentations of BP are fairly common (such as eczema-like and prurigo-like lesions). The progress of the disease is slow and if untreated, it may last for several months to several years or be spontaneous regression or aggravation. Prognosis is better than Pemphigus. Risk factors include the consumptive failure for long-term illness, the infection and other complications and multiple organ failure caused by applying long-term, high-dose glucocorticoids and other immunosuppressive agents.

20.2.3 Histopathology and Immunopathology

Key feature of BP is subepidermal blister. The blister is monolocular and often viable epidermis forming the roof. The blisters may contain numerous eosinophils. Around dermal papilla blood vessels there are inflammatory infiltrates containing many eosinophils and neutrophils with lymphocytes (Color Figure 20 – 7 A).

Direct immunofluorescence is found in more than 90% of patients with IgG and C3 present in the basement membrane zone. IgM and IgA are occasionally present (Color Figure 20 – 7 B). Immuno-fluorescence testing on salt-split skin shows IgG and C3 deposit in epidermis of salt-split skin. Immune electron microscopy shows IgG and C3 deposit at the hemidesmosomes of basement membrane zone, which located in the upper portion of the lamina lucida. Anti-BP antigen antibody could be detected in peripheral blood. Indirect immunofluorescence also shows linear IgG deposit at basement membrane zone.

20.2.4 Diagnosis and Differential Diagnosis

According to typical clinical manifestations and immunopathological features, BP can be diagnosed. BP should be differentiated from pemphigus, eczema, prurigo, diabetic bullae and other diseases. Eczema, prurigo and BP could be distinguished by immunological tests. Anti-BP antigen antibodies could be detected in serum of patients of BP. IgG and C3 deposition can be noted at basement membrane. Histopathology can also be identified. To the patients with diabetic bullae, history of diabetes can be found. Histopathology of diabetic bullae shows subepidermal blisters without inflammatory infiltration of eosinophils and immunological tests are all negative.

20.2.5 Treatment

Treatment aims to control the occurrence of new lesions and lessen the severity of symptoms. In addition, to prevent secondary lesions caused by excessive tense blisters and erosion surface is also important. Medications include glucocorticoid hormone and other immunosuppressive agents

20.2.5.1　General therapy

Support therapy. Supply nutritious and digestible diet. To patients with a lot of blisters and bullae, add defined amount of plasma or albumin to prevent and correct the hypoproteinemia.

20.2.5.2　Local nursing

It can be possible to cut through the bottom of the bullae with sterile scalpel and scissor or to extract the fluid out of the blister with syringe.

20.2.5.3　Drug treatment

(1) Glucocorticoid

Glucocorticoid is the top choice to the drug treatment of BP. It includes systemic and topical therapy.

1) Systemic therapy: Based on scope of damage to determine dosage. Some scholars observed the difference between the treatment of BP with prednisone 0.75 mg/(kg · d) and 1.25 mg/(kg · d), the result of which is that there is no difference in curative ratio on the 21st day and 51st day, but in mortality rate the former was significantly lower than the latter. BP patients are often elderly, so it must be noted to observe and prevent the common adverse reactions of glucocorticoid during the course of treatment.

2) Topical therapy: BP is mainly in the elderly and the reasons of death are often hormone-related complications and multiple organ failure. In abroad, topical therapy is gradually replacing of the systemic treatment. Its methods include intensive topical therapy with very potent corticosteroids creams such as clobetasol propionate or halometasone. According to weight and the number of blisters of newly present, the dose (maximum dose of 40 g/d) and frequency (1 or 2 times per day to 2 times per week) can be determined. Equably spread the cream on the whole body besides the head. Although topical treatment reduces the adverse drug reactions and side effects of glucocorticoid on each system of the whole body, there are still side effects of the skin thinning, telangiectasia and increased opportunities for local infection.

(2) Other immunosuppressive drugs

Cytotoxic drugs combining with glucocorticoid can reduce the steroids dosage and can also be used alone (application methods can refer to "Pemphigus").

20.2.5.4　Other treatment

In less severe BP patients, it can be applied by antibiotic tetracycline or erythromycin with anti-inflammatory effects 1 – 2 g per day or minocycline 0.1 g/d for 1 – 2 months. Combining with a large dose of nicotinamide 1.5 – 2.0 g/d may be better. DDS may also be effective. These drugs above can also be combined with glucocorticoids.

20.3   Dermatitis Herpetiformis

Dermatitis herpetiformis (DH) is characterized by polymorphous lesions, intensely pruritic. Most patients have an associated gluten-sensitive enteropathy. Histopathology shows vesicle formation at the subepidermal. Direct immunofluorescence (DIF) shows granular IgA localized in the dermal papillary tips.

20.3.1   Etiology
The cause of the disease is unclear. Gluten sensitive, genetic factor, viral infection and other factors may contribute.

20.3.2   Clinical Features
DH mostly occurs in young adults. DH often distributes symmetrically on shoulder, back and extensor surfaces of extremities, especially on the elbows and knees. Typical lesions are densely papules, papulovesicle, vesiculobullous on the erythema or wheal, arranged in a ring, semi-circular or map-like. The diameter of vesicles is 0.5 - 1.0cm. Blister wall is thick, in tension, not easy to break, Nikolsky's sign is negative(Color Figure 20 - 8).

Intense itch is characteristic symptom of DH, scratching blisters burst to erosion and crusting, secondary infection, eczema-like change. After the rash subsided it leaves pigmentation.

DH alternates rash onset and remission, very few of which will be self-healing and generally could not associate with systemic symptoms. After eating gluten food lesions will increase, which can be alleviated after the closure.

20.3.3   Histopathology
The initial changes are first noted at the tips of the dermal papillae, where edema and eosinophilic and neutrophilic exudates occur to produce a subepidermal separation. Eventually vesicle formation at the dermoepidermal junction and infiltration of dermal papillary tips with neutrophils are seen. DIF shows granular IgA localized in the dermal papillary tips of perilesional skin(Color Figure 20 - 9).

20.3.4   Diagnosis and Differential Diagnosis
Diagnosis depends on young adults who are with polymorphous lesion to vesiculobullous mainly, Nikolsky sign is negative, with severe itching, and histologically vesicle formation at the dermoepidermal junction, and infiltration of dermal papillary tips with neutrophils are seen. Direct immunofluorescence shows granular IgA localized in the dermal papillary tips of perilesional skin.

DH needs to be differentiated with other bullous diseases and acute or subacute eczema.

20.3.5   Treatment
20.3.5.1   General therapy
Adherence to a gluten-free diet (GFD) improves clinical symptoms in patients with DH.

20.3.5.2   System therapy
Dapsone (DDS) is preferred, 100 - 150 mg/d, divided 2 - 3 times orally, and needed to be used in long term. Other medicine like sulfasalazine(SASP), tetracycline can also be chosen. If patient is not sensitive to the DDS, low-dose systemic corticosteroids 20 - 40 mg can be chosen. Antihistamines to relieve itching may be symptomatic treatment.

20.3.5.3   Topical therapy
Topical corticosteroids, calamine lotion and antibiotic ointment have the effect of anti-inflammatory, antipruritic and prevention of infection.

▪ Summary

Pemphigus is a chronic immunobullous disease characterized by intraepithelial blister formation. Pemphigus is divided into four major types: pemphigus vulgaris (PV), pemphigus vegetans, pemphigus foliaceus (PF), pemphigus erythematosus and several special types: paraneoplastic pemphigus (PNP), drug-induced pemphigus, IgA pemphigus, herpetiform pemphigus. Corticosteroids are the preferred treatment for pemphigus.

Bullous pemphigoid (BP) is a kind of immunobullous disease which is characterized by thick-walled, tense, subepidermal bullae. Histopathology showed subepidermal blisters. Immunopathology showed deposits of IgG and/or C3 at basement membrane zone. Antibody to the basement membrane zone can be found in the blood. Treatment aims to control the primary lesions, lessen the severity of symptoms and prevent secondary lesions. Medications include glucocorticoid hormones and other immunosuppressive agents.

Dermatitis herpetiformis (DH) is a chronic and relapsing bullous dermatosis. The cause is not entirely clear. Most patients are associated with gluten-sensitive enteropathy. Diagnosis depends on the typical symptoms and characteristic histology and immunology. The main treatment methods are strict gluten-free diet, DDS oral and topical drugs to relive the local symptoms.

▪ Questions

1. What are the clinical features of pemphigus and how to diagnose it?

2. What are the clinical features of bullous pemphigoid?

3. What are the clinical and pathological features of dermatitis herpetiformis?

(Guangzhong Zhang 张广中, Li Jin 金力)

Chapter 21

Cutaneous Vascular Disorders

▪ Objectives

To master the pathogenesis, clinical features, diagnosis and treatment of anaphylactoid purpura, erythema nodosum, allergic cutaneous vasculitis and Behcet's disease.

▪ Key concepts

Anaphylactoid purpura is a multisystem vasculitis which involves small blood vessels. It is characterized by non-thrombocytopenic purpura.

Erythema nodosum presents painful, red, erythematous subcutaneous nodules, usually distributed over pretibial areas bilaterally, occasionally elsewhere, it may be accompanied by fever, arthralgias and malaise, usually fade over several weeks.

Allergic cutaneous vasculitis presents polymorphous eruption, including palpable purpura, urticarial lesions, hemorrhagic macules or vesicles. Lesions favor the lower extremities (especially the ankles), only involves small vessels. Histologically, leukocytoclastic vasculitis of the small dermal blood vessels is seen. Occasionally, extracutaneous involvement occurs, but it is usually mild.

Behcet's disease is a multisystem and polysymptomatic disease, synonymy is oculo-oral-genital syndrome. Its diagnosis is based on International Study Group criteria, which contains recurrent oral and genital ulceration, ocular abnormalities (e.g. iridocyclitis, choroiditis) and skin lesions.

▪ Introduction

Cutaneous vascular disorders represent the inflammation of the blood vessel wall, any organ of the body can be involved. Although vasculitis can be idiopathic, parts of patients secondary to a medication, infection, neoplasm or systemic inflammatory disease. It can represent a skin-limited disease or serious systemic involvement.

21.1 Anaphylactoid Purpura

21.1.1 Pathogenesis
The disease has a complex pathogenesis. It frequently follows an upper respiratory tract infection or exposure to allergen or drug, therioma and autoimmune diseases can also cause it. Immune complex deposition within the vascular wall is likely an early event in the disease, complement activation, secondary to immune complex deposition, may result in endothelial cell damage and activation, then increases vascular dilation and permeability, can result in purpura.

21.1.2 Clinical Features
The disease is about 10% of those affected children, and are more common in boys. The rash is characterized by palpable purpura, typically 2 – 10 mm diameter and most commonly affects the legs and buttocks. However, any site can be involved including the upper limbs and trunk (Color Figure 21 – 1). Occasionally, confluent ecchymoses may evolve from confluent small lesions, rarely necrosis and hemorrhagic bullae develop. Paroxysmal colicky abdominal pain accompanied by melena or occult bleeding intussusception may occur. Pain and swelling of the large joints (e. g. knees and ankles) can occur. Vasculitis may also involve vessels in the kidney, lung, and central nervous system. About 5% – 10% of patients can recur for up to several months, but these episodes are usually mild. The visceral disease is self-limiting in most cases. However, intussusception can complicate vasculitis in the acute bowel and renal failure, which develops rarely.

21.1.3 Investigations
Haematuria and proteinuria can always present. Platelet count, prothrombin time, bleeding time and thrombin time are normal.

21.1.4 Pathology
Classic histological findings include endothelial swelling, fibrin deposition within and around the vessels, neutrophilic infiltrate within the vessel walls, and nuclear dust (scattered nuclear fragments from neutrophils). Vascular destruction with hemorrhage may be prominent. Fresh biopsies demonstrate IgA and C3 deposition around the dermal blood vessels.

21.1.5 Diagnosis and Differential Diagnosis
Diagnosis depends on clinical features. A normal blood and platelet count and coagulation examinations can help to differentiate anaphylactoid purpura from other causes of purpura. Identification of typical clinical findings and course, histopathology, and other screening studies [e. g. antinuclear antibodies (ANA), rheumatoid factor] can exclude lupus erythematosus and other connective tissue disorders.

21.1.6 Treatment
Because the cutaneous and musculoskeletal symptoms of anaphylactoid purpura are generally self-limited, the treatment is symptoms-relieving and supportive. Systemic corticosteroids may be of benefit in abdominal pain and arthritis, and reducing the duration of skin lesions. Corticosteroids and/or cytotoxic medications are often used to treat severe renal disease. The prognosis is excellent. Most patients recover within 4 – 6 weeks.

21.2 Erythema Nodosum

21.2.1 Pathogenesis
Erythema nodosum has been considered a delayed hypersensitivity response to a variety of antigenic stimuli, including bacteria, viruses and chemical agents. A wide variety of precipitating factors has been linked with erythema nodosum. Infectious causes are common, including tuberculosis, viral pharyngitis, streptococcal pharyngitis, histoplasmosis, coccididodomycosis, and other deep fungi and atypical mycobacteria. Other commonly reported causes include inflammatory bowel disease, sarcoidosis and certain medications.

21.2.2 Clinical Features
Erythema nodosum appears bilateral, painful, red, subcutaneous erythematous nodules.

These eruptions arise in crops and the most common site is shins (Color Figure 21 – 2). But lesions may also involve the thighs and forearms, and rarely the trunk, neck and face.

Systemic symptoms may occur, which include arthritis, arthralgia, fever and malaise.

Nodules usually fade over several weeks, but recurrences are frequent.

21.2.3   Pathology

The characteristic of erythema nodosum is septal panniculitis. Neutrophilic inflammation can predominate in early lesions. Lymphocytes, histiocytes and giant cells predominate in late stage. Vessels show endothelial cell swelling, inflammation in the vascular walls.

21.2.4   Diagnosis and Differential Diagnosis

An acute eruption of tender subcutaneous nodules over both shins in young person is highly characteristic of erythema nodosum. Erythema nodosum should be distinguished from other forms of panniculitis such as erythema induratum, allergic cutaneous vasculitis and lupus panniculitis. The diseases can be differentiated by pathology.

21.2.5   Treatment

In most patients it is self-limiting, if necessary, treatments include bed rest, salicylates, and non-steroidal. Anti-inflammatory drugs most often recommended for reducing pain. Systemic corticosteroids have been used for severe patients. Improvement may be seen within 2 weeks.

21.3   Allergic Cutaneous Vasculitis

21.3.1   Pathogenesis

The pathogenesis is not definite, but immune complex deposition within the vascular wall is likely an early event in it. Infection agents, drugs and autoimmune disease can form immune complexes. Complement activation, secondary to immune complex deposition, can result in endothelial cell damage and activation, and result in mast cell degranulation. Mast cell degranulation can result in increased vascular dilation and permeability, which are important for leukocyte tethering to endothelium and immune complex deposition.

21.3.2   Clinical Features

Allergic cutaneous vasculitis occurs at all ages and in both sexes, but is more common in the adult people, typically presents with polymorphous lesions consisting of erythematous papules, palpable purpura, vesicles or urticarial lesions after exposure to an inciting agent for 7 to 10 days. The initial lesion is often an urticarial papule or purpuric macule. The lesion's di-

ameter can range from 1mm to several centimeters. The most common site is legs and buttocks, but lesions may also involve the forearms and trunk. The lesions can be associated with pain, burning, or pruritus (Color Figure 21-3). Systemic symptoms such as fevers, weight loss, arthralgias and myalgias may appear. Some patients can accompany visceral disease such as gastrointestinal, genitourinary or neurologic symptoms, which should raise the suspicion of systemic vasculitis. The prognosis of patients with allergic cutaneous vasculitis depends on the severity of systemic involvement, most patients will have spontaneous resolution of cutaneous lesions within several weeks to months, while few will have chronic or recurrent disease at intervals of months to years.

21.3.3   Investigations

Although there are no specific diagnostic findings in this disease, anemia, an elevated erythrocyte sedimentation rate (ESR) and C-reactive protein, a decreased platelet count and an increased globulin fraction are frequently seen. Rheumatoid factor can be positive.

21.3.4   Pathology

The classic histological features of allergic cutaneous vasculitis are referred to as leukocytoclastic vasculitis and consist of transmural infiltration of the walls of small vessels by neutrophils undergoing karyorrhexis of their nuclei, as well as fibrinoid necrosis of the damaged vessel walls. Other findings include leukocytoclasis (degranulation and fragmentation of neutrophils, leading to the production of nuclear dust), extravasated erythrocytes, and signs of endothelial cell damage. Direct immunofluorescence (DIF) frequently demonstrates deposition of C3, IgG, IgM and/or IgA in a granular pattern within the vessel walls.

21.3.5   Diagnosis and Differential Diagnosis

Polymorphous eruption, including palpable purpura, urticarial lesions, hemorrhagic macules or vesicles is highly characteristic of allergic cutaneous vasculitis. Diagnosis is confirmed by histopathology and immunofluorescence. The disease is differentiated from anaphylactoid purpura, the latter has lesions characterized by purpura, urticarial lesions and accompanied arthralgia, abdominal pain and hematuresis and proteinuria.

21.3.6   Treatment

Suspicious medication should be stopped. If existing chronic infectious conditions, patients need an anti-infectious treatment. Dapsone has been reported to induce excellent improvement of skin lesions. Other therapies include NSAIDs, tetracyclines, niacinamide, colchicine and chloroquine. Intralesional corticosteroids may be helpful for mild cases, systemic corticosteroids may be of benefit in treating severe cases.

21.4   Behcet's Disease

21.4.1   Pathogenesis

The pathogenesis is not definite, but genetic, abnormality of immune system, infection and environment factors may contribute to the development of the disease. The HLA-B5 allele is positive among about 61%-88% patients. The patients of Behcet's disease have autoimmune responses. About 50% patients have increased circulating immune complexes and C3. Immunofluorescences present IgA, IgG, IgM and complement 3 deposited on the vessel wall. Infectious etiology (viral or bacterial) may be associated with the disease, such as HSV, hepatitis C virus, streptococcus and tubercle bacillus.

21.4.2   Clinical Features

21.4.2.1   Aphthous stomatitis

Aphthous stomatitis is the major criterion, and is almost always the first symptom of Behcet's disease (98% of patients). It is frequently present during the course of this disease. Oral ulcers locate in the tongue, mucobuccal fold, gums and palate, and begin as painless erythematous papule, which gradually develops a painful non-scarring ulcer with a yellowish pseudomembrane on the centre of the lesions (Color Figure 21 - 4), which heals in about 1 - 2 weeks without scarring.

21.4.2.2   Eye involvement

Eye involvement occurs in 90% of patients. Iridocyclitis, conjunctivitis, hypopyon and corneitis are the most characteristic ocular findings; however, some severe patients can present neuropapillitis, optic atrophy and choroiditis, secondary glaucoma, cataracts and blindness occur as well.

21.4.2.3   Genital aphthae

The genital aphthae occurs in 80% of patients, which primarily involves the penis and scrotum in men and the vulva in women. The anogenital aphthae are more painful than oral lesions, and may be larger and deeper, having irregular margins (Color Figure 21 - 5).

21.4.2.4   Cutaneous lesion

The cutaneous lesions present erythema nodosum-like lesions and folliculitis-like lesions. Erythema nodosum-like lesions appear on the legs and buttocks mostly, presenting several pale red, dark red or purple subcutaneous nodules, with tenderness. The lesions last about 1 month, but new eruptions appear continuously. Folliculitis-like lesions can be seen on the head, face, chest, back and so on, which present sterile vesicopustules and pustular(Color Figure 21 - 6), antibiotics is of no effect. Pathergy test can be seen in about 40%-70% of patients, which can be help to diagnose this disease. Pathergy test positive reaction is as performed on the flexor forearm by aslant inserting a sterile hypodermic needle to an intradermal injection of 0. 1 ml of physiological saline, papule or pustule can develop.

21.4.2.5   Other systemic involvement

Arthritis, gastrointestinal involvement, heart, kidney and neurologic involvement can be seen in some patients.

21.4.3   Investigations

Anemia is frequent, white cell count is often raised and is about $(10-20) \times 10^9 /L$, haematuria and proteinuria can always present. Platelet count, prothrombin time, bleeding time and thrombin time are normal.

21.4.4   Pathology

The histopathology of the cutaneous lesions in part due to the age of the lesion sampled and can involve all sizes of blood vessels within the dermis and subcutis. It presents with vasculitis characterized by angiocentric, neutrophilic infiltrates with leukocytoclasis and erythrocyte extravasation, or as a leukocytoclastic vasculitis with or without mural thrombosis and necrosis. An angiocentric lymphocytic infiltrate characterizes older lesions.

21.4.5   Diagnosis and Differential Diagnosis

Diagnosis is confirmed by aphthous stomatitis, eye involvement, genital aphthae, cutaneous lesion and pathergy test. In the early stage of the disease, when only present with aphthous stomatitis, the ulcers are differentiated from those that occur with complex aphthosis, herpetic stomatitis and pemphigus vulgaris, and cutaneous lesions must be indistinguishable from erythema nodosum and folliculitis.

21.4.6 *Treatment*

Systemic treatment: Dapsone has obvious effect for mucocutaneous involvement, the dose of which is 50 – 150 mg po qd (or sulfapyridine equivalent). Non-steroid anti-inflammatory drugs (NSAIDS) (such as indometacin, ibuprofen and acetosalicylic acid) are effective for the pain of genital aphthae, cutaneous ulcers and arthralgia. Corticosteroids can help severe cases, patients can take prednisone or methylprednisolone. Immunosuppressive agents (e. g. cyclophosphamide, cyclosporine A and azathymine) can be used to those patients who have vital organ involvement. Other treatments include levamisole, colchicin and interferon-γ. Topical treatment: according to different mucocutaneous involvement, we can select different topical agents (e. g. topical corticosteroid, topical antibiotics).

▪ Summary

Cutaneous vascular disorders represent an idiopathic inflammation of the blood vessel wall. Vasculitis may be primary or secondary to infection, medication, neoplasm or systemic inflammatory disease. It can occur in any organ system of the body. In vasculitis, small, medium-sized or large vessels of the arterial and/or venous systems all can be involved. Small vessels reside within the superficial and mid dermis of the skin. Medium-sized vessels are found in the deep dermis or subcutis. Large vessels include the aorta and named arteries. Cutaneous vascular disorders represent common clinical symptoms such as purpura, urticarial lesions, hemorrhagic macules, vesicles, nodules and ulcers as well as systemic symptoms. Histopathologically, dermatoses characterized by intense dermal neutrophilic infiltrates.

▪ Questions

1. How to differentiate anaphylactoid purpura from other causes of purpura?

2. What are pathological features of allergic cutaneous vasculitis?

3. What are clinical features of Behcet's disease?

(**Lin Ma** 马琳)

Disorders of the Skin Appendages

▪ Objectives

To master the knowledge of the causes and clinical features of disorders of the skin appendages.

To have an intimate knowledge of diagnosis and management of acne vulgaris, seborrheic dermatitis.

▪ Key concepts

Acne is a chronic inflammation of the pilosebaceous units in certain areas (face and trunk) that occurs in adolescence and manifests as comedones, papules, papulopustules, nodules, or cystic lesions, and often, but not always followed by pitted or hypertrophic scars.

Seborrheic dermatitis is a chronic, superficial, inflammatory disease of the skin, with a predilection for the scalp, face, chest and back, where skin lipids are significantly higher(in which the seborrheic glands are most active).

Alopecia areata is characterized by rapid and complete loss of hair without any visible inflammation on the scalp skin or any skin symptoms.

Androgenetic alopecia(male pattern alopecia) is the common progressive balding which occurs through the combined effect of a genetic predisposition and the action of androgen on the hair follicles of the scalp.

Rosacea is a centrofacial disease particularly prevalent in middle-aged. The hallmarks of rosacea are papules and papulopustules, vivid red erythema, and telangiectases.

▪ Introduction

Skin appendages include hair, sebaceous glands, sweat glands and nails. The disorders of skin appendages are often used to describe a group of skin diseases associated with skin appendages. Acne vulgaris, seborrheic dermatitis, alopecia areata, androgenetic alopecia and rosacea were described in this chapter. Among this group of diseases, acne vulgaris and seborrheic dermatitis are most common seen. Diagnosis is mainly based on the clinical features.

22.1   Acne Vulgaris

Acne is a chronic inflammation of the pilosebaceous units of certain areas (face and trunk) that occurs in adolescence and manifests as comedones, papules, papulopustules, nodules, or cystic lesions, often, but not always followed by pitted or hypertrophic scars.

22.1.1   Etiology and Pathogenesis
Multiple factors cause acne vulgaris, such as androgenic stimulation of sebaceous glands, proliferation of Propionibacterium acnes, formation of keratinous plug in the infundibulum of the hair follicle. Other factors contributing to the formation of acne vulgaris are hereditary factors, immunological factors and endocrine factors.

Androgen secretion increases in puberty. High level of androgen enlarges the sebaceous glands and thereby increases sebum production. Large amount of sebum benefits the propagation of Propionibacterium acnes in pilosebaceous unit. Bacteria converts lipid into fatty acids, causing an inflammatory response in the pilosebaceous unit. Fatty acids result in hyperproliferation and hyperkeratinization of the lining of orifice of the follicle which cause the block of the discharge of sebum. Comedo formation is caused by "stickness" of the horny cells and sebum, which fail to be properly discharged at the follicular orifice. The distended follicle walls may break and the contents may enter the dermis, provoking the further inflammation and forming a series of clinical manifestations from papules to cysts.

22.1.2   Clinical Features
Acne is mostly a disease of the adolescent. It occurs with greatest frequency between the ages of 10 and 17 years in females; 14 and 19 in males. The primary site of acne is the face and to a lesser degree the back, chest, and shoulders. On the trunk, lesions tend to be numerous near the midline.

The disease is characterized by a great variety of clinical lesions. The lesions may be either noninflammatory or inflammatory. The noninflammatory lesions are comedones, which may be either open (blackheads) or closed (whiteheads). The open comedo appears as a flat or slight raised lesion with a central dark-colored follicular impaction of keratin and lipid. The closed comedones appear as pale, slightly elevated, small papules and do not have a clinically visible orifice. The closed comedones are potential precursors for the large inflammatory lesions.

The inflammatory lesions vary from small papules with an inflammatory areola to pustules to large, tender, fluctuant nodules or cystic lesions, which have been used to describe severe cases of inflammatory acne. Whether the lesion appears as a papule, pustule, or nodule depends on the extent and location of the inflammatory infiltrate in the dermis.

In addition to the above-described lesions, patients may have scars of varying size. The characteristic scar of acne is a sharply punched-out pit. Less commonly, broader pits may occur, and in rare instances, especially on the trunk, the scars may be hypertrophic (Color Figure 22 – 1).

22.1.3   Diagnosis and Differential Diagnosis
The diagnosis of acne vulgaris is usually made from the finding of a mixture of lesions of acne (comedones, pustules, papules, nodules) on the face, back, or chest. Diagnosis is usually easy, but acne may be confused with rosacea, and lupus miliaris disseminatus faciei.

Rosacea is a centrofacial disease particularly prevalent in middle age. The hallmarks of rosacea are papules and papulopustules, vivid red erythema, and telangiectases without significant discomfort.

Lupus miliaris disseminatus faciei consists of multiple, smooth-surfaced, brownish red, 1-to 3-mm papules or nodules that occur over the face, including the eyelids and upper lip. It develops rapidly, has a self-limited course of several months to 2 years, and may leave behind pitted scars.

22.1.4   Treatment
22.1.4.1   Topical treatment
(1) Topical vitamin A acid
Topical vitamin A acid is used extensively for its comedolytic activity, and it can be a slightly irritant reaction at the beginning of treat. Beginning with lower concentration of vitamin A acid reduces the irritant reaction. Most patients can use the 0.025% vitamin A acid cream or gel daily without developing an irritant reaction. Two new synthetic third generation retinoids have been introduced for the treatment of acne. 0.1% adapalene gels and 0.1% tazarotene

gels are reported to be equivalent to vitamin A acid in efficacy and to have less irritancy.

(2) Benzoyl peroxide

Benzoyl peroxide preparations are among the most common topical medications. Benzoyl peroxide is a powerful antibacterial agent, and its effect is probably related to a decrease in the bacterial population and an accompanying decrease in the hydrolysis of triglycerides. Benzoyl peroxide preparations are available in both lotion and gel forms, the latter generally being considered more active. The compound can produce significant dryness and irritation, and allergic contact dermatitis may occur, but it is an uncommon event.

(3) Topical antibiotics

Topical antibiotics are also used for the treatment of acne, the most popular preparations containing erythromycin, and benzoyl peroxide, or clindamycin. Increased levels of Propionibacterium acnes resistance have been reported in patients who are being treated with erythromycin. However, resistance is not seen in patients who are treated with a combination of benzoyl peroxide/erythromycin. Therefore, this combination drug is preferable.

(4) Azelaic acid

Azelaic acid has been shown to have an effect on the process of keratinization. It causes a significant decrease in the follicular bacterial population. 15%-20% azelaic acid cream is effective to treat acne. The side effect is slight skin erythema and irritancy.

22. 1. 4. 2   Systemic treatment

(1) Antibiotics

Oral administration of tetracycline decreases the concentration of free fatty acids. This decrease in free fatty acids is seen with dosages ranging from 250 mg/d to 1 g/d. The free fatty acids are probably not the major irritants in sebum, but their level is an indication of the metabolic activity of the organism and its secretion of other inflammatory products. The decrease in free fatty acids may take several weeks to become evident. Antibiotic therapy is often required for several weeks for maximal clinical benefit. Tetracycline may act through direct suppression of the number of Propionibacterium acnes, but part of its action may also be due to its anti-inflammatory activity. Decreases in free fatty acid formation also have been reported with erythromycin, demethylchlortetracycline, clindamycin, and minocycline.

(2) Isotretinoin

The use of isotretinoin has revolutionized the management of severe treatment-resistant acne. The remarkable aspects of isotretinoin therapy are the completeness of the remission in almost all cases and the longevity of the remission, which lasts for months to years in the great majority of patients.

The drug produces profound inhibition of sebaceous gland activity. The propionibacterium acnes population is also decreased during isotretinoin therapy. Isotretinoin also has anti-inflammatory activity and probably has an effect on the pattern of follicular keratinization. The recommended daily dosage of isotretinoin is in the range of 0.5 to 1 mg/kg per day.

Side effects related to the skin and mucous membranes are cheilitis, xerosis, conjunctivitis, and pruritus. The laboratory abnormalities include elevation of triglycerides. The greatest concern during isotretinoin therapy is the risk that the drug being administered during pregnancy and thereby inducing teratogenic effects in the fetus.

(3) Antiandrogens

1) Cyproterone acetate: Cyproterone acetate is an antiandrogen that blocks the androgen receptor. It is combined with ethinyl estradiol in an oral contraceptive formulation that is widely used for the female patient whose menses is irregular or degree of acne turns worse before menses.

2) Spironolactone: Spironolactone functions also as an androgen receptor blocker. In doses of 50 to 100 mg twice a day, it has been shown to reduce sebum production and improve acne. Side effects include potential hyperkalemia, irregular menstrual periods, and low blood pressure.

(4) Glucocorticoids

Because of their anti-inflammatory activity, systemic glucocorticoids may be of benefit to acne. In practice, their use is usually restricted to the severely involved patient. Furthermore, because of the potential side effects, these drugs are ordinarily used for limited periods of time, and recurrences are common after therapy is discontinued. Prolonged use may results in the appearance of steroid acne.

22. 1. 4. 3   Intralesional corticosteroids

Intralesional corticosteroids are especially effective in reducing inflammatory nodules and cystic lesions. 1% triamcinolone acetonide is best diluted with sterile normal saline solution. Injection often has to be repeated every two weeks. Efficiency is usually obtained after 3 – 4 times of injections.

22. 1. 4. 4 Surgical treatment

Local surgical treatment is helpful in bringing about quick resolution of the comedoes and pustules as well as the cystic lesions. The contents of the comedo are expressed with a comedo extractor. Incising and draining of pustules and cystic lesions avoid the possibility of scar formation.

22. 2 Seborrheic Dermatitis

Seborrheic dermatitis is a chronic, superficial, inflammatory disease of the skin, with a predilection for the scalp, face, chest and back, where skin lipids are significantly higher(in which the seborrheic glands are most active).

22. 2. 1 Etiology

The etiology of seborrheic dermatitis remains unsolved. Investigations have confirmed the presence of the lipophilic yeast Pityrosporum ovale in large numbers in the scalp lesions. Skin sebum production in individuals with seborrheic dermatitis is significantly higher compared with control subjects. All of these mechanisms may promote the propagation of lipophilic organisms, produce inflammation, and possibly precipitate the condition.

Psychology factors, food habits, shortage of Vitamin B and alcohol may contribute to the process and development of the disease.

22. 2. 2 Clinical Features

Seborrheic dermatitis involves infancy and adults, majority between 20 and 50 years, more common in males. The distribution of the disease is mainly on scalp, face, upper trunk, axillae, submammary folds, and groins. The disease is characterized by dry, loose, moist, or greasy scales, and by pink or yellow patches of various shapes and sizes. Pruritus is variable. The disease is chronic with remissions and exacerbations.

On the scalp, the most common form manifests itself as a dry, branny desquamation, beginning in small patches and rapidly involving the entire scalp, with a profuse amount of fine, powdery scales. Hairs are dry, soft, and loose. Another type of seborrheic dermatitis on the scalp is more severe and is manifested by greasy patches, exudation, and thick crusting. The disease frequently spreads to the forehead, ears, postauricular region, and neck(Color Figure 22 - 2).

On the forehead and eyebrow region, grey-white scales and yellowish crust are seen, and the underlying skin is erythematous. In the postauricular region, the skin often becomes erosive, fissured with thick yellow crust. In the nasolabial creases, there may be dark reddish greasy patches. The lesions on the trunk show round, oval patches covered by tiny and greasy scaling. Multiple lesions may turn into annular patches or multi-annular patches. Yellowish and reddish scaling patches are generally seen in axillae and groin, where its appearance may closely simulate eczema because of the body fold and erosion.

Seborrheic dermatitis may progress to a generalized exfoliative state which is known as erythroderma. Generalized eruptions may be accompanied with adenopathy and may mimic other kinds of erythroderma.

22. 2. 3 Diagnosis and Differential Diagnosis

Diagnosis depends on the typical clinical features. Important differential diagnoses include psoriasis and pityriasis rosea.

Psoriasis is characterized by sharply marginated erythema, heavy scales, whose removal discloses bleeding points. Predilection for involvement of the scalp margin, elbows, knees and absence of itching are also suggestive. Herald plaque which followed by fine scaling macules and papules is seen in pityriasis rosea. The long axes of the lesions follow the lines of cleavage. Lesions usually confined by trunk and proximal aspects of the arms and legs.

22. 2. 4 Treatment

In general, therapy is directed toward loosening or removal of scales and crusts, inhibition of yeast colonization, control of secondary infection, and reduction of erythema and itching. Patients should be informed about the chronic nature of the disease and understand that therapy works by controlling the disease rather than by curing it.

22. 2. 4. 1 Topical therapy

Selenium sulfide, tar, and ketoconazole shampoo are all excellent. Corticosteroid solutions or corticosteroids in combination with coal tar are all effective. The most efficacious agents on glabrous skin are the corticosteroid creams. In severe cases, corticosteroids in combination with topical antibiotic agents could be used in which bacterial infection is prominent.

22. 2. 4. 2　Systemic therapy

In generalized or severe cases, systemic corticosteroids and antibiotics for secondary infection may be necessary and effective. Good results are achieved with systemic application of antifungal agents, such as itraconazole, 0. 1 g/d, two to three weeks, in fungal infection cases.

22. 3　Alopecia Areata

Alopecia areata is characterized by rapid and complete loss of hair without any visible inflammation on the scalp skin or any skin symptoms.

22. 3. 1　Etiology

Although the precise etiology of alopecia areata remains unknown, various factors have been suspected of contributing to this condition. These include genetic factors, psychogenic factors, maladjustment of endocrine, and autoimmune diseases such as systemic lupus erythematosus, thyroiditis, diabetes, and vitiligo.

22. 3. 2　Clinical Features

Alopecia areata is characterized by rapid and complete loss of hair in one, or several round or oval patches, usually on the scalp, bearded area, eyebrows, and eyelashes. Often the patches are from 1 to 10 cm in diameter. In affected area, the skin appears smooth and normal. Although the hair loss is patchy in distribution, however, cases may present in a diffuse pattern(Color Figure 22 - 3). During progression period of alopecia areata, the loosing hairs at the periphery of the bald patch pulled out have a tapered, attenuated bulb. In some patients the disease can be progressive, with total loss of scalp hair (alopecia totalis). When hair has been lost over entire body, the designation is alopecia universalis. Alopecia areata can persist several months or several years. Spontaneous recovery is seen in most alopecia areata patients. The regrowing hairs are soft and light in color; later they are replaced by stronger and darker hair. Poor prognosis is associated with childhood onset, widespread involvement, and longer duration.

22. 3. 3　Diagnosis and Differential Diagnosis

Diagnosis depends on the typical clinical features. The sharply circumscribed patch of alopecia with normal skin and the absence of scarring are indicative of alopecia areata.

Important differential diagnoses include tinea capitis. Tinea capitis is characterized by multiple scaly lesions with incomplete alopecia, stubs of broken hair. Fungus could be found under microscopic examination in broken hairs.

22. 3. 4　Treatment

Education about the disease process and prognosis, cosmetically acceptable alternatives (especially information about wigs), prevention the development of new patches all is made available to patient.

22. 3. 4. 1　Topical therapy

High-strength topical steroid creams may be used as first-line therapy. Topical 1%- 3% minoxidil may be combined with the above treatment trials or utilized as a single agent. Intra-lesional injections of corticosteroid suspensions are the treatment of choice for localized cosmetically conspicuous patches such as those occurring in the eyebrow.

22. 3. 4. 2　Systemic therapy

The oral prednisone could be used in rapidly progressing widespread disease (including alopecia totalis and alopecia universalis). However, long-term treatment is frequently needed to maintain growth. Side-effect of corticosteroid should be considered for long-term use. Vitamin B helps the hair growth. Some traditional Chinese medicine could also be chosen to treat the disease.

22. 4　Androgenetic Alopecia

Androgenetic alopecia(male pattern alopecia) is the common progressive balding which occurs through the combined effect of a genetic predisposition and the action of androgen on the hair follicles of the scalp.

22. 4. 1　Etiology

Patients may have family history of androgenetic alopecia, with polygenic or autosomal dominant in males and autosomal recessive in females.

The hair loss seen in androgenetic alopecia is dihydrotestosterone-dependent. The transformation of testosterone to dihydrotestosterone requires the enzyme 5α-reductase. 5α-reductase is found in outer root sheath of hair follicles. That 5α-reductase may be involved in male pattern baldness is suggested the increased expression of 5α-reductase type in the frontal or balding scalp versus the occipital or nonbalding scalp, and the results in animal models of androgenetic alopecia showing reversal of hair loss with 5α-reductase inhibitors.

22.4.2 Clinical Features

Male pattern alopecia shows itself during the twenties or early thirties by gradual loss of hair. Most patients present with complains of gradually thinning hair or baldness. In males, there is a receding anterior hair line, especially in the biparietal regions, which results in an M-shaped recession. The forehead becomes high. Following this the entire top of the scalp may become devoid of hair. Vellus hairs on the scalp continue to grow and become more prominent because of the absence of terminal hairs. (Color Figure 22 – 4)   In females, parietal and temporal recession is not a major feature and severe thinning is not common. Women generally have diffused hair loss throughout the midscalp. The rate of hair loss varies among individuals and it's usually slow. If androgenetic alopecia progresses rapidly, some patients also complain of increased falling out of hair.

22.4.3 Diagnosis and Differential Diagnosis

Clinical diagnosis made on the history, especially family incidence of androgenetic alopecia, and the pattern of alopecia.

Differential diagnosis includes other diffused pattern of hair loss, such as alopecia areata, telogen effluvium, secondary syphilis, SLE, iron deficiency, hypothyroidism, and hyperthyroidism. In young women, such manifestations of endocrinological abnormality should be sought as significant: androgenetic alopecia, acne, hirsutism, or virilization.

22.4.4 Treatment

There is no highly effective therapy to prevent the progression of androgenetic alopecia.

Topically applied minoxidil is helpful in reducing the rate of hair loss, or in partially restoring lost hair in some patients. Antiandrogens such as spironolactone, given as 40 – 60 mg/d, 1 – 3 months, which bind to androgen receptors and block the action of dihydrotestosterone have been reported to be effective in treating women with androgenetic alopecia who have elevated androgens. Finasteride, a new 5α-reductase inhibitor, recedes the lever of dihydrotestosterone in the serum and hair follicle of treated patients to prevent further hair loss and increase the hair growth. Finasteride is given 1 mg/d for 6 – 12 months. Side effects are infrequent. Treat-

ment is not as satisfactory as with men as finasteride is contraindicated in women.

22.5 Rosacea

Rosacea is a centrofacial disease particularly prevalent in middle age. The hallmarks of rosacea are papules and papulopustules, vivid red erythema, and telangiectases.

22.5.1 Etiology

Although the precise etiology of rosacea remains a mystery, various factors have been suspected of contributing to this condition. These include gastrointestinal disturbances, including dyspepsia with gastric hypochlorhydria and infestation with the microaerophilic gram-negative bacterium Helicobacter pylori, hypertension, demodex folliculorum mites, and psychogenic factors. Alcohol, spice food, sunlight, heat and emotion tension are contributing factors.

Rosacea is considered by some authors as a seborrheic disease. The majority of patients with rosacea, however, do not show signs of excessive sebaceous activity, and there is no significant association between rosacea and seborrhea.

22.5.2 Clinical Features

Rosacea is classified into three stages, which may develop successively. In some affected individuals, there is progression through all stages, but this succession does not necessarily occur.

Stage Ⅰ

The erythema persists for hours and days. Telangiectases become progressively more prominent, forming sprays on the nose, nasolabial folds, cheeks, and glabella. Most of these patients complain of sensitive skin that stings and burns after application of a variety of cosmetics, fragrances, and certain sunscreens.

Stage Ⅱ

Inflammatory papules and pustules crop up and persist for weeks. Comedones do not occur. The deeper inflammatory lesions may heal with scarring, but scars are small and tend to be shallow. Facial pores become more prominent. The papulopustular attacks become more and more frequent. Finally, rosacea may extend over the entire face(Color Figure 22 – 5).

Stage Ⅲ

A small proportion of patients go on to develop

the worst expressions of the disease, namely, large inflammatory nodules, furunculoid infiltrations, and tissue hyperplasia. These derangements occur on the cheeks and nose particularly, less often on the chin, forehead, or ears. Finally the patient shows inflamed and thickened edematous skin with large pores, resembling the surface of an orange. Along with folds and ridges, the appearance may mimic the leonine facies of leprosy or leukemia. The ultimate deformities are the phymas, e. g. rhinophyma.

22. 5. 3 Diagnosis and Differential Diagnosis
Diagnosis depends on the typical clinical features. Important differential diagnoses include acne vulgaris and seborrheic dermatitis.

Acne vulgaris affects a younger age group and often has an extensive distribution over the face, neck and trunk whereas extra-facial rosacea is rare. Typical acne vulgaris lacks the redness, telangiectasia and flushing of rosacea while rosacea lacks the comedones of acne vulgaris.

The pattern of the rash in seborrheic dermatitis defers markedly from that of rosacea. The former characteristically involves the scalp, retroauricular area, eyelids and nasolabial folds. The scaling is not normally a feature of rosacea but is the rule in seborrheic dermatitis may also be helpful.

22. 5. 4 Treatment
Rosacea is difficult to treat. All sources of local irritation, such as soaps, alcoholic cleansers, abrasives and peeling agents, must be avoided. Dietary limitations relate only to factors that provoke erythema and flushing, such as alcoholic beverages, hot drinks, and spicy food. Long time sun exposure should be avoided.

22. 5. 4. 1 Topical therapy
Antibiotics are sometimes effective. Topical clindamycin and erythromycin, usually in concentrations from 0. 5 to 2. 0%, are commercially available. Metronidazole is available as a 1% aqueous gel or cream and has shown to be safe and effective in moderation to severe rosacea. Lotions with 2% to 5% sulfur have been used successfully with a very thin application at night recommended. There is preliminary evidence that 0. 2% isotretinoin in a bland cream is helpful. It is less irritating than tretinoin.

22. 5. 4. 2 Systemic therapy
Tetracycline, doxycycline, and minocycline are usually quite effective in controlling papulopustular rosacea. It is important to start with full doses, e. g,

1. 0 tetracycline per day. Likewise, 50 mg of minocycline or doxycycline can be given twice daily. After 2 weeks, daily maintenance doses of 500 mg tetracycline or 50 mg of minocycline or doxycycline are generally sufficient. Metronidazole is a synthetic nitroimidazole-derived antibacterial and antiprotozoal agent. The usual dose is 600 mg daily for 2 weeks. Isotretinoin may be appropriate for all forms of severe or therapy resistant rosacea. Before using isotretinoin, one has to consider indications, contraindications, and all risks. The dose required for the control of severe rosacea varies. The standard dose is 0. 5mg/kg bodyweight per day.

22. 5. 4. 3 Surgical Treatment
A variety of techniques are available including scalpel or razor modeling, electrocoagulation, argon laser, CO_2 laser, and pulsed dye laser.

▪ Summary

Acne is a chronic inflammation of the pilosebaceous units of face and trunk that occurs in adolescence and manifests as comedones, papules, papulopustules, nodules, cystic lesions, and scars. Multiple factors cause acne vulgaris, such as androgenetic stimulation of sebaceous glands, proliferation of Propionibacterium acnes, formation of keratinous plug in the infundibulum of the hair follicle. Topical treatment includes topical vitamin A acid, benzoyl peroxide, topical antibiotics and azelaic acid. Systemic treatment includes antibiotics, isotretinoin, and antiandrogens. Intralesional corticosteroids and surgical treatment are used to deal cystic lesions.

Seborrheic dermatitis is a chronic, superficial, inflammatory disease of the skin, with a predilection for the scalp, face, chest and back, where skin lipids are significantly higher. The etiology of seborrheic dermatitis remains unsolved. In general, therapy is directed toward loosening removal of scales and crusts, inhibition of yeast colonization, control of secondary infection, and reduction of erythema and itching.

Alopecia areata is characterized by rapid and complete loss of hair without any visible inflammation on the scalp skin or any skin symptoms. Genetic factors, psychogenic factors, maladjustment of endocrine and such autoimmune diseases contribute to the causes of alopecia areata. Prevention the development of new patches all is made available to patient.

Androgenetic alopecia is the common progressive balding which occurs through the combined effect of a genetic predisposition and the action of androgen on the hair follicles of the scalp. In males, parietal and temporal recession is a major feature and severe thinning is common. Women generally have diffused hair loss throughout the midscalp. There is no highly effective therapy to prevent the progression of androgenetic alopecia.

Rosacea is a centrofacial disease particularly prevalent in middle age. The hallmarks of rosacea are papules and papulopustules, vivid red erythema, and telangiectases. Rosacea is classified into three stages, which may develop successively. Antibiotics and isotretinoin could be used topically or systemically.

▪ Questions

1. Describe the clinical feature of acne vulgaris and how to diagnose and treat it.

2. Describe the clinical feature of seborrheic dermatitis and how to manage it.

3. Describe the clinical feature of alopecia areata.

4. Describe the cause of androgenetic alopecia and how to treat it.

5. Describe the clinical feature of three stages of rosacea.

(**Mei Di** 狄梅)

Chapter 23

Disorders of Pigmentation

▪ Objectives

To master the knowledge of the causes and clinical features of disorders of pigmentation.

To have an intimate knowledge of diagnosis and management of vitiligo, chloasma and melanosis.

▪ Key concepts

Vitiligo is a common mucocutaneous depigmentation disease and can be categorized as localized, pervasive and generalized. A higher incidence is found among people of dark skin than those of light-colored skin. The domestic prevalence is about 0. 1% to 2%. It is easy to diagnose based on its typical clinical presentation along with pathological examination. The major treatment includes medication, surgery and physical therapy.

Chloasma is the skin pigmentation disease most commonly seen on the faces of young and middle-aged women. The diagnosis can be made based on the history and appearance of typical skin lesions. Current treatment for chloasma includes medication, Chinese herbs and physical therapy.

Melanosis is grey-brown skin pigmentation that primarily affects the face. Its diagnosis can be established easily by history and typical clinical presentation. Currently, the treatment of melanosis includes medication, traditional Chinese medicine and physical therapy.

▪ Introduction

Vitiligo is a commonly acquired localized or pervasive depigmentation of skin, and its cause is unknown. The disease has cosmetic consequences. It is easy to diagnose but difficult to treat. Chloasma is commonly seen in young and middle-aged individuals, affecting significantly more female than male patients. The disease manifests as altered of abnormal pigmentation on the face. The practitioners of traditional Chinese medicine categorize all abnormal facial skin pigmentation as "black spot." It is also called "liver sport", which is attributed to the stagnation of "Qi" in the liver or liver disease. The disease is more commonly seen in pregnant or menopausal women. Melanosis is altered skin pigmentation appearing in colors such as light brown, dark brown, and dark grey, often affecting the face. It is a disease of complicated causes, and its mechanism has yet not to be fully understood. Melanosis in many patients cannot be explained by any identifiable causative or inductive factor. Treatment strategies of Western medicine mainly include sun avoidance, vitamin supplementation and topical depigmentation agents, whose effects are unsatisfactory. Currently, the use of laser and intense pulsed light (IPL) has become a therapy worthy of further clinic research.

23.1 Vitiligo

Vitiligo is a commonly acquired localized or pervasive depigmentation of skin and its cause is unknown. The disease has cosmetic consequences. It is easy to diagnose but difficult to treat.

23.1.1 Etiology

The causes of the disease are unknown and the mechanism may be influenced by multiple external factors, resulting in loss of intracellular tyrosinase function in cells located in the boundaries of the epidermis and cutis. Tyrosinase oxidation is blocked by dopamine and result in difficulties in melanin formation. Finally, skin depigmentation is the result. Current theories are as follows:

23.1.1.1 Auto-immunity hypothesis

Patients of vitiligo often have autoimmune disease, including thyroid disease, diabetes mellitus, rheumatoid arthritis, and pernicious anemia. Antimelanocyte antibody can be detected in human serum. Psoralen + UVA (PUVA), local and systemic steroid treatment, and even external application of cytotoxic medication such as all-transretinoic acid are effective in vitiligo. These clues hint that vitiligo is associated with autoimmunity.

23.1.1.2 Self-destruction of melanocytes hypothesis

Some scholars think that the development of vitiligo is caused by the hyperfunctioning of melanocytes, leading to the exhaustion and early degeneration of these cells. It may also be due to the overpro-

duction or accumulation of the intermediate components or metabolites during the process of melanin formation in the cells. Recently, further research has indicated that the patients of vitiligo may have a defective oxidative mechanism and be over-sensitive to external oxidants (ultraviolet exposure), which predisposes them to cellular damage under persistent oxidative stress, resulting in the ultimate loss of melanocytes and the onset of vitiligo.

23.1.1.3 Neurochemical hypothesis

Studies have reported that vitiligo is associated with psychological changes and diseases. Changes in psychological status could directly influence the body's neurologic and immune function such as autoimmunity. The skin defect of vitiligo along the nerve ganglion distribution could be associated with increases in neural transmitters around melanocytes and subsequent melanocyte injuries or melanin formation inhibition.

23.1.1.4 Genetic influence hypothesis

Clinical observational and epidemiologic studies have shown that vitiligo has close relationships with genetic factors. Based on statistics analyzed abroad, the prevalence of vitiligo in patients' relatives was 18% to 40% abroad and 3.00% to 17.23% domestically in China. In that report, first-degree relatives in all subjects were at high risk of the disease and the genetic transmission frequency was about 3% to 7%, but the mode of transmission was still unknown.

In addition, there have been hypotheses of the relative deficiency of tyrosine, copper ions and dysfunction of keratocytes. Medication, food and sun exposure may induce or exacerbate the disease.

23.1.2 Clinical Features

This disease occurs often among in all ages. The typical skin lesion is localized depigmented patches, which are porcelain white or milk white, with clear margins and abnormally increased pigmentation on the margins(Color Figure 23 – 1). The patches can be partially merged with no skin changes such as scaling or shrinkage. The skin lesions are not uniform and vary in size and number. At the center of each lesion is the "pigmentation island". Lesions can appear on all parts of the body, but are more commonly seen in the parts of exposure or friction, including the face, neck, back of hands, wrists and waist. Mouth, lips, genital area and labium can be involved. Three lesion types can be determined according to the area of patch involvement:

23. 1. 2. 1 Localized

The skin lesion is single and localized in one area. The subtypes are ① segmented, the lesion is distributed along one side of the neural ganglion; and ② mucosal, only mucosal areas are involved.

23. 1. 2. 2 Pervasive

This is the most common type and the lesions are scattered in multiple areas, often symmetrically. The subtypes include ① ordinary, the skin lesions are distributed on multiple sites of the body; ② limb and facial, the face or fingers or toes are involved; and ③ mixed, a combination of the types mentioned above.

23. 1. 2. 3 Generalized

The skin lesion occupies more than 50% of body surface area or the whole body occasionally accompanied by gray hair.

23. 1. 3 Histopathology

Significant deficiency of melanocytes and melanin is found in the epidermis and the melanocytes on the lesion margin are abnormally enlarged. In the later stage, no melanocytes are found in the skin lesion.

23. 1. 4 Diagnosis and Differential Diagnosis

It is not difficult to diagnose the disease based on typical skin lesions, but the differential diagnoses must include the following:

23. 1. 4. 1 Tinea versicolor

Rash can be seen on the neck, chest, back of the shoulders, axillaries, and other areas with abundant sebaceous glands. Pale white, pale brown round or oval patches have small scales and microscopic fungal exam is positive.

23. 1. 4. 2 Simple rosea

It is commonly seen in children and teenagers, and the face is often involved. The skin lesion is round or irregular macula, pink patch at first and then pale patches covered with minimal chaff-like scales.

23. 1. 4. 3 Idiopathic guttate hypomelanosis

This is a disease mostly seen in people over age 30. The skin lesion is round or white polygonal patches and tear-shaped. The diameter is 2 to 6 mm, less than 1 cm in general, and the surface is smooth without fusion.

Differential diagnoses also include nevus anemicus, amelanotic nevus and depigmentation after inflammation.

23. 1. 5 Treatment

Various types of treatments are applied and the main goal is to increase the number of melanocytes in the skin lesion. Currently, the methods are as follows:

23. 1. 5. 1 Medication

① Glucocorticoids: systemic glucocorticoids are often used for generalized and progressive vitiligo, especially for patients with rapid progression of the disease under stress or with autoimmune diseases. External application of steroids is often used for localized and segmented vitiligo. ② Immunoregulation, including tacrolimus, BCG polysaccharide nucleic acid, pimecrolimus and others. ③ The derivatives of vitamin D_3, such as calcipotriol and tacalcitol cream. These drugs can be used to induce activation of tyrosinase in melanocytes and increase melanocyte activity. ④ Photosensitizing agents, including psoralen potion and compound alizarin tincture. Tyrosinase can be activated effectively and increase the photosensitivity of the skin lesion to improve the cycles in skin lesion and serve the aim of treating vitiligo. ⑤ Chinese herbs.

23. 1. 5. 2 Surgery

① Autologous epidermal transplantation, applicable for smaller skin lesions and scale conditions. In general, 5 to 10 skin patches can be transplanted. ② Microdermabrasion used with electrical abrasion or microcrystal abrasion. After the surgery, melanocytes are sometimes activated and multiplied, causing patches to migrate.

23. 1. 5. 3 Physical therapy, including photochemical therapy and phototherapy

① Photochemical therapy, with oral or external photosensitizers. The photosensitizers produce a photo-complex with thymidine in DNA under UVA and inhibit the duplication of DNA, leading to the inhibition of cell proliferation and inflammation. ② Phototherapy, including narrow band ultraviolet B (NB-UVB), 308 mm eximer laser, and 304 mm ultraviolet B. These can stimulate the proliferation of melanocytes and migration toward the depigmented patches.

23. 2 Chloasma

Chloasma is commonly seen in young and middle-aged individuals, affecting significantly more female than male patients. The disease manifests as altered of abnormal pigmentation on the face. The practitioners of traditional Chinese medicine categorize all abnormal facial skin pigmentation as "black spot." It is also called "liver sport", which is attributed to the stagnation of "Qi" in the liver or liver disease. The disease is more commonly seen in pregnant or menopausal women.

23.2.1 Etiology and Pathogenesis

The pathogenesis of chloasma is complicated and remains to be fully elucidated. Most scholars believe that it is related to the following factors: dysfunction of the endocrine system, gestation, estrogen and progesterone levels, use of oral contraceptive pills, diseases of the ovaries and uterus, genetic factors, free radicals, ultraviolet exposure, serum concentrations of copper and trace elements, hepatitis A and B, cholecystitis, tyrosinase dysfunction, use of make-up, phototoxic drugs, anti-epilepsy medication, and emotional fluctuation. Among these factors, endocrine dysfunction, genetic factors, and ultraviolet exposure are considered to be the main causes and sunshine is an exacerbating factor.

From the perspective of traditional Chinese medicine, chloasma belongs to the category of liver spots, black spots, and butterfly rash. The formation of chloasma is commonly thought to be associated with dysfunctional liver, spleen, and kidneys. Some also think that the disease is caused by the stagnation of "Qi" and blood stasis.

23.2.2 Clinical Features

Chloasma afflicts primarily young and middle-aged women and predominantly occurs symmetrically on the zygomatic areas and cheeks (Color Figure 23 – 2). The discoloration is nail or coin sized and of irregular or butterfly-like shape, and appears pale or dark brown. The lesion may have distinct or indistinct margins and can fuse into a larger patch. The forehead, nose, and perioral areas can be involved. Patches can be located in the central, malar, and mandibular areas of the face. The patient may have no symptoms other than the patch. The skin lesions can become exacerbated in the spring or summer but subdued in the fall and winter. Disease progression is not well defined and the disease may persist for months or years. Sunshine is an exacerbating factor and some patients have gradual relief after gestation or cessation of oral contraceptive pills.

23.2.3 Histopathology

Pigment deposits in the basal layer and the pigment cells do not increase. The upper layer of the cutis contains more melanocytes and free pigment particles. Sometimes, infiltration of lymphocytes will occur in blood vessels and the perifollicular areas.

23.2.4 Diagnosis and Differential Diagnosis

The disease can be readily diagnosed from the appearance of yellow brown patches on the face, predominant occurrence in females, and absence of other noticeable symptoms. Differential diagnoses include the following diseases:

23.2.4.1 Riehl's melanosis

It is commonly seen on the face, and begins in the zygomatic and temporal areas with gradual involvement of the forehead, cheeks, retroauricular regions, and the neck. It appears reticular first and becomes patchy with small perifollicular pigment spots in the margin. The lesion has an indistinct boundary. Apart from pigmented patches, limited dilation of capillaries, keratosis of follicular openings and powder scaling can be seen, producing the skin appearance of powder and dust.

23.2.4.2 Freckles

These brown or reddish-brown spots caused by the red-brown form of melanin, called pheomelanin, begin to develop around 5 years of age, and are seen in female more than male in China. The skin characteristics include pale to dark brown spots, which can be pin or grain-sized. The spots are round or irregular in shape and have a smooth texture without scaling. They have clear margins and do not form patches. They are variable in number and are asymmetrically distributed on the face.

23.2.4.3 Addison disease

This disease has pervasive blue-black or red-brown patches, and can be seen on the face, external genitals, and areola of the nipples. Generalized symptoms include weakness, hypotension, and weight loss. Urine collected for 24 hours has lower amounts of 17-OHCS (17-hydroxycorticosteroids) and 17-KS (17-ketosteroids).

Other differential diagnoses include facial pigmentation such as actinic lichen planus, pigmented cosmetic dermatitis, and nevus fuscocaeruleus zygomaticus.

23. 2. 5 Treatment

Chloasma is a kind of skin disease commonly seen and hardly ever cured. Patients have minimal symptoms, but their psychological stress may be severe. Severe cases may influence work and daily living. For this disease, the causes are firstly determined for appropriate treatment. Sunshine exposure and oral contraceptive pills should be avoided. Various treatment methods are used and the main methods are medication, Chinese herbs, and physical therapy.

First, medication can be separated into oral and external use

External use: ① de-coloring agents have significant effects on epidermal chloasma, and include cream with 10% to 20% anchoic acid, or 4% kojic acid, or 2% to 5% hydroquinone. ② External corticosteroids such as 1% hydrocortisone and prednisolone acetate have minimal adverse effects. ③ All-transretinoic acid (ATRA) is a "retinoid" or chemotherapeutic that is sometimes administered for chloasma. ④ Chemical peeling works or epidermal chloasma including 50% to 95% phenol or 10% to 50% trichloroacetic acid solution. Moreover, usage of hydroxy acid for chemical peeling works better in conjunction with decoloring agents.

Oral medications: vitamin C, vitamin E, carotene, green tea, fish oil, chloroquine, and indomethacin. Large-dose vitamin C by injection may be tried.

Second, Chinese herbs emphasize general adjustment, functioning in multiple links, all directions and multiple targets.

Finally, physical therapy includes the application of liquid nitrogen, microdermabrasion, and laser (such as Q-switched ruby laser, Argon Ion Laser, copper-vapor laser, and pulsed dye laser), which can destroy pigment particles and influence pigment cell's activities.

23. 3 Melanosis

Melanosis is altered skin pigmentation appearing in colors such as light brown, dark brown, and dark grey, often affecting the face. It is a disease of complicated causes, and its mechanism has not yet to be fully understood. Melanosis in many patients cannot be explained by any identifiable causative or inductive factor. Treatment strategies of Western medicine mainly include sun avoidance, vitamin supplementation, and topical depigmentation agents, whose effects are unsatisfactory. Currently, the use of laser and intense pulsed light (IPL) has become a therapy worthy of further clinic research.

23. 3. 1 Etiology

The metabolism of melanin in the skin is a dynamic process. Melanin is formed under the effect of tyrosinase. Given the complexity of melanin synthesis, melanosis has been designated as a skin pigmentation disorder that originates from unknown mechanisms. Currently, it is considered to be a type of pigmented contact dermatitis related to long-term exposure to the coal tar and fragrance components in cosmetic products. Other possible causes include sun exposure, vitamin deficiency, and malnutrition. Melanosis in some patients may be attributed to endocrine dysfunction such as abnormal functioning of sex glands, pituitary gland, adrenal cortex, or thyroid gland.

23. 3. 2 Clinical Features

Based on the underlying cause of clinical presentation, melanosis can be classified into several types, including Riehl's melanosis, post-inflammatory melanosis, friction melanosis, tar melanosis, and erythromelanosis follicularis faciei et firstly. This section focuses on Riehl's melanosis (Color Figure 23-3).

Riehl's melanosis was firstly described during the war time, hence also named "war melanosis." Currently, it is regarded as a stage of toxic melanosis and is commonly seen in adults, with a higher prevalence in women. The face is the most frequently affected area, especially the forehead, cheeks, postaural area, lateral neck, and other sun-exposed areas. Sometimes the chest, arms and forearms may also be involved. The affected skin lesion appears brown or blue-grey, surrounded by a border of small perifollicular pigmentation. In early stage, the lesion presents with pruritus and erythema. Later, it develops into reticular pigmentation, in light- or dark-brown color. Typical lesion development includes the following three phases:

23. 3. 2. 1 Inflammatory phase

Local congestive erythema is found accompanied by mild flushing, swelling, and a few areas of chaff-like scaling. Mild pruritus may be present after sun exposure.

23. 3. 2. 2 Pigmentation phase

As the inflammation wanes, erythema subsides and is replaced by marked patchy or reticular pigmentation covered by fine, "dust-like" scales. Besides the pigmented patch, sometimes circumscribed telangiectasia and dyskeratosis follicularis can also be found.

23.3.2.3 Atrophy phase

Only a few patients enter this phase, in which mild pitted atrophy appears within the area of pigmented skin.

23.3.3 Histopathology

Histopathological findings include mild hyperkeratosis in the epidermis, intracellular edema in the stratum spinosum, liquefaction of basal cells, proliferation of melanophages in the upper dermis, and infiltration of lymphocytes, histiocytes, and melanophages around the dermal vessels. In the later stage, the epidermis becomes normalized and inflammatory infiltration is not present.

23.3.4 Diagnosis and Differential Diagnosis

The diagnosis of the disease can be easily confirmed by history and typical skin lesion. However, it should be differentiated from the following diseases:

23.3.4.1 Chloasma

This disease is characterized by well-defined brown lesions without inflammatory reaction. It has a typical butterfly-like distribution, affecting both cheeks.

23.3.4.2 Skin pigmentation of addison disease

This disease presents with diffuse patches in dark blue or reddish brown color, distributed around the face and skin folds such as the groin and nipples. It is accompanied by systemic symptoms of adrenocortical insufficiency. Abnormal laboratory findings may be found in urinary levels of 17-ketosteroid (17-KS), 17-hydroxycorticosteroid (17-OH), aldosterone (ALD), adrenocorticotropin (ACTH), and water tests.

23.3.4.3 Poikiloderma of Civatte

This disease is often seen in middle-aged women, characterized by light reddish brown or bronze-colored macules with telangiectasia and superficial atrophic white dots. It may sometimes be accompanied by pruritus and burning pain.

23.3.4.4 Tar melanosis

This disease, also called "melanodermatitis toxica lichenoides", is a special chronic pigmentation disease induced by occupational hazards in the working or operating environment. It can be diagnosed by a history of long-term tar and sun exposure followed by the inflammatory process. Meanwhile, come-

done, papules, and scales seen in physical examination can help confirm the diagnosis. Since only a few cases are reported out of a large population with occupational contact, the low incidence of this disease marks a significant relationship with the individual's intrinsic factors.

23.3.5 Treatment

The key to treat melanosis is to look for its causes and remove them or reduce contact. The patient should be advised to avoid contact with suspicious substances, strengthen personal protection, and use protective creams. If instructions are followed, the symptoms will improve gradually.

Medical treatment: ① Topical medication: lesions in the inflammatory phase can be treated with glucocorticoid ointment, and lesions in the pigmentation phase can be treated with 3% hydroquinolone cream, coupled with sun-screening products such as 2.5% titanium dioxide (TiO_2) cream or 5% para-aminobenzoic acid (PABA) ointment. ② Oral medication: oral vitamin C 1.0 g three times per day, or intravenous drip 3 – 5 g/d, 15 days per treatment course.

Traditional Chinese medicine.

Physical therapy: To date, laser therapy is the most studied method, and still being discussed.

▪ Summary

Vitiligo is a type of localized or generalized skin depigmentation and its cause is still unknown. Clinical classification is based on characteristics of the white patches including localized, pervasive, and generalized vitiligo. The methods of treatment vary, including medication, physical therapy, and surgery. The aim is to increase the number of melanocytes in the skin lesion and recover normal color of the skin.

Chloasma is a type of chromatodermatosis, most commonly seen on the faces of young and middle-aged women. The pathogenesis of chloasma is complicated and the real causes are still unclear. The diagnosis can be easily made based on the history and characteristic presentation. A variety of treatments are administered, mainly external and oral medication, Chinese herbs, and physical therapy. In addition, attention should be paid to diet and sun protection.

Melanosis is a skin pigmentation disorder that can occur at any age, most often in middle-aged women. It is a disease of complicated causes and its mechanism remains unknown. In many patients, no causative or inductive factor can be found. Currently, it is considered to be a pigmented contact dermatitis. The diagnosis of this disease can be established on the basis of history, typical clinical presentation, and histopathological findings. Regarding treatment, traditional Chinese medicines and high-dose intravenous vitamin C, and topical exfoliating agents are preferred, but the results have been largely unsatisfactory. A combination of medications, traditional Chinese herbs, and physical therapy can enhance therapeutic effectiveness.

▪ Questions

1. Briefly describe the clinical presentation and treatment of vitiligo.

2. What are the differential diagnoses of vitiligo?

3. Please describe clinical manifestations of chloasma.

4. What diseases are included in the differential diagnosis of chloasma and what are the distinguishing characteristics of chloasma?

5. List the clinical presentation and staging of melanosis.

6. What are the differential diagnoses of melanosis?

(**Junying Zhao** 赵俊英)

Chapter 24

Hereditary Disorders

▪ Objectives

To study the clinical manifestation of ichthyosis, keratosis pilaris and palmoplantar keratoderma.

To have the basic knowledge of the management of these disorders.

▪ Key concepts

Ichthyosis is a genetic skin disorder. All types of ichthyosis have dry, thickened, scaly or flaky skin. In many types it is said to resemble the scales on a fish. There is no effective medication to cure this disorder. The main approach to treatment of both conditions includes hydration of the skin and application of an emollient to prevent evaporation.

Keratosis pilaris presents with numerous small, rough papules primarily on the outer aspect of upper arms. Moisturizing creams are helpful to this disorder.

Palmoplantar keratoderma (PPK) is characterized by excessive formation of keratin on the palms and soles. The acquired and congenital varieties may be present alone, or accompanied with other diseases or be a part of a syndrome.

▪ Introduction

Hereditary skin disorders are those that are passed down from generation to generation through familial genes. Some of these disorders cause symptoms that are limited to the skin, can be effectively managed and do not otherwise affect health; others are responsible for more widespread effects on connective and cutaneous tissue and the neurological system, creating chronic effects throughout the body.

24.1 Ichthyosis

Ichthyosis is a skin disorder which causes the formation of dry, fish-like scales on the skin's surface. The condition often begins in early childhood and is usually lifelong. Types of ichthyosis are classified by their appearance and their genetic causes. Ichthyosis caused by the same gene can vary considerably in severity and symptoms. Some ichthyosis don't appear to fit exactly into any one type. Also, different genes can produce ichthyosis with similar symptoms. The most common or well-known types are ichthyosis vulgaris, X-linked ichthyosis and lamellar ichthyosis. The most common type is ichthyosis vulgaris, accounting for more than 95% of all cases.

24.1.1 Etiology

Hereditary ichthyosis vulgaris is an autosomal dominant genetic disorder first evident in early childhood. Ichthyosis vulgaris is classified as a retention hyperkeratosis. The only known molecular marker affected by hereditary ichthyosis vulgaris is profilaggrin. Profilaggrin is a major component of keratohyalin granules and is converted to filaggrin. Filaggrin is proteolyzed and metabolized, producing free amino acids that may play a critical role as water-binding compounds in the upper stratum corneum. Normal cycles of skin hydration and dehydration contribute to normal desquamation. These cycles are disrupted in ichthyosis vulgaris. In ichthyosis vulgaris, the expression of profilaggrin is absent or reduced in the epidermis. This biochemical abnormality correlates with the decreased numbers of keratohyalin granules and the clinical severity of the condition. Mutations in the gene encoding filaggrin have been identified as the cause of ichthyosis vulgaris.

X-linked ichthyosis is a clinically mild genetic disorder of keratinization, with extracutaneous manifestations in some cases. It is caused by a steroid sulfatase (STS) deficiency resulting from abnormalities in its coding gene.

Lamellar ichthyosis is an autosomal recessive disorder. Patients with lamellar ichthyosis have accelerated epidermal turnover with proliferative hyperkeratosis, in contrast to retention hyperkeratosis. This involves a mutation in the gene for transglutaminase 1 (TGM1).

24.1.2 Clinical Features

Ichthyosis vulgaris is characterized by symmetrical scaling of the skin, which varies from barely visible roughness and dryness to strong horny plates. Pruritus can be caused by dry skin. Scales are small, fine, irregular, and polygonal in shape, often curling up at the edges to give the skin a rough feel. Scales vary in size from 1 mm to 1 cm in diameter and range from white to dirty gray and brown. Different types of scaling may be found in different areas, even in the same patient. Most scaling occurs on the extensor surfaces of the extremities, with a sharp demarcation between normal flexural folds and the surrounding affected areas. The lower extremities are affected more often than the upper extremities. Compared to other sites, the scales overlying the shins are thicker, darker, and arranged in a mosaic pattern. If the trunk is involved, scaling tends to be more pronounced on the back than on the abdomen. The face is seen relative sparing, because of increased sebaceous secretions, although the cheeks and forehead may be involved during early childhood in the hereditary form.

X-linked ichthyosis is seen at birth or in the immediate neonatal period. Most typically, X-linked ichthyosis appears in infancy with scaling on the posterior neck, upper trunk, and extensor surfaces of the extremities. The scalp is often involved. As the child ages, the mild scaling evident in the first few days of life becomes more evident and assumes a dirty yellow or brown color with dark, polygonal, firmly adherent scales. This generalized eruption tends to fade on the head but becomes more prominent on the trunk and extremities, particularly on the extensor surfaces of the legs. Scaling has a tendency to be more noticeable in cold and dry weather, improving in the summer months.

In lamellar ichthyosis, the newborn is born encased in a collodion membrane that sheds within 10-14 days. The shedding of the membrane reveals generalized scaling with variable redness of the skin. The scaling may be fine or platelike, resembling fish skin. Although the disorder is not life threatening, it is quite disfiguring and causes considerable psychological stress to affected patients. In Childhood and adulthood, lamellar ichthyosis is characterized by generalized scales, which range from fine and white to thick, dark, and platelike. The lesions involve the entire body and are increased in flexural surfaces such as the axilla, groin, antecubital fossa, and neck. The individual scales tend to be larger over the legs and, in some areas, are centrally attached and raised at the edges. Keratoderma of the palms may be seen in the patient with lamellar ichthyosis.

24. 1. 3 Diagnosis and Differential Diagnosis

Ichthyosis is diagnosed based on the clinical manifestations.

24. 1. 4 Treatments

The main approach to treatment of both conditions includes hydration of the skin and application of an emollient to prevent evaporation. Hydration promotes desquamation by increasing hydrolytic enzyme activity and the susceptibility to mechanical forces. Emollients should be applied after showering or bathing.

Over-the-counter products often contain urea or propylene glycol. Moisturizers containing urea in lower strengths (10%- 20%) produce a more pliable stratum corneum. Propylene glycol draws water through the stratum corneum by establishing a water gradient. Thick skin is then shed following hydration. Propylene glycol is a common vehicle in both prescription and over-the-counter preparations.

Topical retinoids (e. g. tretinoin) may be beneficial. They reduce cohesiveness of epithelial cells, stimulate mitosis and turnover, and suppress keratin synthesis.

24. 2 Keratosis Pilaris

Keratosis pilaris is a very common condition occurs in many people of all ages. It is a benign condition that presents with numerous small, red, rough papules primarily around hair follicles.

24. 2. 1 Etiology

Keratosis pilaris affects nearly 50%- 80% of all adolescents and approximately 40% of adults. Approximately 30%- 50% of patients have a positive family history. Keratosis pilaris is thought to be a disorder of keratinocytes. Instead of exfoliating, these cells build up around the hair follicles.

Dry skin conditions seem to exacerbate the disease. Symptoms generally tend to worsen in winter and improve in summer. Common associations include a family history of keratosis pilaris, ichthyosis, or atopic dermatitis.

24. 2. 2 Clinical Features

Keratosis pilaris causes numerous papules about the size of a grain of sand. These feel rough or look like goose bumps. The papules may be skin colored, red

or brown. Some of the bumps may be slightly red or have an accompanying light-red halo, indicating inflammation. In some instances, scratching away the surface of some bumps may reveal a small, coiled hair.

The outer aspect of upper arms is the area most commonly affected, but it can also affect the thighs, face and buttocks, and less commonly, the forearms and upper back.

24. 2. 3 Diagnosis and Differential Diagnosis

Keratosis pilaris is diagnosed based on the clinical features. However, keratosis pilaris may be associated with other conditions, such as ichthyosis and atopic dermatitis.

24. 2. 4 Treatment

There is no cure for keratosis pilaris but it can be effectively controlled. Treatment options include:

1. Moisturizing creams to soften the skin. Creams that contain urea and salicylic acid may be most effective. Mild cases of keratosis pilaris may be improved with basic lubrication using over-the-counter moisturizer lotions.

2. Intermittent use of topical retinoids (e. g. weekly or biweekly) is quite effective and well tolerated, but usually the response is only partial. After initial clearing with stronger medications, patients may be placed on a milder maintenance regimen afterward.

24. 3 Palmoplantar Keratoderma

Palmoplantar keratoderma (PPK) constitutes a heterogeneous group of disorders characterized by thickening of the palms and the soles. It is subclassified by clinical features and patterns of inheritance. Genetic mutation is identified in some cases.

24. 3. 1 Etiology

The etiology of PPK remains unknown. Diffused PPK may be related to mutations of keratin 1 and 9.

24. 3. 2 Clinical Features

Diffused PPK is uniform involvement of the palmoplantar surface. This pattern is usually evident within the first few months of life. The second pattern is focal PPK, which consists of localized areas of hyperkeratosis located mainly on pressure points and sites of recurrent friction. The third pattern is punctate keratoderma, which is characterized by multiple small, hyperkeratotic papules, spicules, or nodules on the palms and soles. These tiny keratoses may involve the entire palmoplantar surface or may be restricted to certain areas (e. g. palmar creases).

24. 3. 3 Diagnosis and Differential Diagnosis

PPK is diagnosed based on the clinical manifestations. However, distinctive features such as transgredient spread, distant keratoses and periodontosis are not apparent in infants. Therefore, it may be difficult to make a precise diagnosis until adulthood. Complete skin examination will usually exclude those entities with PPK as a part of a generalized disorder of cornification.

24. 3. 4 Treatment

Treatment is difficult. The most common therapeutic options only result in short-term improvement. The mainstays of treatment include the following:

(1) Topical keratolytics (e. g. salicylic acid 5%, lactic acid 10%, urea 10%–40%) are useful in patients with limited keratoderma.

(2) Topical retinoids (e. g. tretinoin) are effective, but often limited by skin irritation.

(3) Oral retinoids are effective. Most hereditary PPKs require long-term treatment. Results indicate that acitretin is comparable to etretinate. Intermittent therapy should be attempted whenever possible. To decrease unacceptable adverse effects in long-term course, the optimal dosage of acitretin in adults is $30-35$ mg/d [$0.5-1$ mg/(kg · d) for adults and 0.5 mg(kg · d) for children]. Treatment of women of childbearing age results in long-term potential teratogenic effects.

■ Summary

Ichthyosis is a genetic skin disorders. All types of ichthyosis have dry, thickened, scaly or flaky skin. In many types the skin is said to resemble the scales of a fish. The severity of symptoms varies enormously. The most common type of ichthyosis is ichthyosis vulgaris, accounting for more than 95% of cases.

Keratosis pilaris is a very common benign skin condition appearing as small, whitish bumps on the upper arms and thighs, especially of children and young adults. Individual lesions of keratosis pilaris arise when a hair follicle becomes plugged with keratin.

Palmoplantar keratoderma is a rare group of disorders where the skin of the palms and soles is thicker than normal. The thickening may occur in small localized areas of the palms and soles or the whole surface.

Treatments for this group of hereditary skin disorders often take the form of topical application of creams and emollient oils, in an attempt to hydrate the skin. Retinoids are also used for some conditions.

■ Questions

1. What are the clinical manifestations of ichthyosis vulgaris, X-linked ichthyosis and lamellar ichthyosis?

2. What are the clinical manifestations of keratosis pilaris?

3. What are the mainstays of treatment for these patients?

(**Zigang Xu** 徐子刚)

Chapter 25

Metabolic and Nutritional Disorders

▪ Objectives

To have an intimate knowledge of the clinical feature of pellagra, and diagnosis the disease. Get the message the etiology of Pellagra, and how to treat the disease.

To have an intimate knowledge of the clinical feature of erythropoietic protoporphyria and porphyria cutanea tarda, and diagnosis the disease. Get the message the etiology of cutaneous porphyrias, and how to treat the disease.

To have an intimate knowledge of the cause, typing and clinical manifestation of acanthosis nigricans, how to diagnosis and heal the disease.

To have an intimate knowledge of the typing and clinical manifestation of primary cutaneous amyloidosis, how to diagnosis and heal the disease.

▪ Key concepts

A cellular deficiency of niacin leads to pellagra.

The classical triad of pellagra is dermatitis, diarrhea and dementia.

The cutaneous porphyrias are a group of disorders caused by defects in the biosynthesis of hemolysis, characterized by photosensitivity of the skin.

A diagnosis of cutaneous porphyrias can be made on clinical grounds and porphyrin analyses carried out in an experienced laboratory.

Acanthosis nigricans is a skin disorder characterized by dark, thick, velvety skin in body folds and creases.

Acanthosis nigricans is often associated with endocrine, malignant, familial, drug-induced and idiopathic.

Primary cutaneous amyloidosis is a skin disease where a substance called amyloid is deposited in the dermal papilla.

25. 1   Niacin Deficiency (Pellagra)

Pellagra is a chronic disease affecting the gastrointestinal tract, the nervous system, and the skin, resulting from a cellular deficiency of niacin.

25. 1. 1   Etiology

Niacin is required for adequate cellular function and metabolism as an essential component in coenzyme I and coenzyme II, which function in vital oxidation-reduction reactions. Primary pellagra results in a cellular deficiency of niacin, resulting from inadequate dietary nicotinic acid (niacin) and/or its precursor, the essential amino acid tryptophan. Secondary pellagra occurs when adequate quantities of niacin are present in the diet, but other diseases or conditions interfere with its intake, absorption and/or processing, such as prolonged diarrhea, anorexia nervosa, chronic alcoholism, and chronic colitis. In China pellagra today is only rarely encountered, mostly in subjects living on an unbalanced diet, such as chronic alcoholics and patients with gastrointestinal diseases or severe psychiatric disturbances.

25. 1. 2   Clinical Features

Early symptoms of pellagra include lassitude, weakness, loss of appetite, and psychiatric or emotional distress (anxiety, irritability and depression). The classical triad of pellagra is dermatitis, diarrhea and dementia. The symptoms do not have to appear in this order.

25. 1. 2. 1   Skin findings

Initially, there is erythema and swelling after sun exposure, accompanied by itching and burning or pain. In severe cases, the eruption may be vesicular or bullous. Exacerbation follows re-exposure to sunlight. After several phototoxic events, thickening, scaling, and hyperpigmentation of the affected skin occur. The lesions appear on areas exposed to sunlight, heat, friction or pressure (Color Figure 25 – 1).

Scrotal and perineal erythema and erosions are common. The mucous membranes of the mouth and vagina are affected by painful fissures, ulcerations, and atrophy.

25. 1. 2. 2   Gastrointestinal symptoms

Gastrointestinal disturbances include poor appetite, nausea, vomiting, epigastric discomfort, abdominal pain, diarrhea and increased salivation.

25. 1. 2. 3   Neurologic changes

In mild instances, the mental disturbance may pass unnoticed, patients perhaps being slightly depressed or apathetic. Sometimes, there is frank disorientation, restlessness and severe central nervous system symptoms. Peripheral neuritis and myelitis are occasionally encountered.

25. 1. 3   Diagnosis and Differential Diagnosis

Diagnosis is based on the patient's history and physical examination, with the former examining in detail information regarding the patient's diet. When this information points to niacin deficiency, replacement is started, and the diagnosis is then partly made by evaluating the patient's response to increased amounts of niacin. Pellagra should also be differentiated from drug eruptions, subacute lupus erythematosus, polymorphous light eruption, pemphigus vulgaris, and porphyria cutanea tarda.

25. 1. 4   Treatment

Dietary treatment to correct the malnutrition is essential. Animal proteins, eggs, milk, and vegetables are beneficial and should be supplemented with 100 mg nicotinamide four times daily. An improvement in the condition is to be expected within a day or two.

25. 2   The Cutaneous Porphyrias

The cutaneous porphyrias are a group of rare disorders caused by defects in the biosynthesis of hemolysis, characterized by photosensitivity of the skin. In this chapter, erythropoietic protoporphyria (EPP) and porphyria cutanea tarda (PCT) are mainly studied.

25. 2. 1   Etiology

The cutaneous porphyrias all result from a partial deficiency of one of the enzymes required for the biosynthesis of hemolysis. This causes accumulations of porphyrins, and their precursors. The photosensitivity in porphyria is caused by the absorption of ultraviolet radiation in the Soret band (408 nm) by increased porphyrins. The deficiency of the enzymes is either acquired or hereditary. EPP is caused by an inherited deficiency of ferrochelatase. PCT results from deficiency of uroporphyrinogen decarboxylase (UROD), which is either acquired or hereditary.

25. 2. 2   Clinical Features

Different type of porphyrias share similar features.

25. 2. 2. 1   Erythropoietic protoporphyria (EPP)

EPP typically presents early in childhood (2 to 5 years of age), but presentation late in adulthood can occur. Unique among the more commons of porphyria is an immediate burning of the skin on sun exposure. Erythema, edema and wheals can be seen. These lesions appear solely on sun-exposed areas. In severe attacks, purpuric lesions and crusted erosions or vesicles may occur. With repeated exposure, shallow linear or elliptical scars, waxy thickening of the skin have been described.

25.2.2.2 Porphyria cutanea tarda (PCT)

PCT is the most common type of porphyria, which represents a heterogeneous group of disorders that may be acquired (type I), or inherited (type II). Acquired PCT usually presents in the middle age while the inherited form can occur at a younger age. It is characterized by photosensitivity resulting in bullae, especially on light-exposed skin. The dorsal hands and forearms, ears, and face are primarily affected. In addition, fragility skin is usually complicated in affected areas, with minor trauma shearing the skin away to leave sharply marginated erosions. Hyperpigmentation, hypertrichosis and sclerodermatous thickenings are also seen (Color Figure 25 – 2). Liver disease is frequently present in patients with PCT.

25.2.3 Laboratory Test

In EPP, the protoporphyrin concentration in red cell, plasma, or faeces is increased. Most PCT patients have an increased urinary porphyrin concentration.

25.2.4 Histopathology

In all the cutaneous porphyrias, homogeneous material is seen within vessel walls of the upper dermal and papillary vascular plexus.

25.2.5 Diagnosis and Differential Diagnosis

A diagnosis of cutaneous porphyrias can be strongly suspected on clinical grounds. An accurate diagnosis can only be made on the basis of porphyrin analyses carried out in an experienced laboratory. The differential diagnosis of PCT include epidermolysis bullosa acquisita, Hutchinson's summer prurigo, drug-induced photosensitivity.

25.2.6 Treatment

General measures include photoprotection, the identification and avoidance of precipitating factors. For EPP, beta carotene, usually at a dose around 180 mg daily in adults (90 mg daily in children) provides some protection for most cases. Initial treatment of PCT involves removal of all environmental agents such as alcohol and medications. Phlebotomy of 500 ml at 2-week intervals is an effective form of treatment. Low-dose chloroquine, given in the dose of 125 mg twice a week, or hydroxychloroquine, 100 – 200 mg twice a week, is an alternative and recommended by some as a first-line treatment.

25.3 Acanthosis Nigricans

Acanthosis nigricans is a skin disorder characterized by dark, thick, velvety skin in body folds and creases. Most often, acanthosis nigricans affects the posterior and lateral folds of the neck, the axilla, groin, umbilicus, forehead, and other areas.

25.3.1 Etiology

The definitive cause for acanthosis nigricans has not yet been ascertained. It is often associated with endocrine(such as hypothyroidism or hyperthyroidism, acromegaly, polycystic ovary disease, insulin-resistant diabetes, or Cushing's disease), malignant and other causes such as familial, drug-induced and idiopathic.

25.3.2 Clinical Features

Acanthosis nigricans is characterized by symmetrical, hyperpigmented, velvety plaques that may occur in almost any location but most commonly appear on the intertriginous areas of the axilla, groin, and posterior neck. The posterior neck is the most commonly affected site in children.

Acrochordons(skin tags) are often found in and around the affected areas. Occasionally, lesions of acanthosis nigricans may be present on the mucous membranes of the oral cavity, nasal and laryngeal mucosa, and esophagus. The areola of the nipple may also be affected. Eye involvement, including papillomatous lesions on the eyelids and conjunctiva, may occur. Nail changes, such as leukonychia and hyperkeratosis, have been reported.

The lesions of malignant acanthosis nigricans are clinically indistinguishable from benign acanthosis nigricans.

According to the causes, acanthosis nigricans may be divided into the following types Type I: Acanthosis nigricans associated with malignancy;

Type Ⅱ: Familial acanthosis nigricans; Type Ⅲ: Acanthosis nigricans associated with obesity, insulin-resistant states, and endocrinopathy.

25. 3. 3 Laboratory Test
Histopathology: hyperkeratosis, papillomatosis, slight hyperpigmentation.

If the cause of acanthosis nigricans is unclear, blood tests, endoscopy, or X-rays may be necessary to look for possible underlying causes.

25. 3. 4 Diagnosis and Differential Diagnosis
Usually it can be diagnosed by simply looking at a patient's skin. A skin biopsy may be needed in unusual cases.

Acanthosis nigricans need differentiate from ichthyosis and other disorders of reticulated hyperpigmentation.

25. 3. 5 Treatment
There's no specific treatment for acanthosis nigricans. Losing excess pounds if you are overweight may cause the skin changes to fade. Retin-A creams, urea 20%, alpha hydroxy acids prescription can lighten the affected area. Oral isotretinoin or fish oil supplements may be useful. Treatment to just improve the appearance includes Retin-A, urea 20%, alpha hydroxy acids, and lactic or salicylic acid prescriptions.

25. 4 Primary Cutaneous Amyloidosis

Primary cutaneous amyloidosis is a disorder where a substance called amyloid is deposited in the skin resulting in discolored plaques or papules in the skin. No other body organs are involved.

25. 4. 1 Etiology
The etiology is not entirely clear, but it is known that the chemical origin of amyloid protein is the epidermal keratin. The epidermal cells get into the dermis and degenerate into amyloid deposition in the dermal papilla.

25. 4. 2 Clinical Features
It has been divided into two main patterns, macular amyloidosis and lichen amyloidosis, are seen, but other variants exist.

Macular amyloidosis is a cutaneous condition characterized by itchy, brown, rippled macules usually located on upper back, especially the interscapular region. Occasionally the thighs, arms (Color Figure 25 - 3, 25 - 4), shins, breasts, and buttocks may be involved. The lesions appear a "curly grain and pepper" show.

Lichen amyloidosis is a cutaneous condition characterized by the appearance of occasionally itchy lichenoid papules, typically appearing bilaterally on the shins, arms. And the back may be involved. The primary lesions appear small, discrete, brown, slightly scaly papules that group to form infiltrated large moniliform plaques.

25. 4. 3 Laboratory Test
Histopathology: Histologically, both forms of the main primary cutaneous amyloidosis is similar. The red amyloid deposition agglomerate can be seen in the dermal papilla. Congo red staining is positive.

25. 4. 4 Diagnosis and Differential Diagnosis
Diagnosis can be made according to clinical manifestations and histopathology. Macular amyloidosis should be differentiated from poikiloderma and dermatomyositis. And lichen amyloidosis should be differentiated from nodular prurigo, hypertrophic lichen planus, lichen simplex chronicus.

25. 4. 5 Treatment
There is no effective therapy. Local corticosteroid cream and 0. 1% tretinoin cream application may be useful. Injection of local lesions with triamcinolone can be used to lichen amyloidosis. Antihistamines should be applied to the pruritic patients.

■ Summary

Pronounced deficiency of niacin leads to pellagra, which is characterized by the classical triad: dermatitis, diarrhea and dementia. Have a dietary treatment and supplement with nicotinamide it is essential for pellagra treatment. The cutaneous porphyrias are a group of disorders caused by defects in the biosynthesis of hemolysis, characterized by photosensitivity of the skin. The porphyrias are diagnosed by identifying characteristic clinical and laboratory analyses. Photoprotection and symptomatic treatment are major measures. Acanthosis nigricans is a skin disorder that may begin at any age. It causes velvety, light-brown-to-black, markings usually on the neck, under the arms or in the groin. Acanthosis nigricans is most often associated with obesity, malignant and other causes. Primary cutaneous amyloidosis is a skin disease where a substance called amyloid is deposited in the dermal papilla. It has been divided into two main forms, macular amyloidosis and lichen amyloidosis. Diagnosis can be made according to clinical manifestations and histopathology. There is no effective therapy.

▪ Questions

1. Describe the classical triad of pellagra.

2. Describe the clinical feature of erythropoietic protoporphyria and porphyria cutanea tarda.

3. Describe the clinical features of acanthosis nigricans.

4. Describe the clinical features of primary cutaneous amyloidosis.

(**Zhusheng Yang** 杨竹生, **Wenbin Liu** 刘文斌)

Chapter 26

Tumors of the Skin

▪ Objectives

To master the clinical features of the benign tumors of the skin.

To have an intimate knowledge of the clinical and histopathology features of actinic keratosis.

To have an intimate knowledge of the clinical and histopathology features of Bowen's disease.

To have an intimate knowledge of the clinical and histopathology features of Paget's disease.

To master the clinical feature of basal cell carcinoma (BCC) and to have an intimate knowledge of the diagnosis and therapy.

To master the clinical feature of squamous cell carcinoma (SCC). And to have an intimate knowledge of the diagnosis and the therapy.

To master the clinical feature and histopathological changes of melanoma.

▪ Key concepts

Nevocellular nevus is one kind of benign tumor of melanocytes system, caused by proliferation of nevus cells.

Congenital blood vessels malformations and hemangioma, which are abnormal structures that result from errors in vascular development or benign proliferations of blood vessel endothelial tissue. The abnormality may result from a functional alteration or an anatomic malformation.

Nevus flammeus, named as well as "port wine stain (PWS)", is the most common type of vascular capillary malformation (CM), which composed of ectatic vessels in the papillary dermis. It is a slow-flow capillary malformation that is typically present at birth.

Venous malformations(VM)are slow-flow vascular malformations that are present at birth. They are not neoplasms but rather birthmarks composed of anomalous ectatic venous channels.

Infantile hemangiomas (IHs) is a diffuse proliferation of immature endothelial cells, followed by spontaneous regression.

The syringoma with individual small, translucent papules are skin-colored, yellowish, brownish, or pinkish, and 1 to 3 mm in diameter. Microscopically, the syringoma is characterized by dilated cystic sweat ducts, some of which have tail-like strand of cells projecting from one side of the duct into the stroma, giving a resemblance to a tadpole or comma. The lumina contain amorphous debris.

Milium is a benign tumor originated from epidermis or skin appendages. It can be divided into primary type and secondary type. Histopathologically, a small epidermal cyst is located in the dermis.

Both of keloids and hypertrophic scars are benign skin tumors originated from excessive connective tissue in dermis. The typical lesion is a firm, hypertrophic, pink or red plaque. The pathological features are the increased numbers of fibroblasts and the new growth of collagen.

Seborrheic keratosis is also called senile wart. It is a benign tumor composed of epidermal keratinocytes, more common in the elderly.

Actinic keratosis is a precancerous condition, with the feature of atypism of the epidermis.

Bowen's disease (BD) is an in situ squamous cell carcinoma (SCC).

Paget's disease is a rare cutaneous intraepithelial adenocarcinoma.

The most common and least serious skin cancer is the basal cell carcinoma(BCC) which typically appears as a shiny, small lump on sun-exposed skin. It may bleed, develop into a crust, seem to heal, and then bleed again. Although this kind of tumors is a slow growing, destructive skin tumor, it can become very large and penetrate deeply. Basal cell epithelioma or carcinoma usually occurs in persons over age 40; it's more prevalent in blond, fair skinned males and is the most common malignant tumor affecting the white race.

Squamous cell carcinoma (SCC) is the second most common form of nonmelanoma skin cancer following basal cell carcinoma.

Malignant melanoma is a malignant tumor raising from the melanocytes. Melanomas are classified into the following types: nodular, superficial spreading, acral lentiginous and lentigo maligna. All types of the lesions are blackish and vaguely margined.

Malignant melanoma tends to metastasize to other areas of the body such as the lungs and the bone via lymphatics and blood stream. Early diagnosis and surgical removal are essential. Other treatments are largely ineffective.

▪ Introduction

Tumors, whether malignant or benign, should be examined to determine the skin component from which they originate. The clinical features, course of progression, and prognosis differ according to the cells from which the tumor derives. Malignant skin tumors may derive from epidermal or follicular keratinocytes, intradermal mesenchymal cells, skin appendages such as sweat glands, or neural crest cells. Benign tumors may become malignant and have malignant diagnostic names. This chapter introduces benign and malignant tumors that have relatively high incidences.

26.1   Benign Tumors of the Skin

Cutaneous benign tumors are commonly seen. The ability to correctly diagnose and treat cutaneous benign tumors and to distinguish them from malignant lesions is a necessary skill. Diagnosis is usually based on the appearance of the lesions and the clinical history of the patient, the lesions should be biopsied for histopathologic examination to rule out a malignancy. Generally, excision is the main treatment of choice for the majority of cutaneous benign tumors, the other ones are often treated with laser therapy, electrodesiccation and so on. The following, we'll discuss deeply five types of cutaneous benign tumors.

Nevocellular nevus also known as pigmental nevus or melanocytic nevus, is a benign tumor of melanocytes system, caused by proliferation of nevus cells. Nevus cells are usually located in superficial dermis and look like melanocytes in appearance, but they are more similar to Schwann cells in deep dermis. In accordance with the views of Kawamura, nevus cells are derived from neural crests. The latter can produce pigment and is closely related to nerve fibers. The distribution of melanocytes in the skin can be reflected by their morphology. They are dendritic in the junction of epidermis and dermis, spherical in the upper dermis and spindle-shaped in the lower dermis. Nevus cells become nevus during the migration to the epidermis.

Congenital blood vessels malformations are rare disorders representing errors in vascular development. Hemangiomas are benign proliferations of blood vessel endothelial tissue. Now, we discuss the most common types, which are port wine stain (PWS), venous malformation (VM) and infantile hemangioma (IH).

Syringoma is more common in females than males and most likely to appear in adolescence. Familial patterns may occur.

Milium is a benign tumor originated from epidermis or skin appendages. It can occur in any age and there appear to be no gender bias. It can be divided into primary type and secondary type. The cause of primary type is unclear, usually, secondary milium occurs after a blistering disease, burn scarring or radiodermatitis.

Keloids and hypertrophic scars are benign skin tumors originated from excessive connective tissue in dermis. The typical pathological features are the increased numbers of fibroblasts and the new growth of collagen. It is comparatively difficult to be healed.

Seborrheic keratosis can occur on any body site, especially on the chest and back, face, neck, and the back of hands. The most common appearance is that of a very superficial verrucous plaque which appears to be stuck on the epidermis, varying from dirty yellow to black in color and having loosely adherent greasy keratin on the surface. If the lesion appears atypical, it is necessary to offer excision and biopsy.

26. 1. 1 Nevocellular Nevus

26. 1. 1. 1 Clinical features

The majority of nevus begins to appear in childhood or adolescence, appearing as macules, papules, papillary, verrucous, nodular or as polypoid. Nevus can be located in anywhere of the body and from a few millimeters to several centimeters in diameter, or even larger. The color of nevus is usually brown or black, but can be blue, purple or sometimes normal skin color.

Nevocellular nevus can be classified into junctional nevus, compound nevus and intradermal nevus according to the position of the nevus cells in the skin.

(1) Junctional nevus

Junctional nevus is a light to dark brown macule from a few millimeters to several centimeters in diameter. Generally, it has a smooth surface without hair, but can also be slightly elevated. They can ap-

pear on anywhere of the body including palms, soles and genitalia, there appear to be no gender bias(Color Figure 26 - 1).

(2) Compound nevus

Compound nevus is similar to junctional nevus in appearance, but may be slightly elevated(Color Figure 26 - 2).

(3) Intradermal nevus

Intradermal nevus is the most common type of nevus. It can also be found in anywhere of the body, but there is a predilection for head and neck, hardly appear in palms, soles and genitalia. Intradermal nevus always has a regular border and is a light to dark brown macule and varies in size from a few millimeters to several centimeters in diameter. The lesions are dome-shaped papules or nodules, but can be papillary or as polypoid. It maybe accompanied by terminal hair(Color Figure 26 - 3).

Usually, junctional nevus is smooth, compound nevus is slightly elevated, and intradermal nevus is dome-shaped, but can be papillary or polypoid. Histopathological examination is necessary if we cannot make sure in clinical.

26. 1. 1. 2 Histopathology

(1) Junctional nevus

The nevus cell nests exist in the lower epidermis or the bulge adjacent to the dermis, with a large amount of melanin. There is no inflammatory infiltration within the dermis except trauma and malignancy(Color Figure 26 - 4).

(2) Compound nevus

The histopathology of compound nevus is similar to that of junctional nevus, but nevus cell nests extend to the dermis. Nevus cells in the deeper dermis are spindle-shaped, with little or no pigment. There is hardly inflammatory infiltration within the dermis(Color Figure 26 - 5).

(3) Intradermal nevus

The nevus cell nests of intradermal nevus are located in dermis. There is an obvious normal region between nevus cell nests and epidermis. Nevus cells in the superior dermis contain a moderate amount of melanin, whereas in the deeper dermis, nevus cells are spindle-shaped without pigment. There is hardly inflammatory infiltration within the dermis(Color Figure 26 - 6).

26. 1. 1. 3 Diagnosis and differential diagnosis

The diagnosis of nevocellular nevus is not difficult to establish on the basis of history, typical symptoms and histopathological examination.

Nevocellular nevus should be differentiated from freckles, non-melanocytic lesions such as seborrheic keratosis, actinic keratosis, blue nevus, lentigo, malignant melanoma and so on, histopathological examination is important for differential diagnosis.

Any pigmented lesion in adult that is growing or changing in any way should be examined carefully.

26.1.1.4　Treatment

No treatment is required in most cases, surgical removal is the basic treatment if necessary. But even when the histopathological examination is benign, follow-up is necessary.

26.1.2　Congenital Blood Vessels Malformations and Hemangioma

Congenital blood vessels malformations and hemangioma, which are abnormal structures that result from errors in vascular development or benign proliferations of blood vessel endothelial tissue. The abnormality may result from a functional alteration or an anatomic malformation.

Vascular anomalies can be divided into two groups: vascular tumors and vascular malformations. Vascular tumors usually appear after birth; vascular malformations are usually present at birth. Vascular tumors include: ① hemangiomas, infantile type and congenital type (RICH: rapidly involuting congenital hemangioma; NICH: noninvoluting congenital hemangioma), ② Kaposiform hemangioendothelioma, ③ tufted angioma, ④ pyogenic granuloma and ⑤ spindle cell hemangioendothelioma. Vascular malformations include: ① capillary malformations: port wine stain (PWS) and telangiectasis, ② lymphatic malformations, ③ venous malformations, ④ arterial malformations and ⑤ combined malformations.

Now, we discuss the most common types, which are port wine stain (PWS), venous malformations (VM) and infantile hemangioma (IH).

26.1.2.1　Nevus flammeus

26.1.2.1.1　Introduction

Nevus flammeus, named as well as "port wine stain(PWS)", is the most common type of vascular capillary malformation (CM), which composed of ectatic vessels in the papillary dermis, Occurring in 0.3% of newborns and it may persist in at least 5% of the population. It is a slow-flow capillary malformation that is typically present at birth.

26.1.2.1.2　Clinical features

The lesions are usually unilateral and located on the face(glabella, eyelids, nose, and upper lip, Color Figure 26-7) and neck, although they may be widespread and involved as much as half the body. The mucous membrane of the mouth may be involved, appearing as well-defined red macular stains. They vary in color from pink to dark or bluish red. Although the surface of a nevus flammeus is usually smooth, small vascular nodular outgrowths or warty excrescences may be present or develop in the course of life. These lesions often become more bluish or purple with age; however, they sometimes become fainter but rarely disappear. Several reports document multiple basal cell carcinomas occurring in adult life over sites of long-standing nevus flammeus.

Port-wine stains are components of many rare congenital disorders. Clinical syndromes associated with nevus flammeus include: Sturge-Weber syndrome, Klippel-Trenaunay syndrome, Cobb's syndrome and so on. Such as the Beckwith-Wiedemann syndrome, which may comprise facial portwine stain, macroglossia, omphalocele, visceral hyperplasia, hemihypertrophy, and hypoglycemia.

26.1.2.1.3　Histopathology

There are dilated capillaries and ectasias that occupy the papillary dermis. When the lesion is raised or nodular, dilation appears not only in the superficial capillaries but also in some of the blood vessels in the deeper layers of the dermis and in the subcutaneous layer.

26.1.2.1.4　Diagnosis

Nevus Flammeus are diagnosed on the basis of their clinical appearance, appearing as well-defined pink or bluish red patches stains.

Histological features might be helpful.

26.1.2.1.5　Treatment

Currently, the pulsed dye laser (PDL) is the standard care for patients with port wine stains. The lasers used most commonly employ a wavelength that selectively targets oxyhemoglobin(585,595 nm) and results in intravascular coagulation, and a pulse duration that limits destruction and heat dissipation to the targeted vasculature without causing damage to the surrounding structures in the epidermis or dermis. Treatment on patients before school age is often desirable to reduce the psychological impact of a cosmetically significant congenital blood vessels malformation.

26.1.2.2　Venous malformation(VM)

VMs are slow-flow vascular malformations that are present at birth. They are not neoplasms but rather birthmarks composed of anomalous ectatic venous channels. The old term for this lesion was cavernous hemangioma.

26. 1. 2. 2. 1 Clinical features

They usually present as rounded, bright red or deep purple, spongy masses that enlarge when the affected area is in a dependent position or with physical activity. These lesions arise sporadically at all sites, including the mucous membranes, which occur frequently on the head and neck. Familial VMs can occur and are inherited in an autosomal dominant manner(Color Figure 26 - 8)

There are two rare conditions in which numerous venous malformations occur: Maffucci's syndrome and the blue rubber bleb nevus. Maffucci's syndrome shows the outstanding features in multiple vascular malformations with dyschondroplasia, resulting in defects in ossification. The blue rubber bleb nevus have a distinct appearance which most of them are protuberant, dark blue, soft, and compressible, occurring also in the oral mucosa, the gastrointestinal tract. They may subsequently increase in size and number.

26. 1. 2. 2. 2 Histopathology

VMs reveal in the deep dermis and subcutis with large, irregular spaces containing red blood cells and fibrinous material. The spaces are lined by a single layer of thin endothelium. Calcification of the walls and phlebolith-like calcific bodies in the lumina may be present.

26. 1. 2. 2. 3 Diagnosis and differential diagnosis

Diagnosis of VM is based on the clinical and histological features. MRI will help confirm the diagnosis of a VM and delineate the extent of involvement, as well as it can detect the developmental venous anomalies of the brain and may see more commonly in patients with head and neck VMs than in the general population. They should be identified and differentiated from true cerebral VMs because they do not lead to the complications associated with the latter. Sometimes, the breast lesions can be confused with angiosarcoma, according to histopathological characteristics, different diagnosis might be confirmed.

26. 1. 2. 2. 4 Treatment

The general goals of therapy are to prevent distortion of facial features, limit bony deformation, preserve function, and minimize painful swelling. VMs may be treated with surgical excision, sclerotherapy, or a combination of both.

26. 1. 2. 3 Infantile hemangioma

Infantile hemangioma (IH), also known as strawberry hemangioma, is its dramatic growth after birth, by diffuse proliferation of immature endothelial cells, followed by spontaneous regression. The growth and involution of infantile hemangioma is quite different from other vascular anomalies, which do not regress and can occur at any time during life.

26. 1. 2. 3. 1 Etiology

Risk factors include premature infants(especially if <1500 g in weight), Caucasian race, multiple gestation pregnancy and chorionic villous sampling. Girls are affected two to four times more often than boys.

26. 1. 2. 3. 2 Clinical features

Infantile hemangioma(IH) is a benign endothelial proliferation. The majority of IHs (80%) appear between 2 and 5 weeks of age.

These soft, raised, strawberry-red marks are actually tufts of extra blood vessels; they can be as small as a freckle or as large as a coaster (Color Figure 26 - 9). Seen mostly on the chest, upper back, and head, mucous membranes are involved in 10%.

40% of the lesions are associated with complications such as ulceration, bleeding, infection, pain, cardiac failure, airway compromise or eye impairment. There are clinical subtypes defined according to the depth of soft tissue involvement: superficial, deep, and mixed. The superficial type hemangioma has bright red-dish and bumpy appearance. The deep type can present with normal to bluish skin. Some types might ulcerate and appear hemorrhagic, and can demonstrate atrophic or hypertrophic scarring, hypopigmentation, telangiectasis and residual fatty tissue. On the other hand, up to 70%-90% of IHs might be disappear spontaneously at age 5 - 7years.

26. 1. 2. 3. 3 Histopathology

During their period of early growth, the histological features show considerable proliferation of their endothelial cells. Numerous normal mitotic figures and many perivascular mast cells are present. Intralesional nerves often show perineural and endoneural "pseudoinvasion". This feature is helpful for diagnosis, because it is very rarely present in other benign vascular tumors. In mature lesions, some of the capillary lumina may be greatly dilated, and the lining endothelial cells appear flatter.

26. 1. 2. 3. 4 Diagnosis and differential diagnosis

Diagnosis of IH can be confirmed by clinical and histological features. These soft, raised, strawberry-red marks are actually tufts of extra blood vessels. Numerous normal mitotic figures and many perivascular mast cells are present. Intralesional nerves often show perineural and endoneural "pseudoinvasion", according to these, different diagnosis with vascular malformations might be identified.

26. 1. 2. 3. 5   Treatment

In most cases, it is not necessary to immediate therapy because of the anticipated spontaneous regression of IHs. Treatment should be taken in cases of large lesions causing cosmetic disgustion, ulcerated lesions and lesions preventing normal feeding, respiration or vision.

X-ray therapy may be accepted, intralesional steroids (triamcinolone acetonide10 mg/ml administered every 4 weeks, not to exceed 3 - 5 mg/kg per treatment session), and oral steroids (1. 5 - 2 mg/kg per day of prednisone for 4 - 8 weeks) had been the treatment of choice for a long time. Sometimes, except for surgical excision, 585 nm or 595 nm pulsed dye laser (PDL) also can be used.

26. 1. 3   Syringoma

26. 1. 3. 1   Clinical features

It is more common in females than males and most likely to appear at adolescence. Familial patterns may occur. The individual small, translucent papules are skin-colored, yellowish, brownish, or pinkish, and 1 to 3 mm in diameter (Color Figure 26 - 10). The surface may be rounded or flat-topped. In most cases, they are multiple and tend to have a bilateral symmetry in distribution on the eyelids and upper cheeks. Other sites of involvement include the chest, forehead, abdomen, axilla, penis and vulva, and they may rarely be found in unilateral or linear groupings. They develop slowly and persist indefinitely without symptoms.

26. 1. 3. 2   Pathology

Microscopically, the syringoma is characterized by dilated cystic sweat ducts, some of which have tail-like strand of cells projecting from one side of the duct into the stroma, giving a resemblance to a tadpole or comma. The lumina contain amorphous debris. Strands of epithelial cells may occur independently of the ducts. Two rows of epithelial cells usually line the duct walls (Color Figure 26 - 11).

26. 1. 3. 3   Diagnosis and differential diagnosis

With the typical symptoms and characteristic histopathology, diagnosis of syringoma can be confirmed. It is most likely to be confused with tricho-

epithelioma on the face, xanthelasma on the lids, or disseminated granuloma annulare on the trunk.

26. 1. 3. 4   Treatment

The main reason for treatment is cosmetic. Careful destruction with electrodesiccation, laser ablation, or cryotherapy with liquid nitrogen may help.

26. 1. 4   Milium

26. 1. 4. 1   Clinical features

Milium is more common in women. A small, firm, white to yellowish-white papule of 1mm to 2mm in diameters occurs immediately below the epidermis. Primary milium occurs most frequently on the eyelids, followed by the cheeks, penis and labia. Secondary milium occurs on the ear, back of the hand, forearm and traumatic skin. White keratinous contents are discharged by incision (Color Figure 26 -12).

26. 1. 4. 2   Histopathology

A small epidermal cyst is located in the dermis.

26. 1. 4. 3   Diagnosis and differential diagnosis

Diagnosis of milium depends on the typical symptoms and histopathological examination. Milium should be differentiated from syringoma, acne and so on, histopathological examination is important for differential diagnosis.

26. 1. 4. 4   Treatment

No treatment is required in most cases. A small incision using a scalpel, or a puncture with a hypodermic needle is conducted to remove the spherical white substance.

26. 1. 5   Scars (Keloids and Hypertrophic Scars)

26. 1. 5. 1   Etiology

The cause is unknown. Trauma is usually the immediate causative factor, but this induces scars only in those with a predisposition for its development. Some races, notably Afro-Caribbeans, are more prone to develop keloids than others. A positive family history is obtained in 5% - 10% of Europeans with keloids, particularly severe lesions.

26. 1. 5. 2   Clinical features

The most common location of keloids is the sterna region, while the neck, ears, or trunk are frequently involved. A scar at any site has the potential to become hypertrophic. The early, the lesion is a small, firm, pink or red papule, and grow slowly, then become round or irregular, thickened, hypertrophic and smooth plaque (Color Figure 26 - 13). A keloid often sends out clawlike prolongations while a hypertrophic scar remains confined to the initial injury. The former is often irritable and hypersensitive, and sometimes exquisitely tender, and tends to regress after several years. The latter shows signs of regression after a few months(Color Figure 26 - 14).

26. 1. 5. 3   Pathology

The epidermis is normal, or thinned by the underlying lesion. In the early stages, keloids and hypertrophic scars exhibit increased cellularity (Color Figure 26 - 15). In keloids, there is a dense and sharply defined new growth of myofibroblasts and collagen in the dermis with a whorl-like arrangement of hyalinized bundles of collagenous fibers. In hypertrophic scars, the new collagen bundles in the dermis lie parallel to the epidermis. Mucinous material is deposited focally in keloids but not in hypertrophic scars.

26. 1. 5. 4   Diagnosis and differential diagnosis

With the typical symptoms and characteristic histopathology, diagnosis of scars can be confirmed. For keloids and hypertrophic scars, the most pronounced distinction is the clawlike projections of the former that are absent in the latter. Lesions which can cause diagnostic difficulty include sclerotic basal cell carcinoma, scar sarcoid or dermatofibrosarcoma.

26. 1. 5. 5   Treatment

It is comparatively difficult to cure keloids. When the keloid is young, radiotherapy including superficial X-rays can be chosen. Intralesional injection of glucocorticoid is frequently sufficient, but local atrophy should be avoided. The surgical removal by excision cooperated with local injection of glucocorticoid and X-rays radiotherapy, can be effective. Laser treatments have a high recurrence rate.

26. 1. 6   *Seborrheic Keratosis*

26. 1. 6. 1   Etiology

The cause is unknown. Multiple seborrheic keratoses may be a familial trait. Solarization and chronic inflammatory stimulation may relate to it. It can occur as a manifestation of visceral malignancy, usually cancer of the gastrointestinal tract. This is known as the sign of Leser - Trélat.

26. 1. 6. 2   Clinical features

Seborrheic keratoses occur on any body site, especially on the chest and back, face, neck, and the back of hand. They are multiple, oval, slightly raised, light brown to black, sharply demarcated papules or plaques, rarely more than 3 cm in diameter. The most common appearance is that of a very superficial verrucous plaque which appears to be stuck on the epidermis, varying from dirty yellow to black in color and having loosely adherent greasy keratin on the surface (Color Figure 26 - 16). On the hand and face, seborrheic keratoses may remain superficial for a long period, and can be mistaken for melanocytic lesions. They are usually asymptomatic but may be itchy.

They may increase in number over the years, and some elderly patients have very large numbers. There rarely is malignancy in them.

26. 1. 6. 3   Pathology

The essential change is an accumulation of normal keratinocytes between the basal layer and the keratinizing surface of the epidermis. There exist six histologic types: hyperkeratotic, acanthotic, adenoid or reticulated, clonal, irritated, and melanoacanthoma. The common histologic characteristics of the six types include hyperkeratosis, acanthosis, papillomatosis and small horn pseudocyst (Color Figure 26 - 17). There is usually some inflammatory reaction in the dermis.

26. 1. 6. 4   Diagnosis and differential diagnosis

With the typical symptoms and characteristic histopathology, diagnosis of Seborrheic keratoses can be confirmed. Lesions which can cause diagnostic difficulty include AK, melanocytic nevus, malignant melanoma, pigmented BCC or SCC.

26. 1. 6. 5   Treatment

Usually seborrheic keratoses don't need therapy. Satisfactory results can be obtained by freezing with liquid nitrogen, or cauterizing with CO_2 laser. If the lesion appears atypical, it is necessary to offer excision and biopsy.

26. 2   Precancerous Dermatosis

26. 2. 1   *Actinic Keratosis*

Synonyms: Senile keratosis, solar keratosis.

26. 2. 1. 1   Introduction

UV exposure induces keratinocytic atypia, particularly in the basal cell layer. The atypical keratinocytes proliferate in the epidermis. It is the early stage of squamous cell carcinoma in situ.

Asymptomatic, vaguely margined erythema or keratotic lesions accompanied with scaling and crusting occur in the elderly, on sun-exposed sites of the body.

Horn-like protrusions (cutaneous horns) form in cases with marked keratinization. Cryotherapy, excision and topical anti-cancer agents are the main treatments.

26.2.1.2 Clinical features

A light-pink erythematous plaque several millimeters to 1 cm in diameter occurs on sun-exposed areas of the body, such as the face or dorsal hand. The plaque is covered with scales and crusts (Color Figure 26 – 18). The margin of the plaque is often vague. Keratinization is usually intense. Grayish-white keratotic nodules or horn-like protrusions (cutaneous horns) may form. The skin lesion occurs singly or multiply, most frequently in persons over age 60. Nearly all elderly Caucasians are affected. Actinic keratosis occurs in infancy in patients with xeroderma pigmentosum.

26.2.1.3 Pathogenesis

Epidermal keratinocytes that are damaged by UV proliferate abnormally in the dermis.

26.2.1.4 Histopathology

There are three histological types of actinic keratosis. Malignant changes are localized in the covering epidermis and follicular and sweat pore regions remain normal. Atypism is found in the lower epidermal basal layer(Color Figure 26 – 19).

26.2.1.5 Diagnosis, Differential diagnosis

Skin biopsy is conducted when it is difficult to differentiate actinic keratosis from seborrheic keratosis and senile lentigo.

26.2.1.6 Treatment

The main treatments are surgical removal, cryotherapy and topical application of anticancer agents such as 5-FU and bleomycin.

26.2.1.7 Prognosis

Some cases progress to squamous cell carcinoma. Aggravation and enlargement of the peripheral erythema and rapid enlargement of ulcers often indicate progression of actinic keratosis.

26.3 Malignant Tumors of the Skin

26.3.1 Bowen's Disease

Bowen's disease (BD) is an in situ squamous cell carcinoma (SCC) which was first described in 1912 by JT Bowen and it has the potential to progress to invasive carcinoma. BD is very common in the Caucasian population with an incidence of 1. 42 per 1000 in some populations.

26.3.1.1 Etiology

Several etiological factors of BD have been re-

ported, such as irradiation (ultraviolet irradiation, radiotherapy, photochemotherapy), carcinogens (e. g. arsenic), immunosuppression (e. g. after organ transplantation, AIDS), viral (strong association of perianal and genital lesions with HPV; 47% of acral and 24% of nonacral extragenital BD contain HPV genome) and some others like chronic injury or dermatosis.

26.3.1.2 Clinical features

Clinically a typical BD is a slowly enlarging erythematous patch or plaque which is well demarcated and has a scaling or crusted surface. In some cases it can be pigmented or verrucous. It is commonly located on the lower limbs and on the head and neck. But BD is also seen subungual or periungual, palmar, genital and perianal. Usually BD is a solitary lesion, but in 10% to 20% it occurs at multiple sites. The risk of progression into an invasive carcinoma is 3% to 5% in extragenital lesions and about 10% in genital lesions.

26.3.1.3 Histopathology

Histological examination revealed full-thickness involvement of the epidermis by atypical keratinocytes. There was acanthosis with thickening of the rete ridge, overlying parakeratosis and hyperkeratosis. The dermis shows no invasion of tumor cells and it sometimes contains a dense infiltrate of lymphocytes or histiocytes.

26.3.1.4 Differential diagnosis

The differential diagnosis of Bowen's disease includes seborrheic keratosis, actinic kerclinical and basal cell carcinoma, bowenoid papulosis. These diseases can be differentiated on the basis of their clinical features and histopathological findings.

26.3.1.5 Treatment

The choice of treatment should be guided by efficacy, location and size of BD, number of lesions, availability of the therapy, the clinicians' expertise, patients' factors (age, immune status, concomitant medication, comorbidities and compliance), cosmetic outcome and the patients' preference.

The different treatment options for BD are cryotherapy, curettage with cautery, excision, 5-fluorouracil (5-FU), radiotherapy, laser, photodynamic therapy (PDT), imiquimod and some other therapies that were described in some case reports or small numbers of patients.

26.3.2 Paget's Disease

Paget's disease is a rare cutaneous intraepithelial

adenocarcinoma involving primarily the epidermis but occasionally extending into the underlying dermis. Paget's disease is divided mammary Paget's disease and extramammary Paget's disease. Mammary Paget's disease was first described by James Paget in1874. Extramammary Paget's disease was originally described in 1889 by Crocker.

26. 3. 2. 1　Etiology

The prevailing view is that most, if not all, cases of mammary Paget's disease originate from in situ or invasive ductal carcinoma in the underlying breast tissue. The origin of extramammary Paget's disease is less well defined, and the findings in mammary Paget's disease were initially extrapolated in an attempt to explain the development of the extramammary form. It was therefore proposed that all cases of extramammary Paget's disease arose as epidermotropic spread from an in situ or invasive neoplasm arising in an adnexal gland within the dermis, analogous to mammary Paget's disease arising from ductal carcinoma in situ.

26. 3. 2. 2　Clinical features

Mammary Paget's disease occurs exclusively on the nipple/areola complex from where it may spread on to surrounding skin. The clinical appearance is usually a demarcated, thickened, eczematoid, erythematous sweeping or crusted lesion with irregular borders. Nipple discharge and ulceration may occur. An associated breast tumor may be palpable. A small proportion of cases of mammary Paget's disease are clinically occult and only detected histologically when a representative section of the nipple and areola is submitted from a mastectomy.

The most common presenting symptom of extramammary Paget's disease is pruritus. The clinical appearance is similar to mammary Paget's disease. Lesions occasionally show hyperpigmentation or hypopigmentation. In the anogenital region atypical appearances occur; ulceration or areas of leukoplakia have been reported. Extramammary Paget's disease is a slow growing tumor and the appearances of long standing lesions may be modified by repeated traumatisation/excoriation or superimposed infection. An associated tumor may be palpable. The features can be so non specific that misdiagnosis as an inflammatory or infective skin condition (eczema, psoriasis, moniliasis) is common, and lesions may be advanced before appropriate treatment is instigated.

26. 3. 2. 3　Histopathology

The histopathological findings are similar in mammary and extramammary Paget's disease. Paget's cells are large cells with abundant basophilic or amphophilic, finely granular cytoplasm, which tend to stand out in contrast to the surrounding epithelial cells. On close inspection the nucleus is usually large, centrally situated, and sometimes contains a prominent nucleolus. Pronounced nuclear atypia and pleomorphism are present. Signet ring cells might be present in small numbers and mitotic figures are frequent. The Paget's cells might be dispersed singly or form clusters, glandular structures, or solid nests. There may be infiltration into upper strata of the epidermis, but most cells are concentrated in the lower portion, often being observed in the pilosebaceous apparatus. Cells might be presenting sweat gland ducts, leading to confusion as to whether the lesion has arisen within the epidermis or has spread from a local apocrine neoplasm. A dense inflammatory infiltrate is often seen associated with the epidermal malignancy.

26. 3. 2. 4　Differential diagnosis

Differential clinical diagnoses include generalized inflammatory skin conditions such as eczema and psoriasis, as well as erosive adenomatosis, a condition specific to the nipple.

26. 3. 2. 5　Treatment

Surgical excision with margins and radiotherapy has been shown efficacious in treating Paget's disease of the nipple. Mastectomy may be required.

There are scattered Paget's cells with large, clear cytoplasm.

26. 3. 3　Basal Cell Epithelioma (Carcinoma)

26. 3. 3. 1　Etiology

Prolonged sun exposure is the most common cause of basal cell epithelioma, but arsenic ingestion, radiation exposure, burns, immunosuppression and, rarely, vaccinations are other possible causes. Although the pathogenesis of basal cell epithelioma is uncertain, some experts now hypothesize that it originates when, under certain conditions, undifferentiated basal cells become carcinomatous instead of differentiating into sweat glands, sebum, and hair.

26. 3. 3. 2　Clinical features

Three types of basal cell epithelioma occur:

(1) Noduloulcerative lesions occur most often on the face, particularly the forehead, eyelid margins, and nasolabial folds. In early stages, these lesions are small, smooth, pinkish, and translucent papules. Telangiectatic vessels cross the surface, and

the lesions are occasionally pigmented. As the lesions enlarge, their centers become depressed and their borders become firm and elevated. Ulceration and local invasion eventually occur. These ulcerated tumors, known as "rodent ulcers," rarely metastasize; however, if untreated, they can spread to vital areas and become infected. If they invade large blood vessels, they can cause massive hemorrhage. Characteristic of noduloulcerative BCE:

1) Early stage lesions: Small, smooth pinkish translucent popular lesions with telangiectatic vessels on the surface and occasionally pigmentation.

2) Late stage lesions: enlarged, center depressed, borders firm and elevated, eventually ulcerating and becoming locally invasive.

3) "Rodent ulcers": ulcerated tumors, which rarely spread. These occur if late-stage lesions are not treated. They can spread, if untreated, to vital areas and become infected or cause massive hemorrhage if they invade large blood vessels

(2) Superficial basal cell epitheliomas are often numerous and commonly occur on the chest and back. They're oval or irregularly shaped, lightly pigmented plaques, with sharply defined, slightly elevated threadlike borders. Because of superficial erosion, these lesions appear scaly and have small, atrophic areas in the center that resemble psoriasis or eczema. They're usually chronic and don't tend to invade other areas. Superficial basal cell epitheliomas are related to ingestion of or exposure to arsenic containing compounds.

Characteristic of superficial BCE: Oval shaped, light-colored plaques with sharply defined, slightly elevated threadlike borders. Scaly, with small atrophicareas in the center that resemble psoriasis or eczema. Usually chronic and noninvasive

(3) Sclerosing basal cell epitheliomas (morphealike epitheliomas) is the most difficult to diagnose, and is prone to recur after apparently adequate surgery. They look like a skin-colored, rather waxy, thickened scar.

Waxy, sclerotic, yellow to white plaques without distinct borders. Often resemble small patches of scleroderma.

26.3.3.3　Diagnosis and differential diagnosis

All types of basal cell epitheliomas are diagnosed by clinical appearance, an incisional or excisional biopsy, and histologic study.

26.3.3.4　Treatment

Depending on the size, location, and depth of the lesion, treatment may include curettage and electrodesiccation, chemotherapy, surgical excision, irritation, cryotherapy, or chemosurgery.

(1) Curettage and electrodesiccation offer good cosmetic results for small lesions.

(2) Shave, curettage, and cautery (and other types of minor surgery). Many small, well defined nodular or superficial BCCs can be successfully removed by removing just the top layers of the skin. The wound usually heals within a few weeks without needing stitches. Topical fluorouracil is often used for superficial lesions. This medication produces marked local irritation or inflammation in the involved tissue but no systemic effects.

(3) Microscopically controlled surgical excision carefully removes recurrent lesions until a tumor-free plane is achieved. After removal of large lesions, kill grafting may be required.

(4) Irradiation is used if the tumor location requires it and for elderly or debilitated patients who might not withstand surgery.

(5) Cryotherapy with liquid nitrogen freezes and kills the cells.

(6) Chemosurgery is often necessary for persistent or recurrent lesions. Chemosurgery consists of periodic applications of a fixative paste (such as zinc chloride) and subsequent removal of fixed pathologic tissue. Treatment continues until tumor removal is complete.

(7) Imiquimod cream. This is applied to superficial BCCs three to five times each week (Monday to Friday) for six to sixteen weeks. The imiquimod results in an inflammatory reaction, maximal at three weeks. Up to 85% of suitable BCCs disappear, with minimal scarring.

26.3.3.5　Prevention

People who have had a basal cell carcinoma should have a skin exam every six months to one year.

Advise the patient to relieve local inflammation from topical fluorouracil with cool compresses or corticosteroid ointment.

Sun exposure and sunbathing produce gradual skin damage even if sunburn is avoided. Ten to forty years can pass between the time of sun exposure and the development of skin cancer.

Instruct the patient to eat frequent small meals that are high in protein. Suggest eggnog, pureed foods, or liquid protein supplements if the lesion has invaded the oral cavity and caused eating problems.

BCC cells arrange in a palisading pattern, the

cells have a large oval nucleus, a small amount of cytoplasm, and low atypicality.

26. 3. 4　Squamous Cell Carcinoma

Squamous cell carcinoma (SCC) is the second most common form of nonmelanoma skin cancers following basal cell carcinoma. Together with basal cell carcinoma, the most common skin cancer, it is referred to as nonmelanoma skin cancer. Squamous cell carcinoma rarely causes further problems when caught and treated early. Untreated, squamous cell carcinoma can grow large or spread to other parts of your body, causing serious complications.

26. 3. 4. 1　Etiology

Most cases of SCC will be caused by exposure to the sun's harmful ultraviolet (UV) rays. The risk of developing SCC increases when a person also has one or more of these risk factors:

(1) Fair skin.

(2) Blonde or red hair; blue or green eyes.

(3) History of indoor tanning.

(4) Diagnosed with actinic keratoses (AKs).

(5) Family history of skin cancer.

(6) Weakened immune system (immunosuppression).

(7) Received radiation therapy.

(8) History of exposure to coal tar products or arsenic.

The risk of developing SCC also increases with age because each exposure to harmful UV rays causes more damage to the skin. As this damage accumulates, the risk of developing skin cancer grows.

26. 3. 4. 2　Clinical features

The main symptom of squamous cell skin cancer is a growing bump that may have a rough, scaly surface and flat reddish patches.

The bump is usually located on the face, ears, neck, hands, or arms, but may occur on other areas. A sore that does not heal can be a sign of squamous cell cancer. Any change in an existing wart, mole, or other skin lesion could be a sign of skin cancer(Color Figure 26 - 26, 26 - 27).

26. 3. 4. 3　Diagnosis and treatment

Before SCC can be treated, the diagnosis must be confirmed with a biopsy(Color Figure 26 - 28). This simple procedure can be performed in the office and involves removing a small amount of tissue so that it can be examined under a microscope. If the diagnosis is SCC, a variety of surgical and non-surgical treatment options are available. The dermatologist will choose an appropriate treatment after considering the location of the tumor, size, microscopic characteristics, health of the patient, and other factors.

Most treatment options are relatively minor, office-based procedures that require only local anesthesia. These include:

(1) Simple surgical excision

Removes the cancer and some of the surrounding healthy tissue. The removed specimen is examined under a microscope to determine if all of the skin cancer has been removed.

(2) Mohs micrographic surgery

Performed by a specially trained dermatologic surgeon, Mohs allows the surgeon to spare as much normal skin as possible while simultaneously removing the cancer.

(3) Electrodesiccation and curettage

Removes the cancerous tumor by scraping (curetting) it off. The base of the tumor is burned (cauterized) with an electric needle (electrodesiccation).

(4) Cryosurgery

Removes the tumor by freezing it with liquid nitrogen.

(5) Radiation therapy

Damages or kills the cancerous cells with high-energy X-rays, which also help to prevent continued growth.

(6) Topical therapy

Medications such as imiquimod and 5-fluorouracil can be applied at home to treat the cancer.

Squamous cell carcinoma demonstrates invasive cancer with atypical keratinocytes

26. 3. 5　Malignant Melanoma

Melanoma is a malignant tumor of melanocytes. It begins when melanocytes change and grow uncontrollably. Melanocytes located predominantly in the skin, but also be found in the eyes, ears, GI tract, leptomeninges, and oral and genital mucous membranes. Melanoma is one of the less common types of skin cancers. However, it causes the greatest number of skin cancer—related deaths worldwide.

26. 3. 5. 1　Etiology and pathogenesis

The etiology and pathogenesis of melanoma are unknown. The epidemiologic studies reveal that exposure to solar radiation is the major cause of melanoma. Melanoma is a greater problem in light-skinned whites (skin types I and II), and sunburns during childhood and intermittent burning exposure seem to have a higher impact than cumulative UV exposure over time. Other predisposing and risk factors are the presence of precursor lesions (atypical melanocytic nevi and congenital melanocytic nevi) and a family history of melanoma.

Epidemiologic studies demonstrate a role for genetic predisposition and sun exposure in melanoma development. The major gene involved in melanoma development resides on chromosome 9p21. This gene, known as CDKN2A, encodes two separate gene products that are negative regulators of cell cycle progression.

26.3.5.2 Clinical features

Melanoma is classified by clinical features and pathology into superficial spreading, nodular, acral lentiginous, and lentigo malignant melanoma. All types begin as horizontal proliferation of tumor cells in the epidermis. At this phase, a dark brown or black patch is clinically observed. After the patch enlarges to a certain size, the tumor cells begin to proliferate vertically. The patch partially elevates and forms a black nodule, erosion and ulcer. When the patch infiltrates beyond the dermis, the risk of metastasis sharply increases. Metastasis is lymphatic in most cases; satellite lesions form around the primary location and metastasize to the regional lymph nodes, resulting in distant metastasis. Melanomas occur not only in skin, but also in the eyeballs, oral cavity and nasal mucosa. Melanocytes continue to produce melanin after they become malignant; the skin lesion in most cases becomes blackish brown.

There are five characteristic clinical features of melanoma, whose initials read ABCDE, which are as follows:

A: Asymmetry.

B: Borderline irregularity.

C: Color variegation.

D: Diameter enlargement (over 6 mm).

E: Elevation of surface.

In rare cases, melanoma cells lack melanin production. This is called amelanotic melanoma and has an even worse prognosis.

(1) Nodular melanoma (NM)

A dome-shaped nodular lesion occurs, often accompanied with ulceration. They are sharply delimited nodules with a variable degree of pigmentation ranging from black to light brown or totally amelanotic. In the last instance they may be red and mistaken for hemangiomas. They start as papules that grow rapidly and ulcerate. Occasionally they may be pedunculated. Only about 10% of all melanomas are

nodular but they have the highest mortality rates.

(2) Superficial spreading melanoma (SSM)

It is the most common type of melanoma, perhaps as many as 70% of all melanomas fall in this category. It is seen more often on the upper back and legs of young to middle age men and women. The lesions are usually over 1cm in diameter and present as an irregular macule with different shades of color, ranging from black to brown, red, pink and white. The variegation indicates regression. If a nodule can be palpated invasion may be suspected. This tumor may grow in the area of a previously existing nevus.

(3) Acral lentiginous melanoma (ALM)

This type of melanoma is found on the palms, soles, nail matrix and mucous membranes. It is the most common type of melanomas in orientals, blacks, and other individuals with darker skin. It usually has a poor prognosis(Color Figure 26 – 29).

(4) Lentigo maligna melanoma (LMM)

A blackish-brown spot first appears. Usually seen on the face of older patients, it can be seen also on the arms and upper trunk. It presents as an irregularly shaped, highly pigmented macule that enlarges gradually to reach a diameter often in excess of 3 or 4 cm. If regression has taken place, the appearance is mottled, with different shades of brown, red, black and even depigmentation.

26.3.5.3 Histopathology

The atypical melanocytes of melanoma in situ are confined to the epidermis. These atypical melanocytes are in a variety of morphology, and the infiltrate is dispersed or clustered. There is a distinct inflammatory response consisting of patchy aggregations of lymphocytes and melanophages within the papillary dermis(Color Figure 26 – 30A).

Malignant melanoma usually occurs in the epidermal-dermal junction, the tumor cells can invade downward into the dermis. The atypical melanocytes infiltrate as nests or diffusely in the dermis and adipose layer. These atypical melanocytes vary in shape and size, and the majority of the tumor cells are spindle-shaped and epithelioid. They have atypical hyperchromatic nuclei, large nucleoli and abundant cytoplasm. Mitoses are easily found. Immunohistochemically, the atypical melanocytes express S100 protein, HMB-45 and Mart-1(Color Figure 26 – 30B and C).

26.3.5.4 Diagnosis and differential diagnosis

The diagnosis of MM can be established according to the clinical features and histopathological changes, but it is almost always necessary to do an immunohistochemical staining.

A wide variety of skin should be differentiated from MM. Junctional nevus is a light to dark brown macule or maculopapule, several millimeters in diameter. It has a regular border, a smooth surface without hair. However, MM is usually > 6 mm in diameter, with irregular border, and change in the appearance, symptoms such as pain, pruritus, bleeding, crusting and so on. Seborrheic keratoses are multiple, oval, slightly raised, light brown to black, sharply demarcated papules or plaques. It is a hyperplasia of the epidermis and without atypical melanocytes.

26. 3. 5. 5   Treatment

Treatments are chosen according to the stage of melanoma. If the tumor is shallower than 2 mm, it should be removed with a 1cm margin. When the tumor is thicker than 2 mm, total resection with 2 cm margin should be conducted. Dissection of the regional lymph node and amputation of fingers, toes or other extremities may be conducted. In recent years, sentinel node biopsy has been frequently conducted to measure the necessary range of surgery.

In progressive cases with distant metastasis, surgery is rarely performed; instead, chemotherapy, radiation therapy and immunotherapy are conducted. Interferon may also be used. The patient responds to chemotherapy in fewer than 30% of cases.

▪ Summary

"Nevus" is Latin for "maternal impression" or "birthmark". It denotes a circumscribed, non-neoplastic skin or mucosal lesion. The term is qualified according to the cell or tissue of origin. Nevi may be caused by hereditary or embryologic factors and may appear at any time in life (Unna, 1894). They progress extremely slowly.

Examination of a skin tumor is for determination not only of malignancy or benignancy but also of the skin component from which the tumor derives.

A tumor may originate from epidermal keratinocytes, from cells of appendages such as those in sweat glands, or from neural crest cells or mesenchymal cells. The epidemiology, pathology and course of tumors vary depending on the origin of the cells. Benign tumors may become malignant and have malignant diagnostic names.

▪ Questions

1. What is the clinical feature of nevocellular nevus and how to diagnose and treat it?

2. Briefly describe the clinical characteristics of nevus flammeus.

3. How to diagnose and treat the nevus flammeus?

4. What are the clinical features of venous malformation and how to diagnose and treat it?

5. Briefly describe the clinical characteristics of infantile hemangioma.

6. How to diagnose and treat the infantile hemangioma?

7. Describe the clinical and pathological features of syringoma.

8. What is the clinical feature of milium and how to diagnose and treat it?

9. Describe the clinical and pathological features of scars.

10. What are the clinical and pathological features of Seborrheic keratoses?

11. What are the typical pathological changes of actinic keratosis?

12. Describe the clinical feature of BCC.

13. Describe the treatment options of SCC.

14. Describe the histopathological changes of melanoma

15. Describe the characteristic clinical features of melanoma

(**Dong Lan** 兰东, **Fang Liu** 刘方,
Xiuying Zhang 张秀英, **Yanling He** 何焱玲)

Chapter

27

Sexually Transmitted Diseases

▪ Objectives

To master the knowledge of clinical manifestations, diagnosis and treatment of syphilis and gonorrhea.

To grasp the preliminary knowledge about genital chlamydial trachomatis infection, condyloma acuminatum, genital herpes and AIDS.

▪ Key concepts

Syphilis is one of the chronic sexually transmitted disease caused by *Treponema pallidum* subspecies pallidum. It is a multistage disease with diverse and wide-ranging manifestations.

Gonorrhea is caused by *Neisseria gonorrhoeae*, and mainly manifested as the genitourinary suppurative infection.

Chlamydial trachomatis genital infection is often responsible for urethritis and cervicitis in sexually active adults and may result in serious sequelae such as epididymitis in males, and pelvic inflammatory disease (PID), ectopic pregnancy and sterility in females.

Condyloma acuminatum (CA), also known as genital warts, is a sexually transmitted disease caused by the human papillomavirus (HPV), and mainly spread through skin-to-skin contact during sexual activity and mostly often occur in the external genitalia, anus and other parts.

Genital herpes (GH) is a herpes simplex virus infection in the genital and perianal mucocutaneous sites. It is a chronic recurrent sexually transmitted disease and difficult to be cured. Genital herpes is more commonly caused by herpes simplex virus type 2 (HSV-2) infection.

Acquired immunodeficiency syndrome (AIDS) is caused by the human immunodeficiency virus (HIV). HIV infects the human CD4$^+$ T lymphocytes and kills them. Although there is so far no treatment available to cure people with HIV or AIDS, HAART (highly active antiretroviral therapy) is very effect to suppress the viral replication, restore the immune system and prolong their life.

Chancroid is a sexually transmitted disease caused by the Gram-negative streptobacillus *Haemophilus ducreyi* and characterized by painful genital ulcers and painful inguinal lymphadenopathy.

Lymphogranuloma venereum (LGV) is a sexually transmitted disease caused by Chlamydia Trachomatis.

▪ Introduction

Sexually transmitted diseases (STDs) refer to a group of contagious diseases and mainly spread through sexual contact and indirect way. They are not only involved in urogenital organs, but also infect the local lymph nodes, or even cause systemic infection through blood spread. STDs have become serious social problems and public health issues.

27.1　STDs General Introduction

27.1.1　Pathogen

The sexually transmitted diseases (STDs) are common and present serious health problem. The classic STDs include syphilis, gonorrhea, chancroid, condyloma accuminatum (CA), genital herpes, lymphogranuloma venereum (LGV), nongonococcal urethritis (NGU), and general STDs' pathogens include the following forms (Table 27 – 1).

Table 27 – 1　The general STDs' pathogens

Pathogens		Diseases
Viruses	Herpes simplex virus (HSV)	Herpes genitalis (HSV-1,2)
	Human papilloma virus	Condyloma acuminatum
	Human immunodeficiency virus (HIV)	Acquired immune deficiency syndrome (AIDS)
	Cytomegalovirus (CMV)	Genital CMV infection
	Hepatitis B virus (HBV)	Hepatitis B
	Hepatitis C virus (HCV)	Hepatitis C
	Molluscum contagiosum virus	Genital smolluscum contagiosum
Chlamydia	*Chlamydia trachomatis* (CT)	Cervicitis/urethritis (D – K)
		Lymphogranuloma venereum; (L)
Mycoplasma	*Ureaplasma urealytium* (UU)	Cervicitis/urethritis
	M. hominis (MH)	Cervicitis/urethritis
	M. genitalium (GU)	Cervicitis/urethritis
Bacteria	*Gonococcus* (NG)	Gonorrhea
	Calymmatobacterium granulomatis	Granuloma inguinale
	Haemophilus ducrey (HD)	Chancroid
	Gartner Haemophilus (GV)	Bacterial vaginosis
Spirochaeta pallida		Syphilis
Fungal	*Candida albicans*	Candidal vulvovaginitis
		Balanoposthitis
Protozoan	*Trichomonas vaginalis*	Trichomonas vaginitis
Parasites	*Pediculus inguinalis*	Crab lousiness
	Sarcoptes mites	Scabies

27.1.2　Common Venereal Syndromes

27.1.2.1　Urethral discharge in men

The syndromes include urethral discharge, dysuria (pain on urination) and frequent urination. The common causes of the syndromes are: *Gonorrhoea*, *Chlamydia trachomatis* (CT), *Ureaplasma urealytium* (UU), and *M. genitalium* (GU).

27.1.2.2　Vaginal discharge and/or lower abdominal pain in women

The syndromes include unusual vaginal discharge, vaginal itching, dysuria, dyspareunia, lower abdominal pain, tenderness on palpation. The common causes of the syndromes are: trichomoniasis, candidiasis, gonorrhoea, chlamydia infection, mixed anaerobes, ureaplasma urealytium (UU), and M genitalium (GU).

27. 1. 2. 3   Genital ulceration in men and women

The syndromes include genital sore, genital ulcer,and enlarged inguinal lymph nodes. The common causes of the syndromes are: syphilis, chancroid, and genital herpes.

27. 1. 2. 4   Genital warts

Most condition is condyloma acuminatum.

27. 1. 3   STDs Transmission

27. 1. 3. 1   Infective agents

Infective agents include patients and carriers.

27. 1. 3. 2   The STDs' routes of transmission

(1) Sexual behavior including intercourse and close contact.

(2) Blood and blood products.

(3) Mother-to-children:including inside uterus, birth canal, breast-feeding.

(4) Iatrogenic infection, artificial insemination, organ transplantation.

27. 1. 3. 3   Susceptible population

All persons are susceptible to STDs.

27. 1. 3. 4   High risk populations

Including prostitute, homosexuality, drug abuser, and having multiple sexual partners.

27. 1. 4   STDs Laboratory Diagnosis

27. 1. 4. 1   Specimen collection:

(1) Discharge:including urethra,vagina,cervix, pharyngeal portion,and anal canal.

(2) Blood.

(3) Cerebrospinal fluid.

(4) Other: biopsy.

27. 1. 4. 2   Pathogen detection

(1) Directly detections include staining and cultivation,generally applied for gonorrhea et al.

(2) Indirectly detections include seroimmunity (detecting for antigens and antibodies). Most are applied for detecting viral infection and syphilis,for example: HIV,HSV,Chlamydia,and Spirochaeta pallida.

(3) Nucleic acid detection include pathogen's DNA and RNA. The methods have PCR, LCR and hybridization in situ.

27. 1. 5   Therapeutic Principle

(1) Early discovering.

(2) Early treatment.

(3) Enough dosage.

(4) Enough course of treatment.

(5) Following up on time.

27. 1. 6   STDs' Prevention

This aim is to protect healthy persons from infecting and to discover early the patients and the suspects for decreasing their infectivity and complication. Theses measures include below:

(1) To popularize the knowledge of STDs and to improve self-protection awareness.

(2) To use condom.

(3) To prohibit strictly risky sexual behaviors, for example: multiple sexual partners, intercourse not to use condom.

(4) To prevent vertical transmission and blood Transmission.

(5) Managements of sex partners include examination and treatment.

27. 1. 7   STDs' Hazard

(1) STDs make a hazard of individual' physical and mental health. It makes the illness of body but also makes the stress of mental. If patients miss the suitable opportunity of treatment, STDs can cause the serious complications. For example: male's Epididymitis, chorditis, infertility, female's pelvic inflammation, salpingitis, endometritis, ectopic pregnancy,abortion,and barren.

(2) It can transmit to sexual partner and spouses.

(3) Some STDs are transmitted from the infected mother to her unborn child,and the infection is passed from infected mother through the placenta into the fetus. The syphilitic mother may have miscarriage and stillbirths. HIV can be transmitted by HIV positive mother to her child. The infected child can have congenital syphilis and HIV infection.

27.2   Syphilis

Syphilis is a chronic, contagious, sexually transmitted disease caused by *Treponema pallidum* (*T. pallidum*) subspecies pallidum. *T. pallidum* enters through the skin or mucous membranes, where the spirochete produces a non-painful ulcer known as a chancre. In congenital syphilis,the *T. pallidum* crosses the placenta and infects the fetus. Syphilis is a multistage disease with diverse and wide-ranging manifestations.

27. 2. 1   Etiology

The pathogenic *Treponema* for humans includes *T.*

pallidum subspecies *pallidum*, which causes venereal syphilis; *T. pallidum* subspecies *pertenue*, which causes yaws; *T. pallidum* subspecies *endemicum*, which causes endemic syphilis or bejel; and *T. carateum*, which causes pinta. *T. pallidum* subspecies *pallidum* (hereafter referred to in this chapter simply as *T. pallidum*), a thin delicate organism with 4 to 14 spirals and tapered ends, measures 6 to 15 μm in total length and 0. 2 μm in width. The structure of these organisms is somewhat different: the cells have a coating of glycosaminoglycans, which may be host-derived, and the outer membrane covers the three flagella that provide motility. The motility is characteristic, consisting of three movements: a projection in the direction of the long axis, a rotation on its long axis, and a bending or twisting from side to side. It cannot be cultured on artificial media but it can be propagated in organ culture, such as rabbit testis. *T. pallidum* is anaerobic, and it is very sensitive to drying, sunlight and heat, and also to soap and weak disinfectants. However, it has a strong tolerance for low temperature.

    T. pallidum rapidly penetrates intact mucous membranes or microscopic abrasions in skin and within a few hours enters the lymphatics and blood to produce systemic infection and metastatic foci long before the appearance of a primary lesion. The infection of endothelial cells leads to endarteritis obliterans and periarteritis with plasmacytic infiltration.

    Syphilis immunity is probably a combination of both humoral and cell-mediated defenses. The host with normal immune system is possibly in the main of TH1 cell-mediated response during the whole infection, which causes regression of early lesions and continuance of latency. Due to immunity impaired, HIV alters the natural history of syphilis, and initial presentation may be more varied, and increases the rate of neurosyphilis in co-infected patients.

    Treponema possess a complex antigenic makeup that is difficult to determine, including immune shield, immune privilege, anti-phagocytosis and induce macrophage function down-regulation. In addition, the cells have a high lipid content (cardiolipin, cholesterol), which is unusual for most bacteria.

    Genital sores (chancres) caused by syphilis make it easier to transmit and acquire HIV infection sexually. There is an estimated 2-to 5-fold increased risk of acquiring HIV if exposed to that infection when syphilis is present. Ulcerative STDs that cause sores, ulcers, or breaks in the skin or mucous membranes, such as syphilis, disrupt barriers that provide protection against infections. The genital ulcers caused by syphilis can bleed easily, and when they come into contact with oral and rectal mucosa during sex, increase the susceptibility to HIV.

27. 2. 2 Transmission

Syphilis is passed from person to person through direct contact with syphilis sore. Sores occur mainly on the external genitals, vagina, anus, or in the rectum. Sores also can occur on the lips and in the mouth. Transmission of the organism occurs during vaginal, anal, or oral sex. Pregnant women with the disease can pass it to the babies they are carrying. Syphilis cannot be spread through contact with toilet seats, doorknobs, swimming pools, hot tubs, bathtubs, shared clothing, or eating utensils.

27. 2. 3 Clinical Features

Syphilis includes acquired syphilis and congenital syphilis according to different transmissions, and according to the courses there are early syphilis and late syphilis.

    27. 2. 3. 1   Acquired syphilis

    (1) Primary syphilis

    The typical primary chancre usually begins as a single painless papule that rapidly becomes eroded and usually becomes indurated, with a characteristic cartilaginous consistency on palpation of the edge and base of the ulcer(Color Figure 27 - 1). It appears at the spot where syphilis entered the body. The time between infection with syphilis and the start of the first symptom can range from 10 to 90 days (average 21 days). In heterosexual men the chancre is usually located on the penis, whereas in homosexual men it is often found in the anal canal or rectum, in the mouth, or on the external genitalia. In women, common primary sites are the cervix and labia. Consequently, primary syphilis goes unrecognized in women and homosexual men more often than in heterosexual men. Multiple primary lesions may be more common among men with concurrent HIV infection. The chancre lasts 3 to 6 weeks, and it heals without treatment. However, if adequate treatment is not administered, the infection progresses to the secondary stage.

    Regional lymphadenopathy usually accompanies the primary syphilitic lesion, appearing after 1 week of the onset of the lesion. The nodes are firm, non-suppurative, and painless. Inguinal lymphadenopathy is unilateral and may occur with anal as well as with external genital chancres. Lymphadenopathy may persist for months.

(2) Secondary syphilis

1) Mucocutaneous lesions

Syphilids: The mucocutaneous manifestations of secondary syphilis are called syphilids and occur in 80% of cases. The early eruptions are symmetrical, more or less generalized, macular; later they are maculopapular or papular eruptions, which are usually polymorphous, and less often scaly, pustular, or pigmented. Maculars are apt to be distributed over the trunk and proximal extremities. They are pink or rose or brownish red and round or oval rash with 1 – 2 cm in diameter, and fading by pressed with no fusion. The presence of lesions on the palms (Color Figure 27 – 2) and soles (Color Figure 27 – 3) is strongly suggestive. They are invasive, copper red macular or maculopapular and like soy bean in size with collar-like scaling generally. The papular types of eruption usually arise a little later than the macular. The fully developed lesions are of a raw-ham or coppery shade, round, and from 2 to 5 mm or more in diameter. They are often only slightly raised, but a deep, firm infiltration is palpable. The surface is smooth, sometimes shiny, at other times covered with a thick, adherent scale. Papules are frequently distributed on the face and flexures of the arms and lower legs but are often distributed all over the trunk. The pustular syphilids usually occur in debilitating patients. The pustule arises on a red, infiltrated base. Involution is usually slow, resulting in a small, rather persistent, crust-covered, superficial or deep ulceration. The early eruptions may result in post-inflammatory hyper-pigmentation. The syphilids may disappear within 4 to 12 weeks.

Condyloma latum: Condylomata lata are papular lesions, relatively broad and flat, located on folds of moist skin, especially about the genitalia and anus; they may become hypertrophic and instead of infiltrating deeply, protrude above the surface, forming a soft, red, often mushroom like mass 1 to 3 cm in diameter, usually with a smooth, moist, weeping, gray surface. It may be lobulated but is not covered by the digitate elevations characteristic of venereal warts (condylomata acuminate).

Syphilitic alopecia: Syphilitic alopecia is an uncommon manifestation of secondary syphilis, occurring in only 4 percent of these individuals. It is non-inflammatory and non-cicatricial hair loss that can present in a diffuse pattern, a mouth-eaten pattern, or a combination of both. The scalp is the most commonly affected area. Syphilitic alopecia often accompanies other mucocutaneous symptoms of secondary syphilis, but it can be the only presenting symptom.

2) Mucous lesions: Mucous patches occur on the tonsils, tongue, pharynx, gums, lips, and buccal areas, or on the genitalia. They are macerated, flat, rounded erosions covered by a delicate, grayish, soggy membrane.

3) Systemic involvement: The lymphatic system in secondary syphilis is characteristically involved. The lymph nodes most frequently affected are the inguinal, posterior cervical, postauricular, and epitrochlear. The nodes are shotty, firm, slightly enlarged, and nontender.

Acute glomerulonephritis, gastritis or gastric ulceration, proctitis, hepatitis, acute meningitis, sensorineural hearing loss, iritis, anterior uveitis, optic neuritis, Bell's palsy, multiple pulmonary nodular infiltrates, periostitis, osteomyelitis, polyarthritis, or tenosynovitis may all be seen in secondary syphilis.

Relapsing secondary syphilis: The early lesions of syphilis undergo involution either spontaneously or with treatment. Relapses occur in about 25% of untreated patients, 90% within the first year. Such relapses may take place at the site of previous lesions, on the skin or in the viscera. Recurrent eruptions tend to be more configurate or annular, larger, and asymmetrical.

(3) Late syphilis

Late syphilis is defined by the WHO as greater than 2 year's duration.

1) Tertiary cutaneous syphilis: Tertiary syphilids most often occur 3 to 5 years after infection. Sixteen percent of untreated patients will develop tertiary lesions of the skin, mucous membrane, bone, or joints. Two main types of tertiary syphilids are recognized, the nodular syphilid and the gumma.

2) Nodular syphilid: The nodular or tubercular type consists of reddish brown or copper-colored firm papules or nodules, 2 mm or larger. The individual lesions are usually covered with adherent scales or crusts. The lesions tend to form rings and to undergo involution as new lesions develop just beyond them, so that they produce characteristic circular or serpiginous patterns enduring for many years. These often occur on the extensor surfaces of the arms and on the back of the trunk. Such patches are composed

of nodules in different stages of development so that it is common to find scars and pigmentation together with fresh and also ulcerated lesions.

3) Syphilitic gumma: Gummas may occur as unilateral, isolated, or single lesions, or in serpiginous patterns. They may be restricted to the skin or originating in the deeper tissues, break down and secondarily involve the skin. The individual lesions, which begin as small, painless nodules, slowly enlarge to several centimeters. Central necrosis is extensive and may lead to the formation of a deep punched-out ulcer with steep sides and a gummy base. Again, progression may take place in one area while healing proceeds in another. The most commonly involved sites include the skin and skeletal system, the mouth and upper respiratory tract, the larynx, the liver, and the stomach; however, any organ may be involved.

4) Late osseous syphilis: Skeletal syphilids occur most commonly on the head and face, then on the tibia. Late manifestations of syphilis may produce periostitis, osteomyelitis, osteitis, and gummatous osteoarthritis. Osteocope—bone pain, most often at night—is a suggestive symptom.

5) Late ocular lesions: Ocular lesions that suggest late syphilis include otherwise-unexplained pupillary abnormalities, optic neuritis, and a retinitis pigmentosa syndrome as well as the classic iritis (especially granulomatous iritis) or uveitis.

6) Cardiovascular syphilis: cardiovascular manifestations include uncomplicated aortitis, aortic regurgitation, saccular aneurysm, or coronary ostial stenosis, with symptoms usually appearing 10 to 30 years after infection. Symptomatic cardiovascular complications developed in 10% of persons with late untreated syphilis.

7) Neurosyphilis: Neurosyphilis, usually appearing 3 to 20 years after infection, include asymptomatic neurosyphilis, Tabes dorsalis, dementia paralytica, and meningovascular syphilis. 10 percent of persons with late syphilis will become neurosyphilis.

27. 2. 3. 2 Congenital syphilis

The manifestations of congenital syphilis can be divided into three types according to their timing: ① early manifestations, which appear within the first 2 years of life (often between 2 and 10 weeks of age); ② late manifestations, which appear after 2 years and are noninfectious; and ③ congenital latent syphilis.

(1) Early congenital syphilis

Children often have premature birth, poor growth and nutrition, weight loss, dehydration, loose skin, looking like the elderly, feeding difficulties, low weak hoarse cry, and irritability

1) Mucocutaneous lesions: Cutaneous lesions of congenital syphilis, which generally appear after 3 weeks of age and few at birth, resemble those of acquired secondary syphilis. The fissures often occur on the perioral and perianal with a characteristic radial scar after healing.

2) Syphilitic rhinitis: Syphilitic rhinitis generally appears within 1 to 2 months of age. Rhinitis begins as symptoms of the nasal catarrh, and followed by ulcers on the nasal mucosa, discharging bloody sticky secretions, breathing and sucking difficulty caused by blocked nose after the aggravation of the disease. It can lead to nasal septum perforation, nasal collapse, and the formation of saddle nose in severe cases.

3) Osseous syphilis: Bone lesions occur in 70% to 80% of cases of early congenital syphilis, which include osteochondritis, osteomyelitis, periostitis and syphilitic dactylitis. Epiphysitis is common and apparently causes pain on motion, leading to the infant's refusing to move (Parrot's pseudoparalysis).

In addition, lymphadenopathy, hepatosplenomegaly, nephrotic syndrome, meningitis, and hematological system's changes are common.

(2) Late congenital syphilis

Late congenital syphilis generally appears after 5 to 8 years of age, and a variety of manifestations will occur at the age of 13 to 14. Keratitis, bone lesions and neurosyphilis are common, however, cardiovascular manifestations are rare.

1) Mucocutaneous lesions: Late mucocutaneous lesions have a low incidence, and gummas are more common. They most frequently occur on palatum durum and nasal septum mucosa, which can cause the perforation of the palate and nasal septum, and saddle nose.

2) Ocular lesions: About 90% of persons are interstitial keratitis, which begins as the obvious inflammation around the cornea, then followed by the characteristic diffuse corneal opacity, which can lead to permanent lesions, such as blindness by repeated attacks.

3) Osseous syphilis: Periostitis is common, and saber shin and perisynovitis (Clutton's joints) can occur. Clutton's joints affect the knees, leads to symmetrical, painless swelling, slight rigidity, and arthroedema.

4) Neurosyphilis: In late congenital syphilis,

asymptomatic neurosyphilis is present in about one-third to an half of untreated patients, and clinical neurosyphilis are found at up to adolescent age, which frequently affects cerebral nerves, especially the auditory nerve and the optic nerve. Few children appear Tabes dorsalis and dementia paralytica.

5) Characteristic stigmata

Hutchinson's teeth: They are a malformation of the central upper incisors that appears in the second or permanent teeth. The characteristic teeth are cylindrical rather than flattened, the base is narrower than the cutting edge, and in the center of the cutting edge a half-moon notch may develop.

Mulberry molars: The first molar usually appears smaller with poorly developed cusps, and it has a deflexion to the centrum, which looks like a mulberry.

Articulatio sternoclavicularis hyperplastic: It is due to bone warts which occur at the junction of the sternum and the clavicle.

Interstitial keratitis.

Nerve deafness: It usually begins as vertigo, then followed by hearing loss, which generally occurs in the preschool child.

Hutchinson's teeth, nerve deafness, and interstitial keratitis have since become known as the Hutchinson triad.

27.2.3.3   Latent syphilis

The absence of clinical manifestations of syphilis, together with positive serologic tests for syphilis indicates a diagnosis of latent syphilis. To establish a diagnosis of latent syphilis, strict criteria are called for. Clinical evidence of active, early, late or congenital syphilis must be absent, CSF must be normal and a chest X-ray must also be normal (view aorta at a right angle).

27.2.4   Laboratory Tests

Laboratory tests mainly contain tests for direct detection of *T. pallidum*, serologic tests for syphilis, detecting techniques of molecular biology and CSF examination.

27.2.4.1   Tests for direct detection of *T. pallidum*

Treponema pallidum can be identified by dark-field microscopy or silver stain method.

27.2.4.2   Serologic tests for syphilis

It can be divided into two parts.

(1) Standard non-treponemal tests

The tests are often used for screening and are quantitative. They are useful in assessing response to treatment, condition of relapse or reinfection. There are three tests available including the Venereal Disease Research Laboratory (VDRL), the rapid plasma reagin (RPR) test and the unheated serum reagin (USR) test.

(2) Treponemal antigen tests

Specific treponemal antibody tests are used for confirmatory testing. They are qualitative procedures and are not helpful in assessing treatment response. They mainly include the fluorescent treponemal antibody absorption (FTA-ABS) test, the treponema pallidum haemagglutination test (TPHA) and so on.

27.2.4.3   Detecting techniques of molecular biology

For example, polymerase chain reaction (PCR) can detect DNA of T. pallidum. The test is very sensitive and specific, it's an advanced method in diagnosis however, it is not recommended for the diagnosis of neurosyphilis.

27.2.4.4   CSF examination

CSF examination is used for the diagnosis of neurosyphilis, including white blood cell count, protein concentration, VDRL and so on. There are nonspecific abnormalities in the CSF when suffering from neurosyphilis, such as raised cell count and increased protein. However, VDRL is specific evidence in diagnosing neurosyphilis.

27.2.5   Diagnosis and Differential Diagnosis

To diagnose syphilis duly, doctors should ask a history in detail, carry out a complete physical examination and do laboratory tests repeatedly because of its complex and diverse clinical manifestations.

The diagnosis of primary syphilis is based on a history of exposure, the incubation period, and the typical clinical manifestations, together with laboratory tests, which include dark-field microscopic examination, silver stains, Giemsa stains, and the direct fluorescent antibody T. pallidum (DFA-TP) test, or negative reactive serum treponemal tests in the early period and seropositive in the late period. A non-reactive serum test can not be used to rule out syphilis. The genital lesions that most commonly must be differentiated from those of primary syphilis include those caused by chancroid, genital herpes, fixed drug eruption, and Behcet's disease.

The diagnosis of secondary syphilis is based on a history of exposure, the typical clinical manifestations, especially mucocutaneous lesions, together with laboratory tests, which include a dark-field-positive ulcerative lesion and a strong positive reactive serum test. Secondary syphilis must be differentiated from pityriasis rosea, psoriasis vulgaris, viral exanthema, and tinea cruris.

The diagnosis of late syphilis is based on a history of exposure, the typical clinical manifestations, together with laboratory tests, which include typical histopathology, positive nontreponemal antibody tests, or a positive treponemal test with a negative nontreponemal test. Neurosyphilis have CSF abnormalities including lymphocytes values $\geqslant 10$/ml, protein values > 50 mg/dl, and reactive CSF-Venereal Disease Research Laboratory (VDRL) tests. Late syphilis must be differentiated from cutaneous tuberculosis, leprosy and cutaneous tumor.

The diagnosis of congenital syphilis is based on a history of a syphilitic mother, the typical clinical manifestations, together with laboratory tests. A positive dark-field examination and a positive reactive serum test (specific antitreponemal Igm) indicate a diagnosis of syphilis.

27.2.6 Treatment

Penicillins is the first line drug, adequate treatment requires the maintenance of serum concentrations in excess of 0.03 U/ml for at least 10 days. Benzathine penicillin G, procaine benzylpenicillin, penicillin G crystalline are usually used. Benzathine penicillin G is not the preferred drug in the treatment of cardiovascular syphilis. In penicillin-allergic patients, the preference alternative drug is ceftriaxone sodium, tetracycline and doxycycline are two other alternative drugs.

(1) Early syphilis

Patients with primary, secondary, or early latent syphilis known to be of less than 2 year's duration can be treated with 2.4 million units of benzathine penicillin G intramuscularly weekly for 2 to 3 weeks, or procaine benzylpenicillin 0.8 million units once daily for 10 to 15 days. In penicillin-allergic, ceftriaxone sodium 1g intravenous drip daily for 10 to 14 days, tetracycline 500 mg orally 4 times daily or doxycycline 100 mg orally twice daily for 2 weeks is recommended.

(2) Late syphilis

The recommend treatment of late or late latent syphilis of more than 2 year's duration is benzathine penicillin G 2.4 million units intramuscularly weekly for 3 to 4 weeks, or procaine benzylpenicillin 0.8 million units once daily for 20 days. In penicillin-allergic patients, tetracycline 500mg orally four times daily or doxycycline 100mg orally twice daily for 30 days is recommended.

(3) Neurosyphilis

To avoid a Jarisch-Herxheimer reaction, patients could oral prednisone. Recommended treatment regimens for neurosyphilis include penicillin G crystalline, 2 to 4 million units intravenously every 4 hours for 10 to 14 days; or penicillin G procaine, 2.4 million units intramuscularly daily plus probenecid 500 mg orally four times daily, both for 10 to 14 days. Most experts recommend benzathine penicillin G, 7.2 MU, divided in three weekly intramuscularly doses, after completion of the above. In penicillin-allergic patients, the treatment is the same as above.

(4) Pregnant women

According to the different stages of syphilis in pregnant patients, the corresponding treatment regimens are recommended, of which the usage and dosage is the same in other patients. However, patients should be carried out a course of treatment both on the first trimester and the third trimester of pregnancy. Penicillin-allergic patients could take oral erythromycin.

(5) Congenital syphilis

After the patient has had an LP for examination of the CSF to be abnormal, infants with early congenital syphilis should be given penicillin G crystalline, 100,000 to 150,000 U/(kg·d) (administered as 50,000 U/kg intravenously every 12 to 8 hours for 10 to 14 days); or penicillin G procaine, 50,000 U/kg intramuscularly daily in a single dose for 10 to 14 days. Benzathine penicillin G, 50,000 U/kg intramuscularly may be used to treat infants with a completely normal evaluation. In late congenital syphilis, patients should be treated with penicillin G crystalline, 200,000 to 300,000 U/(kg·d) intravenously or intramuscularly (50,000 U/kg every 4 to 6 hours for 10 to 14 days); or penicillin G procaine, 50,000 U/(kg·d) intramuscularly for 10 to 14 days as a course or followed by a course again. Older children's usage of penicillin should not exceed adults' usage with the corresponding stage. Penicillin-allergic patients could take oral erythromycin, 10 to 15 mg/(kg·d) (every 6 hours for 30 days).

Points for attention:

Syphilis should be treated early, adequately and regularly, and as much as possible to avoid the cardiovascular syphilis, neurosyphilis and serious complications. Meanwhile, partners should be treated against a sex during the treatment to prevent further infection and others to be infected.

Follow-up for clinical and serological assessment should be done, testing is repeated every 3 months in the first year, every 6 months in the second year, and repeated at the end of the third year. Patients with documented neurosyphilis should also have a repeat CSF evaluation at 6 months and at 6-month intervals. Patients with maternal syphilis should have a repeat follow-up at every month before delivery. The infants should have a repeat follow-up at 1st month, 2nd month, 3rd month, 6th month, and 12th month.

Patients with the disease course of more than 1 year, relapsed patients, serofast patients, patients with hearing impairment, patients with abnormal vision, they should accept examination of cerebrospinal fluid to confirm if neurosyphilis exist or not.

In cases of serological or clinical relapse, re-treatment with double doses is recommended.

Jarisch-Herxheimer reaction: The Jarisch-Herxheimer reaction is an acute febrile reaction that occurs in many patients who received treatment. It is mediated by cytokines and occurs within several hours after treatment. It consists of shaking chills, fever, headache, accelerated breathing, tachycardia, malaise, and exacerbation of primary disease. An increase of inflammation in a vital structure may have serious consequences, as when there is an aneurysm of the aorta. A short course of corticosteroids helps preventing Jarisch-Herxheimer reaction. Cardiovascular syphilis treatment should start from small amounts of penicillin, and to increase the dose gradually until the fourth day, the treatment according to normal dose. If chest pain happened, or heart failure worsened, or the changes of ST-T in ECG became more markedly during the treatment, treatment should be suspended.

27.3 Gonorrhea

27.3.1 Etiology

N. gonorrhoeae was discovered by Albert Neisser in 1879. It is a Gram-negative, aerobic diplococcus, with oval or kidney form, it principally infects host columnar epithelium. Outside the human host it is delicate, it is very sensitive to drying, heat, and also general disinfectants, but within the host body it has a huge capability to effect antigenic variation that helps it escape the host immune response and to evolve antimicrobial resistance.

27.3.2 Transmission Way

Gonorrhea mainly through sexual contact with an infective person, human is the only natural host of the gonococci. Gonorrhea patients is the main source. A few cases can be infected because of contacting with drench coccus of secretions or contaminated equipment, such as clothing, bedding, towel, bathtub, toilet etc.

27.3.3 Clinical Features

It occur in all ages, especially in young people. The incubation period is short, usually 2 - 10 days, averagely 3 - 5 days, Typical symptoms may occur after sexual contact.

27.3.3.1 Uncomplicated gonorrhea

(1) Male gonorrhea

In males, the normal presentation is acute urethritis, with urgency of micturation and disuria, after 1 to 2 days There is often onset of serious burning on urination, odynuria accompanied by a purulent discharge (Color Figure 27 - 4). In MSM, rectal and pharyngeal may also be infected, and can lead to anorectitis and pharyngitis. When posterior urethra is infected, there is onset of terminal bleeding and hemospermia. On occasion bubonadenitis occurs. general symptom is often light, a few man may occur fever and anepithymia.

(2) Female gonorrhea

In females, the initial site of infection is the cervix, but those sites of the urethra, rectum and pharynx should also be tested. There may be onset of those symptoms such as excessive vaginal discharge, dysuria, and intermenstrual bleeding. But most women with early infections report no clinical symptoms.

The female children may be infected after close contact with her infected parents, a few because of sexual abuse, commonly display diffuse vaginitis and vulvitis. Sometimes involving the anus and rectum.

(3) Gonococcal conjunctivitis

In adults, it is usually due to autoinoculation of the organisms from infected anogenital area. It presents as an acutely painful red eye accompanied by a purulent discharge that may develop into panophthalmitis and loss of sight.

It occurs more frequently in newborn babies as ophthalmia neonatorum, which normally occurs in the first week after birth, which is essential that prompt recognition and treatment to prevent permanent visual damage.

27. 3. 3. 2   Complications

This may occur in both sexes, as a result of local abscess, from ascending infections and from haematogenous spread. It is mostly due to those factor of malpractice, intemperance, or sex, and ascending infection may causes posterior urethritis, prostatitis, vesiculitis, epididymitis, and pelvic inflammation, which repeatedly occur may lead to urethral stricture, Vas deferens and fallopian tube stenosis or block, even progress to infertility.

In men, acute prostatitis may occur with symptoms of fever, urinary frequency, stranguria and perineal pain, prostate enlargement and distinct tenderness on digital rectal examination. Chronic prostatitis may present no obvious subjective symptom, only the urinary meatus are sealing at the first urinasanguinis.

In women, the major complication is pelvic inflammatory disease, which is usually acute in onset, include acute salpingitis, endometritis, secondary tubo-ovarian abscess and pelvic abscess, peritonitis which due to abscess burst. It may present as fever, lower abdominal and pelvic pain, and distinct adnexal and cervical motion tenderness on bimanual pelvic examination. It easily develop into pelvic and adnexal infection upon misdiagnose and malpractice patients. Repeated recurrence may lead to fallopian tube stenosis or block, thus may cause chronic lower abdominal pain, ectopic pregnancy, infertility.

27. 3. 3. 3   Disseminated gonococcal infection (DGI)

It occurs in 1%-3% of gonorrhea patients from haematogenous spread and in either sex. But it is more common in women than men. In women it normally occurs in menstruation, pregnancy and recent childbirth, with the following symptoms as fever, chill, general malaise. There often appear a few of dispersed lesions in peripherally near affected joints, it may also occur arthritis, tenosynovitis, infective endocarditis, pericarditis, pleurisy, liver perihepatitis and pneumonia, etc. It may occur severe bacteremia, if not timely treatment it can be life-threatening. Diagnosis is on the basis of the clinical features and positive joint fluid, blood, and lesions culture of *Neisseria gonorrhoeae*.

27. 3. 4   Diagnosis and Differential Diagnosis

According to the history including of sexual contact, sex partner infection, and contaminated equipment contact, clinical features and laboratory results, it can be diagnosed. Laboratory examination includes microscopy, culture and NAATs (nucleic acid amplification tests). The gold standard for diagnosing gonorrhoea is culture of gonococcus.

This should be identified from chlamydia urethritis, a vaginal yeast infection and trichomonad vaginitis, etc. Chlamydia urethritis without drench coccus on clinical features, combining laboratory results can be identified. But the two pathogens often coexist, which should be paid attention to.

27. 3. 5   Treatment

The gonococcus has an observable propensity to develop antimicrobial resistance. The WHO recommends that only antimicrobial regimens that can assure >95% cure rates are employed. In most parts of the world, this means that penicillin, tetracycline, some macrolides and quinolones are no longer first-line therapy.

Until 1976 penicillin was the first-line therapy of gonorrhea. Since 1976, penicillin-resistant gonococcal strains were detected for the first time, gonococcal resistance to other antibiotics has been reported.

27. 3. 5. 1   Treatment of uncomplicated gonorrhea

(1) gonococcal urethritis, cervicitis, proctitis

Ceftriaxone 250 mg IM in a single dose, or spectinomycin 2 g (cervicitis 4 g) IM in a single dose, or cefotaxime 1 g IM in a single dose, or cefixime 400 mg orally in a single dose, or other third-generation cephalosporins.

Plus treatment for *Chlamydia* if *Chlamydial* infection is not ruled out.

(2) Children gonorrhea

Recommended regimens for children who weight >45 kg, treat with one of the regimens recommended for adults (see Gonococcal infections). Recommended regimens for children who weight ≤45 kg, treat with ceftriaxone 125 mg IM in a single dose or spectinomycin 40 mg/kg, IM in a single dose.

Plus treatment for *Chlamydia* if *Chlamydial* infection is not ruled out.

Tetracycline is forbidden for those children aged

< 8 years. Fluoroquinolones should not be recommended for persons aged <18 years。

27.3.5.2 Treatment of complicated gonorrhea

(1) Gonococcal epididymitis, vesiculitis, prostatitis

Ceftriaxone 250 mg IM in a single daily dose for 10 days, or spectinomycin 2 g IM in a single daily dose for 10 days, or cefotaxime 1 g IM in a single daily dose for 10 days, or cefixime 400 mg orally in a single daily dose for 10 days.

Plus treatment for *Chlamydia* if *Chlamydial* infection is not ruled out.

(2) Gonococcal pelvic inflammation

Treat with one of the regimens recommended for gonococcal epididymitis, plus metronidazole 400 mg orally twice daily for 14 days.

Collaboration with the gynecologist in adnexitis or pelvic inflammation and with the urologist in epididymitis is recommended.

27.3.5.3 Treatment of special gonorrhoea

(1) gonococcal pharyngitis

Ceftriaxone 250 mg IM in a single dose, or cefotaxime 1 g IM in a single dose.

Plus treatment for Chlamydia if Chlamydial infection is not ruled out.

(2) Gonococcal-ophthalmia

For newborns: Ceftriaxone 25 - 50 mg /kg(total dose ≤125 mg) IM or IV in a single dose, or spectinomycin 40 mg/kg IM in a single dose.

For adults: Ceftriaxone 1 g IM in a single dose, or spectinomycin 2 g IM in a single dose.

At the same time, irrigate eyes with physiological saline, once per hour.

Plus treatment for *Chlamydia* if *Chlamydial* infection is not ruled out.

The eyedrops of 1% silver nitrate should be used to prevent gonococcal ophthalmia of newborns.

(3) Gonorrhea in pregnancy

Pregnant women can be treated with a recommended or alternate cephalosporin, and should not be treated with quinolones or tetracyclines. Those women who cannot tolerate a cephalosporin should be administered a single 2 g dose of spectinomycin IM. Either azithromycin or amoxicillin should be given for treatment of Chlamydial Infection during pregnancy.

27.3.5.4 Treatment of DGI

(1) DGI in newborns

Ceftriaxone 25 - 50 mg/(kg · d) IV or IM in a single daily dose for 7 days, with duration of 10 - 14 days, if meningitis is documented.

Cefotaxime 25 mg/kg IV or IM every 12 hours for 7 days, with a duration of 10 - 14 days, if meningitis is documented.

The mothers of baby who have gonococcal infection and the mothers' sex partners should be evaluated and treated according to the recommendations for treatment of gonococcal infections in adults (see Gonorrhoea.).

(2) DGI in adults

Ceftriaxone 1 - 2 g IV or IM twice daily dose with a duration ≥ 10 days, or spectinomycin 2 g IM twice daily dose with a duration ≥ 10 days, the duration should be 14 days, if meningitis is documented.

27.3.6 Follow-Up Examination and Confirmation of Cure

The subjective feelings of patients after therapy are not standard for the healing of gonorrhoea, sexual intercourse is prohibited until healing has been established. Microscopic examination is at least necessary, if possible a culture of gonococcus should be performed.

In man, the follow-up examination should be carried out at least once 3 - 7 days after completion of therapy. In women, it should be carried out on the seventh day after completion of therapy, and at 5 days after the next menstrual period.

Patients with gonorrhoea should be fully evaluated and screened for other STDs and HIV, asked to assist with partner notification efforts, and be offered non-judgmental education, counseling and support.

27.4 Chlamydia Trachomatis Genital Infection

Chlamydia trachomatis is a type of intracellular parasitic organisms. *Chlamydia pathogenicity* in humans has been a great concern, especially in recent years, the classic sexually transmitted diseases such as gonorrhea and syphilis incidence remained a stable situation, in some Western countries, caused by the *Chlamydia trachomatis* sexually transmitted diseases, their incidence rate has exceeded number 1 in all sexually transmitted diseases than gonorrhea.

27.4.1 Etiology

Chlamydia trachomatis is the most common pathogen in NGU, chlamydia is intra cellular microorganism between the bacteria and viruses, Gram-negative bacteria, diameter 250 – 500 nm, Chlamydia trachomatis host only human and mice. Chlamydia trachomatis has A, B, Ba, C-K in 12 serotypes, including B, D, Da, E, F, G, H, I, Ia, J, K can cause infection of the genitourinary system. Chlamydia is sensitive to heat, in 56 – 60 ℃ can survive only 5 – 10 minutes, at 37 ℃ 48 hours decreased significantly, in 4 ℃ chlamydia can well survive about 24 hours, can be stored for several years at – 70 ℃. 0. 1% formaldehyde solution, 0. 5% phenol can kill chlamydia in the short term, 75% ethanol to have very strong killing power, half a minute that is effective and can be inactivated ether at room temperature for 30 minutes.

27. 4. 2 Clinical Features

Generally, majority of *Chlamydia trachomatis* infection is asymptomatic or mild sign, the onset period is not urgent as gonorrhea attack. The latent period is 7 – 21 days. The clinical symptoms of *Chlamydial trachomatis* infection is similar with bacterial urethral tract infection (UTI), but may milder with frequency, itching, burning and difficulty of urination. There are milder red, less excretion, characterized serous or purulent fluid on the urethra open, be visualized vie hand squeezing on the open area. There is often discharge show on the underwear or less serous excretion sealed open during the morning wake. 50% of patients are ignored or misdiagnosed during the first consultation. 10%– 20% patients are co-infection with gonorrhea in female outreach to other location from cervical, present with more discharge (leucorrhea), cervical swelling, erosion, mild difficulty of urination and frequency, asymptom are also common.

The *Chlamydia trachomatis* could develop to be epididymitis in male if without proper treatment or mis-treatment. Acute epididymitis is common, unilateral and present with local painful on epididymis, enlarging and sore while palpation. It will present with swelling scrotum, redness painful and seminal duct getting thick once combine with testitis. The Reiter's syndrome present with urethritis, conjunctivitis and arthritis--triple symptom complex, and also can combine with Prostatitis, endometritis, PID, Fertility problems and ectopic pregnancy. The new born can be infected to be conjunctivitis or pneumonia by *Chlamydia trachomatis* exposal birth canal during born process.

27. 4. 3 Diagnosis

According to the history of sexual activity, urethritis present with mild symptom, smear each oil secretions under the neutral view mirror, more than 5 polymorph nuclear leukocytes, and no detection of *Neisseria gonorrhea*. Laboratory tests, including antigen detection, monoclonal antibody labeling, immunoassay (enzyme linked immunosorbent assay) and DNA amplification method.

27. 4. 4 Treatment

27. 4. 4. 1 Urethritis (cervicitis)

Doxycycline 200 mg/d, orally 2 times a day, 7 – 10 days; azithromycin 1 g state dose; camino ADM 200 mg/d, orally 2 times a day, erythromycin 2 g/d, orally 4 times a day, 7 – 10 days.

27. 4. 4. 2 Pregnant women

Azithromycin 1 g daily, 7 days; or amoxicillin (amoxicillin) 800 mg, 4 times a day, 7 days; or erythromycin 0. 5 g, 4 times a day.

27. 4. 4. 3 Neonatal chlamydial conjunctivitis

Erythromycin 40 mg/(kg · d), orally 4 times daily for 2 weeks; topical tetracycline, erythromycin or norfloxacin eye drops. System applications can also cure chlamydia erythromycin in the treatment of nasopharyngeal infections, and prevention of chlamydia pneumonia.

27. 4. 4. 4 Neonatal pneumonia

Erythromycin 50 mg/(kg · d), orally 4 times a day, 10 – 14 consecutive days; its efficacy is about 80%.

27. 4. 4. 5 Children

Body weight < 45 kg, erythromycin 50 mg/ (kg · d), orally 4 times a day, 10 – 14 consecutive days, body weight ⩾ 45 kg, but age <8 years old, or age> 8 years old children, treatment with adults, erythromycin/tetracycline 0. 5 g, 4 times a day, 7 days; azithromycin 1 g, single dose.

27. 5 Condyloma Acuminatum

Condyloma acuminatum (CA), also known as genital warts, is caused by a virus called the human papilloma virus (HPV). CA is a sexually transmitted disease, it mainly spread through skin-to-skin contact during sexual activity and mostly often occur in the external genitalia, anus and other parts. Around the world, the incidence of CA increased dramatically in recent years, it is even the most common sexually transmitted disease in some countries.

27. 5. 1   Etiology

At present, it has been found over 100 different types of human papilloma virus. Among them, the viruses which can infect the genitals were divided into high-risk or low-risk type. High-risk-human papilloma virus type (16, 18, 31, 33, 51, 54) related to the occurrence of genital cancer, especially cervical cancer. while low-risk (6, 11, 42, 44) type cause benign lesions. CA is usually low-risk type human papillomavirus infection and approximately 90% of genital warts are related to HPV types 6 and 11. HPVs are addicted to epithelial, they all infect the squamous stratified epithelia and stimulate the growth of it, the process is directly responsible for the characteristics papilloma hyperplasia.

27. 5. 2   Clinical Features

Genital warts have a variety of appearances. The typical genital wart is soft, pink, elongated and sometimes filiform or pedunculated (Color Figure 27 -5). They can be small or large, flat or raised, single or clumped into a group that may look like a cauliflower. In women, the warts appear on the vulva, in or around the vagina or anus, on the cervix. In men, genital warts normally develop on the penis or scrotum or anus. The warts may also develop on mouth as a result of a virus that is transmitted during oral sex. The soaking for 3 to 5 minutes in 3% to 5% acetic acid of the genitalia prior to examination is likely to turn the lesions white (particularly on the mucosal surfaces), which make them easier to be detected when they are small. In most patients they are asymptomatic, but may cause discomfort, discharge or bleeding. Nevertheless, they have a psychosexual impact in a majority of patients. HPV infection appears to be more common and worse in patients with various types of immunologic deficiencies. Recurrence rates, size, discomfort, and risk of oncologic progression are highest among those patients. Latent illness often becomes active during pregnancy.

27. 5. 3   Diagnosis and Differential Diagnosis

Diagnosis of genital warts is made by visual inspection and may be confirmed by biopsy. Histologic examination of the skin lesion demonstrates papillomatosis accompanied by the characteristic features of acanthosis, parakeratosis, and hyperkeratosis. Koilocytosis, which is perinuclear cytoplasmic halos, is commonly observed in the superficial epithelial cells. CA needs to be identified with pseudo-condyloma, pearly penile papules, condyloma latum, Bowen papulosis disease and ectopic sebaceous gland disorders.

(1) Pseudo condyloma

The majority of patients with pseudo-condyloma are symptomless but with harbor roe-like warty papulae distributed symmetrically on both labia minora; acetic acid white test is negative.

(2) Pearly penile papules

The papules appear as one or several rows of small, flesh-colored, smooth, dome-topped to filiform papules situated circumferentially around the corona or sulcus of the glans penis and persist throughout life; acetic acid white test negative.

(3) Condyloma latum

A secondary syphilitic eruption of flat-topped papules, occurring in groups covered by a necrotic layer of epithelial detritus, and secreting a seropurulent fluid; they are found in moist creased areas, as around the anus and external genitalia; dark-field microscopy can be found TP, the syphilis sero-positive.

27. 5. 4   Treatment

Treatment of genital warts should be guided by the preference of the patient, the available resources, and the experience of the health-care provider.

27. 5. 4. 1   Topical treatment

(1) 5% Imiquimod

It induces interferon production and is a cell-mediated immune response modifier. Has minimal systemic absorption but causes erythema, irritation, ulceration, and pain at application site. Patients should apply imiquimod cream once daily at bedtime, three times a week for up to 16 weeks. The treatment area should be washed with soap and water 6 - 10 hours after the application. The safety of imiquimod during pregnancy has not been established.

(2) Podophyllum resin

Extract of various plants, which are cytotoxic. Effective in arresting mitosis in metaphase. Concentration of 20% - 50% applied by physician onto lesions 1 - 2 times per week. Not for application to cervix, vagina, or anal canal where the squamocolumnar junction is prone to dysplastic changes. The drug has teratogenic effects, pregnant women banned.

(3) Podofilox

Purified podophyllotoxin that is antimitotic,

cytotoxic, and available for patient's home use. Patients should apply 5% podofilox to visible genital warts twice a day for 3 days, followed by 4 days of no therapy. This cycle may be repeated, if necessary, for up to four cycles. Slightly higher cure rates can be expected with podofilox than with podophyllin. Additionally, useful for prophylaxis. The safety of podofilox during pregnancy has not been established.

(4) Trichloroacetic or bichloracetic acids

At various concentrations (up to 80%), these agents rapidly penetrate and cauterize skin. Paint treatment onto lesions, avoiding uninvolved skin, repeat treatment q1 - 2week. Although caustic, this treatment causes less local irritation and systemic toxicity. Additionally, has low cost.

(5) Other

5% fluorouracil, bleomycin, etc.

27.5.4.2   Physical treatment

Such as cryotherapy, carbon dioxide laser treatment, electrosurgery, surgical excision etc. can be selected as appropriate.

27.5.4.3   Interferon

Both natural and recombinant, have been used for the treatment of genital warts. Interferon is probably effective because of its antiviral and immunostimulating effects, Interferon therapy is not recommended as a primary modality.

27.6 Genital Herpes

27.6.1   Etiology

Herpes simplex virus contains two serotypes: HSV-1 and HSV-2. HSV-2 is mainly responsible for approximately 60%- 90% of genital herpes, and 10%-40% of GH were caused by HSV-1. HSV can reside in lesion exudate, semen, prostatic fluid, cervical and vaginal secretions. Genital herpes mainly spreads during sexual activity.

27.6.2   Clinical Features

Genital herpes usually occurs in sexually active population aged 15 - 45. A variety of lesions occur in the male or female genital or perineal area, which occasionally are seen in perianal, groin and scrotum, etc. In the male homosexual population, genital herpes can involve the rectum and anus. The severity and the frequency of clinical manifestations are related to the type of HSV and immune status of the patient.

Genital herpes is generally divided into primary genital herpes, recurrent genital herpes, sub-clinical genital herpes, non-typical symptoms genital herpes and so on.

27.6.2.1   Primary genital herpes

It is HSV infection in patients at the first time with clinical symptoms and signs. The average incubation period after the genital acquisition of HSV approximately ranges 2 to 12 days (average, 3 to 5 days). In its classic clinical presentation, primary infection begins with macules and papules and progresses to vesicles, pustules, erosions and ulcers (Color Figure 27 - 6). Early symptoms of the first outbreak can include: itching or burning in the genital or anal area, headache, fever, swollen glands and so on. Such symptoms can last for 2 to 3 weeks.

27.6.2.2   Recurrent genital herpes

HSV-2 infection in the genital area is much more likely to recur than HSV-1. Generally, the first relapse after primary infection occurs in 1 - 4 months. Averagely patients who have a first outbreak can expect to have 3 - 4 outbreaks within a year. Approximately half of patients who recognize recurrences have prodromal symptoms, ranging from mild tingling sensations occurring several hours before the eruption to shooting pains in the buttocks, legs, or hips occurring as long as five days before the eruption. Lesions are usually fewer grouped blisters, asymmetric distribution, which become erosions or shallow ulcers quickly, ranging from mild tingling sensations to itching or burning feeling.

27.6.2.3   Sub-clinical genital herpes

It is HSV infection with no clinical symptoms and signs. However, asymptomatically viral shedding exists, which can be contagious.

27.6.2.4   Unrecognized or atypical genital herpes

It may show tiny fissures, ulcers, erythema, etc. which are easily overlooked.

27.6.2.5   Special type of genital herpes

Herpetic proctitis.

Herpetic cervicitis.

Neonatal herpes.

Disseminated HSV infection can be involved in herpes meningitis, hepatitis, pneumonia and skin infections, and so on.

Genital herpes during pregnancy can result in intrauterine growth retardation, miscarriage, premature delivery or stillbirth, etc.

27.6.3 Diagnosis and Differential Diagnosis

The disease mainly based on medical history (history of sexual contact or history of spouse infection etc.), typical clinical manifestations and laboratory tests for diagnosis. This disease must be differentiated from other diseases such as contact dermatitis, herpes zoster, primary syphilis, chancroid and Behcet's disease, etc. Rash characteristics and laboratory tests for the differential diagnosis of genital herpes have some help.

27.6.4 Treatment

(1) Topical therapy

Keep the infected area clean and dry. 3% acyclovir cream or 1% penciclovir cream and so on can be applied to lesions area.

(2) Systemic therapy

Primary genital herpes is treated with oral acyclovir 200 mg five times a day or 400 mg three times a day, famciclovir 250 mg three times a day, or valacyclovir 300 mg twice a day, all for 7 – 10 days.

Recurrent genital herpes is treated with oral acyclovir 200 mg five times a day or 400 mg three times a day, famciclovir 125 – 250 mg three times a day, or valacyclovir 300 mg twice a day, all for 5 days.

Frequent recurrence of genital herpes (more than 6 to 12 per year) is treated with oral acyclovir, 400 mg twice a day, or valaciclovir 300 mg once a day. Or famciclovir 125 – 250mg, twice a day for 4 months to 1 year.

Primary infection with severe symptoms or extensive lesions is treated with intravenous aciclovir 5 –10 mg/(kg · d) for 5 – 7 days.

27.7 AIDS

27.7.1 Introduction

AIDS stands for acquired immunodeficiency (or immune deficiency) syndrome. It results from infection with a virus called HIV, which refers to human immunodeficiency virus. This virus infects key cells in the human body called CD4-positive ($CD4^+$) T cells. These cells are part of the body's immune system. When HIV invades the body's $CD4^+$ T cells, the damaged immune system loses its ability to defend against diseases caused by bacteria, viruses, and other microscopic organisms. A substantial decline in $CD4^+$ T

cells also leaves the body vulnerable to certain cancers.

By the end of 2009, 33.4 million people worldwide were living with HIV/AIDS, with the vast majority living in developing countries. Through 2009, 2 million people worldwide have died from AIDS. As of the year 2009, nearly 48 thousands people in China were confirmed to be HIV-positive. By the end of 2009, in total 740 thousands Chinese people were living with HIV/AIDS, among them 635 thousands Chineses now carry the HIV virus but do not yet have symptoms.

27.7.2 Etiology

The symptoms of AIDS were first recognized in the early 1980s. In 1984, the responsible virus was identified and given a name. In 1986, it was renamed the human immunodeficiency virus (HIV).

HIV belongs to a special class of viruses called retroviruses. Within this class, HIV belongs to the subgroup of lentiviruses, while HIV is different in structure from other retroviruses. An HIV particle is around 100 – 150 billionths of a meter in diameter. HIV particles surround themselves with a coat of fatty material known as the viral envelope (or membrane). Projecting from this are around 72 little spikes, which are formed from the proteins gp120 and gp41. Just below the viral envelope is a layer called the matrix, which is made from the protein p17. The viral core (or capsid) is usually bullet-shaped and is made from the protein p24. Inside the core are three enzymes required for HIV replication called reverse transcriptase, integrase and protease. Also held within the core is HIV's genetic material, which consists of two copies of single-stranded RNA enclosed by a conical capsid comprising the viral protein p24, typical of lentiviruses. HIV has just nine genes. Three of the HIV genes, called gag, pol and env, contain information needed to make structural proteins for new virus particles. The other six genes, known as tat, rev, nef, vif, vpr and vpu, code for proteins that control the ability of HIV to infect a cell, produce new copies of virus, or cause disease.

Two types of HIV have been identified. HIV-1 is the main cause of HIV infection throughout the world. HIV-2 is a prevalent cause of HIV infection in West Africa and is increasingly being identified in other areas. HIV-2 is less virulent than HIV-1.

27.7.3 Pathogenesis

Like all viruses, HIV must invade the cells of other organisms to survive and reproduce. HIV multiplies in $CD4^+$ T cells of the human immune system and kills vast numbers of the cells it infects. The result is disease symptoms.

How does HIV infection become established in the body? Researchers have found evidence that immune-system cells called dendritic cells may begin the process of infection. After exposure, these special cells may bind to and carry the virus from the site of infection to the lymph nodes, where other immune system cells become infected.

HIV targets cells in the immune system that display a protein called CD4 on their surface. Such cells are called CD4-positive ($CD4^+$) cells. When HIV encounters a $CD4^+$ cell, a protein called gp120 that protrudes from HIV's surface recognizes the CD4 protein and binds tightly to it. Another viral protein, P24, forms a casing that surrounds HIV's genetic material.

27.7.4 Transmission

Studies indicate that HIV transmission requires intimate contact with infected blood or body fluids (vaginal secretions, semen, pre-ejaculation fluid, and breast milk). HIV infection is spread in three ways as follow:

(1) Sexual intercourse

HIV is spread most commonly by sexual contact with an infected partner. The virus can enter the body through the lining of the vagina, penis, rectum, or mouth during sexual relations. Sexual activities that can result in HIV infection include sexual intercourse, anal sex (heterosexual or homosexual) and oral sex (heterosexual or homosexual).

(2) Direct contact with infected blood

HIV can be spread through direct contact with infected blood: a) Through blood or blood products transfusion. b) Through injecting drugs. This happens when needles or syringes contaminated with HIV are shared. c) In a health-care setting. Transmission from patient to health-care worker or vice-versa-via accidental sticks with contaminated needles or other medical instruments-can occur, but this is rare.

(3) From an infected mother to her unborn child

Women can transmit HIV to their fetuses during pregnancy or birth. HIV also can be spread to babies through the breast milk of mothers infected with the virus.

Activities that don't involve the possibility of intimate contact with infected blood or body fluids are regarded as no risk of infection. Research indicates that HIV is NOT transmitted by casual contact such as touching or hugging, having household items such as utensils, towels, and bedding, contact with sweat or tears, sharing facilities such as swimming pools, saunas, hot tubs, coughs, sneezes or toilets with HIV-infected people.

Prevention is the key to personal protection against HIV and AIDS. Prevention involves safer sex practices, drug use and limiting HIV exposure and minimizing HIV exposure from medical procedures.

27.7.5 Clinical Features

There are four stages of HIV infection: primary, a-symptomatic, symptomatic, and AIDS. Knowing what stage an individual is can help physicians to design treatment plans.

Stage 1: Primary HIV infection

The first stage of HIV infection is called primary infection. Primary infection begins shortly after an individual first becomes infected with HIV. This stage lasts for a few weeks. During this period, individuals experience symptoms similar to the flu. Very few individuals seek treatment during this time, and those who do are usually misdiagnosed.

Often, if an HIV test is performed, it will come back negative, since antibodies are not yet being produced by the individual's immune system. Those who believe they have been exposed to HIV should repeat the test again after six months.

Stage 2: Asymptomatic HIV

In the second stage, individuals are free from any symptoms of HIV. Levels of HIV in the blood are very low, but are detectable. If an HIV test is performed, it will come back positive. While the individual is asymptomatic, the HIV in their blood is reproducing constantly. This stage lasts about ten years, but can be much longer or shorter depending on the individual.

Stage 3: Symptomatic HIV

In the third stage, the immune system has become so damaged by HIV that symptoms begin to appear. Symptoms are typically mild at first, and then slowly become more severe. Opportunistic infections, infections that take advantage of the immune system's vulnerable state, begin to occur.

These infections affect almost all the systems of the body and include both infections and cancers. Some common opportunistic infections include tuberculosis, cytomegalovirus, and shingles.

Stage 4: Acquired immune deficiency syndrome

In the fourth and final stage, a person is diagnosed as AIDS. To be diagnosed as AIDS, a person has to exhibit certain opportunistic infections, such as HIV wasting syndrome, pneumocystis pneumonia, or Kaposi sarcoma. Once a person is diagnosed with AIDS, they can never return to a stage of HIV, even if the individual gets better.

27.7.6   Cutaneous Manifestations

Cutaneous manifestations of HIV disease can present as neoplastic, infectious and noninfectious diseases.

27.7.6.1   Infectious diseases

Viral infections: In patients infected with HIV, several viruses of the Herpesviridae family may lead to cutaneous disease, including chronic perianal and perioral herpetic ulcers caused by HSV, recurrent typical zoster caused by herpes zoster virus (HZV), and disseminated CMV infection. Epstein-Barr virus (EBV) has been implicated in the pathogenesis of oral hairy leukoplakia. Widespread or recalcitrant warts may be observed on the oral mucosa, the face, the perianal region, and the female genital tract in patients infected with HIV.

Fungal infections: Recurrent and persistent mucocutaneous candidiasis is common in patients with HIV infection, such as dermatophytosis, or tinea capitis, pityriasis versicolor. Deep fungal infections are rare. Cutaneous cryptococcosis may be observed in patients with HIV infection. Cutaneous histoplasmosis may lead to red papules, ulcerations, acneiform papules, or molluscum like lesions in patients infected with HIV. Systemic coccidioidomycosis may disseminate to the skin, usually as hemorrhagic papules or nodules.

Bacterial infections: Impetigo and folliculitis may be recurrent and persistent in HIV/AIDS, particularly in children. Disseminated furunculosis, gingivitis, gangrenous stomatitis, and abscess formation can occur in patients with HIV infection. Bacillary angiomatosis, which is caused by *Bartonella henselae* and rarely by *Bartonella quintana*, usually manifests as red papules and nodules.

27.7.6.2   Noninfectious diseases

Noninfectious diseases association with HIV include scabies, seborrheic dermatitis, pruritic papular eruption(PPE), atopic disease, and urticaria, thrombocytopenic purpura, vitiligo, alopecia areata, pemphigoid, and other kinds of diseases.

27.7.6.3   Neoplastic diseases

Kaposi sarcoma(KS) was the first reported malignancy associated with HIV infection. The worldwide prevalence of KS in patients with AIDS may approach 34%. KS is believed to be a proliferation of endothelial cells induced by human herpesvirus type 8. KS begins as pink macules that become disseminated and palpable. Purplish or brown macules and plaques may become nodular. Other HIV-associated malignancies include AIDS-related B-cell non-Hodgkin lymphomas, anal carcinoma and cervical intraepithelial neoplasia, squamous cell carcinoma of the anal mucosa, intraoral or multiple squamous cell carcinoma, Bowen disease, metastatic basal cell carcinoma and malignant melanoma.

27.7.7   Diagnosis

The blood tests most commonly used to diagnose HIV infection are measuring the levels of antibodies produced against HIV. Antibody-detecting assays, or tests, include the enzyme immunoassay (EIA), enzyme-linked immunosorbent assay (ELISA), and western blot test. Usually, the first test that laboratories use to detect the presence of HIV antibodies is EIA or ELISA. If the first test manifests a positive result (HIV antibodies appear to be present), then the more sensitive Western Blot test is used to confirm it.

Early diagnosis of HIV infection is important, because it allows people to seek treatment that will suppress HIV's attack on the immune system and prevent opportunistic infections, and because it helps women who are planning a pregnancy or who are already pregnant take steps to reduce the risk of transmitting the HIV infection to the baby.

27.7.8   Treatment

Although there is no treatment currently available that can cure people of HIV/AIDS, a number of therapies have been developed to help them stay healthier and live longer. Some medications target HIV itself, to reduce the virus's assault on the immune system, or to even prevent the virus from entering human immune cells. Other treatments are used to treat or prevent specific opportunistic infections that threaten the health of people with HIV-damaged immune systems.

Four classes of antiretroviral drugs have been developed to interfere with the activity of these viral enzymes and slow down the multiplication of the virus. These are nucleoside analog reverse transcriptase inhibitors (NRTIs), non-nucleoside reverse transcriptase inhibitors (NNRTIs), protease inhibitors(PIs) and fusion inhibitors.

A new treatment approved in the past years works in a completely new way by preventing the virus from entering the human immune cells. Other drugs and therapies are used to prevent or treat opportunistic infections and other AIDS-related conditions.

27.8 Chancroid

Chancroid is a sexually transmitted disease characterized by painful genital ulcerations and inflammatory inguinal adenopathy with abscess formation. It caused by the Gram-negative bacillus *Haemophilus ducreyi*. Chancroid accounts for a large proportion of genital ulcers in the developing countries.

27.8.1 Etiology
H. ducreyi is a small, gram-negative, facultative anaerobic coccobacillus. The organism enters the skin or mucosa through microabrasions during sexual contact. Viable *H. ducreyi* are demonstrable in lesions, but very few organisms have been found within phagocytes. *H ducreyi* infection causes both a delayed type sensitivity response and antibodies to several surface antigens. Chancroid has been shown to facilitate HIV transmission.

27.8.2 Clinical Features
The incubation period is between 3 and 7 days, rarely more than 2 weeks. No prodromal symptoms are known.

Initial lesion at the site of inoculation is a papule. After 24 to 48 hours, the papule evolves into a pustule. The pustule then spontaneously ruptures and forms a classic nonindurated, painful ulcer with a purulent base and ragged, undermined borders. The ulcers are usually covered by grayish, necrotic purulent exudates. Its base is composed of granulation tissues which bleed easily. The diameter varies from 1 to 20 mm. The ulcers can be single or multiple. There may be "Kissing" lesions due to autoinoculation on adjacent cutaneous surfaces.

In men most ulcers are found on the coronal sulcus, frenulum, or glans penis. The shaft of the penis and the anus may also be involved less frequently. In women most lesions occur at the vaginal entrance, including the labia majora and minora, fourchette, vestibule, and clitoris. Cervical and vaginal wall ulcers are rare. Extragenital ulcers have been reported on the breasts, fingers, thighs, and inside of the mouth.

Approximately up to 50% of patients develop painful tender inguinal adenitis, which frequently becomes fluctuant and spontaneously rupture. The adenitis is usually unilateral in most patients.

A number of clinical variants of chancroid have been recognized. ① Giant chancroid: lesion extends peripherally beyond its margins. ② Transient chancroid: small ulcer heals spontaneously in a few days. ③ Follicular chancroid: initial follicular pustule evolves into a classic ulcer. ④ Papular chancroid: ulcerated papule may resemble that of condylomata lata of Secondary Syphilis. ⑤ Phagedenic chancroid: Ulceration causes extensive profound destruction of tissue rapidly. ⑥ Serpiginous chancroid: Multiple ulcers that confluent to form a serpiginous pattern. ⑦ Mixed chancroid: ulcers of chancroid occur together with an indurated nontender ulcer of syphilis.

27.8.3 Laboratory Tests
Culture of *H. ducreyi* currently remains the primary tool for chancroid diagnosis. Specimens for culture should be taken from the purulent ulcer base or active border. Small, yellow-gray, translucent colonies appear in 24 to 48 hours after inoculation. The identification of *H. ducreyi* is performed with some biochemical reactions.

Gram stain of genital ulcer secretions can reveal small, Gram-negative, bipolar-staining rods in a "schools of fish" pattern, but this test lacks both sensitivity and specificity.

Serologic tests to detect antibody to *H. ducreyi* also have been described. Although these methods have limited usefulness in distinguishing recent from past infections, they provide useful screening methods for community-level epidemiologic studies.

27.8.4 Diagnosis and Differential Diagnosis
Chancroid is most prominent in promiscuous person. In most of the cases, the clinical diagnosis for chancroid is mainly based on the manifestation of ulcers in the genital areas.

A probable diagnosis of chancroid can be made

if the next criteria are present: ① the patient has one or more painful ulcers; ② the patient has no evidence of syphilis by darkfield examination or by serologic testing examined at least 7 days after onset of ulcers; ③ the result of a test for herpes simplex virus is negative.

Clinical diagnosis is often inaccurate, and laboratory determination should be attempted in suspected cases. Gram stain of secretions may present a predominance of characteristic gram-negative coccobacilli. Culturing the bacterium—*Haemophilus ducreyi* has been considered the "gold standard" to confirm the symptoms.

Although there are many distinguishing features, there is considerable overlap between the clinical appearances of chancroid and primary syphilis. Table 27 – 1 shows the classic differences in clinical presentation between these two diseases.

Table 27 – 1 The classic differences between chancroid and hard chancre

Diseases	Chancroid	Hard chancre
Etiologic agent	*Haemophilus ducreyi*	*Treponema pallidum*
Incubation period	3 – 7days	3 weeks
Numbers of ulcer	2 or more	Mostly only one
Characteristics of lesion	Painful nonindurated ulcer with irregular undermined edges and a purulent exudative base	Painless, indurated, clean-based ulcer
Lymphadenopathy	Tender, suppurative, painful	Hard but painless, not purulent

27.8.5 Treatment

Azithromycin, 1 g PO in a single dose; or ceftriaxone, 250 mg IM in a single dose; or ciprofloxacin, 500 mg PO twice daily for 3 d; or erythromycin base, 500 mg PO 3 times daily for 7 d.

27.9 Lymphogranuloma Venereum

Lymphogranuloma venereum (LGV) is a rare sexually transmitted disease caused by *Chlamydia trachomatis* strains of the L_1, L_2, and L_3 serovars. Classically, acute LGV is characterized by transient ulcers followed by suppurative inguinal lymphadenopathy. Without treatment, late complications developed after many years include genital elephantiasis and rectal strictures. The worldwide incidence of LGV is decreasing, but the disease is still endemic in Southeast Asia, Africa, Central and South America, and parts of the Caribbean.

27.9.1 Etiology

LGV is caused by *C. trachomatis* serovars L_1, L_2, and L_3. Different from the other serovars that remain confined to the mucosa, L_1, L_2, and L_3 serovars have a high affinity for macrophages. After being inoculated, the organisms multiply in macrophages, and spread to the draining lymph nodes to cause lymphadenitis.

27.9.2 Clinical Features

The incubation period varies from 3 days to 4 weeks. Its clinical presentation varies with three stages.

27.9.2.1 Primary stage

The primary genital lesion may begin as a self-limited small painless papule or ulcer at the site of inoculation. In men, the lesion may usually involve the coronal sulcus, prepuce, or balanus; and in women on the vulva. The primary lesion is transient, often heals in several days to a week before recognition by the patient without scarring.

27.9.2.2 Secondary stage

Occurring days to a few weeks after primary lesion appearance, the secondary stage is systemic and lymph nodes involvement. According to the way of transmission, two major syndromes are important: the inguinal syndrome and the acute anorectal syndrome.

The inguinal syndrome is characterized by painful inguinal and/or femoral lymphadenitis and is the major manifestation in male. At the beginning, the skin overlying the involved discrete LN is erythematous and indurated. Over the following 1 to 2 weeks, the LN enlargement and coalescence occurs to form a tender immovable inflamed mass, which may rupture spontaneously and develop sinus tracts draining through the skin. Unilateral involvement occurs in two-third of the cases. Synchronous enlargement of inguinal and femoral nodes on either side of the inguinal ligament leads to the pathognomonic "groove sign". At this stage, systemic symptoms may appear, including fever, chills, headache, malaise, decreased appetite and myalgias.

The acute anorectal syndrome is characterized by bloody rectal discharge and painful inflammation, progressing to hemorrhagic proctitis. It is the most common manifestation in female and in homosexual men who practice receptive anal intercourse. Patients may complain of anal pruritus, bloody rectal discharge, tenesmus or constipation.

27.9.2.3 Tertiary stage

During the infection, fibrosis may occur. It can lead to different degrees of lymphatic obstruction, chronic edema, and strictures. These results are mostly permanent. This stage is more commonly seen in female and includes rectal strictures and genital elephantiasis. These sequelae may appear years after primary infection in the absence of treatment.

Less commonly, besides the above-mentioned manifestations, meningoencephalitis, polyarthritis, hepatosplenomegaly, iritis and erythema nodosum can occur.

27.9.3 Laboratory Tests

Serology tests are sensitive but non-specific because of cross-reactivity with other chlamydial infections. More over, they do not distinguish current from prior infection. The complement fixation test is the most commonly used method. Titers above 1:64 are highly suggestive of LGV. The microimmunofluorescence test is more specific but more unavailable.

Chlamydia culture can supply direct evidence of *C. trachomatis* infection. But culture does not differentiate between LGV and non-LGV serovars.

Mild leukocytosis, false-positive serologic test for syphilis, and high levels of immunoglobulin A and immunoglobulin G in serum maybe occur.

27.9.4 Diagnosis and Differential Diagnosis

The clinical diagnosis for LGV is predominantly based on the manifestation of genital ulcers followed by inguinal lymphadenopathy. Diagnostic tests include culture and serology tests.

The characteristic LGV primary ulcer differs from the chancre of primary syphilis because the latter usually is bigger with indurated margins. The typical ulcer of chancroid is painful with irregular undermined edges and a purulent exudative base; extensive lymphadenopathy may represent in both LGV and chancroid.

27.9.5 Treatment

Recommended antimicrobial therapy for LGV is a 3-week course of oral doxycycline, 100 mg twice daily, or when contraindicated, erythromycin base 500 mg orally four times daily. Doxycycline is contraindicated in pregnancy. Fluctuant buboes should be aspirated. Surgery is usually necessary in late stages.

All patients should be followed clinically until signs and symptoms have resolved. Fluctuant buboes should be aspirated and may not fully resolve by the completion of the antimicrobial course.

27.9.6 Prognosis

Every patient should be followed clinically until signs and symptoms disappeared. The prognosis for LGV patients is excellent if infection is properly recognized early and treated ahead of the development of severe sequelae.

■ Summary

Syphilis is a chronic, contagious, sexually transmitted disease caused by *Treponema pallidum* subspecies *pallidum*. In congenital syphilis, the treponema crosses the placenta and infects the fetus. It is a multistage disease with diverse and wide-ranging manifestations. The diagnosis of syphilis may involve dark-field microscopy examination of skin lesions, serological nontreponemal test and treponemal-specific test. Syphilis should be treated early, adequately and regularly, and as much as possible to avoid the cardiovascular syphilis, neurosyphilis and serious complications. Penicillins are the first line drugs. In penicillin-allergic patients, the preference alternative drug is ceftriaxone sodium, tetracycline and doxycycline are two other alternative drugs. Serial cerebrospinal fluid examinations are necessary to ensure adequate treatment of neurosyphilis. Follow-up for clinical and serological assessment should be done.

Gonorrhea is a disease caused by *Neisseria gonorrhoeae*, and mainly genitourinary suppurative infection. Diagnosis depends on laboratory examination, clinical features and history. The effective treatment contains systemic administration of ceftriaxone or spectinomycin et al.

Chlamydia trachomatis genital infection is a sexually transmitted disease caused by *Chlamydia trachomatis*, and its incidence rate has exceeded number one in all sexually transmitted diseases. *Chlamydia trachomatis* is the most common pathogen in NGU. According to the history of sexual activity, urethritis present with a mild symptom, diagnosis can be determined with the laboratory tests.

Condyloma acuminatum, also known as genital warts, is caused by the human papillomavirus (HPV). CA is a sexually transmitted disease, it mainly spreads through skin-to-skin contact during sexual activity and mostly often occurs in the external genitalia, anus and other parts. in recent years the incidence of CA increased dramatically Around the world, in some countries it even becomes the most common sexually transmitted disease.

Genital herpes (GH) is a herpes simplex virus infection in the urinary genital, perianal mucocutaneous sites, which is a chronic, recurrent sexually transmitted disease difficult to be cured. Herpes simplex virus contains two serotypes: HSV-1 and HSV-2. Genital herpes infection is usually due to HSV-2. The disease mainly based on medical history (history of high risk behavior or sexual partner infection etc.), typical clinical manifestations for clinical diagnosis. systemic administration and topical use of medicine is needed for proper treatment.

Acquired immunodeficiency syndrome (AIDS) is caused by the human immunodeficiency virus (HIV). When HIV infect the $CD4^+$ T lymphocytes, the damaged immune system loses its ability to defend against microscopic organisms. HIV infection is transmitted by three routes: sexual intercourse, direct contact with infected blood, and mother-to child transmission. Anti-HIV antibody test is used for diagnosis of HIV infection. Although there is no treatment currently available that can cure people of HIV or AIDS, HAART(highly active antiretroviral therapy) has been developed to help them live longer.

Chancroid is a sexually transmitted disease characterized by painful genital ulcers and painful inguinal lymphadenopathy. It is caused by the Gram-negative streptobacillus *Haemophilus ducreyi*. There are many differences and similarities between the syphilitic chancre and chancroid. The treatment for chancroid is a single oral dose of Azithromycin or a single IM dose of ceftriaxone or oral Erythromycin for seven days.

Lymphogranuloma venereum (LGV) is a rare sexually transmitted disease caused by *Chlamydia trachomatis* strains of the L_1, L_2, and L_3 serovars. Acute LGV is characterized by transient ulcers followed by suppurative inguinal lymphadenopathy. Without treatment, late complications developed after many years include genital elephantiasis and rectal strictures. If infection is properly recognized early and treated ahead of the development of severe sequelae, the prognosis for LGV patients is excellent.

▪ Questions

1. What is the clinical feature of syphilis and how to diagnose and treat it?

2. What is the cause of gonorrhea and how to treat it?

3. What is the clinical feature of *Chlamydial trachomatis* genital infection?

4. What is the clinical feature of condyloma acuminate, and the advantages and disadvantages of its treatment?

5. What is the cause of genital herpes and how to treat it?

6. What is the cause of AIDS and how to diagnose and treat it?

(Yanchun Liu 刘彦春, Yanqing Gao 高艳青,
Cuie Liu 刘翠娥, An Liu 刘安,
Xin Sun 孙欣, Chunbo Wei 魏春波,
Yan Wu 吴焱, Yingxue Song 宋映雪)

References

[1] William D James, Timothy G Berger, Dirk M Elston. Andrews' diseases of the skin. 10th ed. Canada: Elsevier Inc, 2006.

[2] Tony Burns, Stephen Breathnach, Neil Cox, et al. Rook's Textbook of Dermatology. 8th ed. Chichester: Blackwell Publishing Ltd, 2010.

[3] Klaus Wolff, Lowell A Goldsmith, Stephen I Katz, et al. Fitzpatrick's dermatology in general medicine. 7th ed. New York: McGraw-Hill Professional, 2007.

[4] Zhang Xuejun. Dermatovenerology. 7th ed. Beijing: The People's Medical Publishing House, 2008.

[5] Hiroshi Shimizu. Shimizu's textbook of dermatology. Nakayama Shoten: Hokkaido University Press, 2007.

[6] Lawrence CM. An Introduction to Dermatological Surgery. 2nd ed. St Louis: Mosby, 2002.

[7] Elsaie ML. Cutaneous remodeling and photorejuvenation using radiofrequency devices. Indian J Dermatol, 2009, 54(3): 201 – 205.

[8] Akdis CA, Akdis M, Bieber T, et al. Diagnosis and treatment of atopic dermatitis in children and adults: European Academy of Allergology and Clinical Immunology/ American Academy of Allergy, Asthma and Immunology/PAACTALL Consensus Report. J Allergy Clin Immnol, 2006, 118(1): 152 – 169.

[9] Zhao Bian. Clinical Dermatology. 3rd ed. Nanjing: Jiangsu Science and Technology Publishing House, 2001.

[10] Akdis CA, Akdis M, Bieber T, et al. Diagnosis and treatment of atopic dermatitis in children and adults: European Academy of Allergology and Clinical Immunology/American Academy of Allergy, Asthma and Immunology/PAACTALL Consensus Report. J Allergy Clin Immnol, 2006, 118(1): 152 – 169.

[11] Jean L Bolognia, Joseph L Jorizzo, Ronald Prapini, et al. Dermatology e-dition: Text with Continually Updated Online Reference, 2 – Volume Set. Louis: Mosby Inc, 2007.

[12] O'Connor NR, McLaughlin MR, Ham P. Newborn skin: Part I. Common rashes. Am Fam Physician, 2008, 77(1): 47 – 52.

[13] Minoru Hasegawa, Manabu Fujimoto, Kazuhiko Takehara Shinichi Sato. Pathogenesis of systemic sclerosis: Altered B cell function is the key linking systemic autoimmunity and tissue fibrosis. Journal of Dermatological Science, 2005, 39: 1 – 7.

[14] Lorinda Chung, Jan Lin, Daniel E Furst, et al. Systemic and localized scleroderma. Clinics in Dermatology, 2006, 24: 374 – 392.

[15] Carlson JA, Ng BT, Chen KR. Cutaneous vasculitis update: diagnostic criteria, classification, epidemiology, etiology, pathogenesis, evaluation and prognosis. Am J Dermatopathol, 2005, 27: 504 – 528.

[16] Harper J, Oranje A, Prose N. Textbook of Pediatric Dermatology. 2nd ed. Chichester: Blackwell Publishing Ltd, 2006.

[17] Maria C Garzon, Jennifer T Huang, Odile Enjolras, et al. Vascular malformations. J Am Acad Dermatol, 2007, 56: 353 – 359.

[18] Zeina Tannous, Nelly Rubeiz, Abdul-Ghani Kibbi. Vascular anomalies: portwine stains and hemangiomas. J Cutan Pathol, 2010, 37 (Suppl. 1): 88 – 95.

[19] Coovadia H. Current issues in prevention of mother-to-child transmission of HIV-1. Curr Opin HIV AIDS, 2009, 4(4): 319 – 324.

[20] WHO. Prioritizing second-line antiretroviral drugs for adults and adolescents: a public health approach report of a WHO working group meeting. Geneva: WHO, 2007.

[21] DiClemente RJ, Wingood GM, Del Rio C, et al. Prevention interventions for HIV positive individuals. Sex Transm Infect, 2002, 78(6): 393 – 395.

1

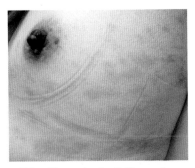

Color Figure 4 - 1　Inflammatory
hyperemia

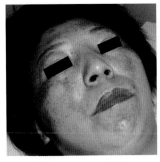

Color Figure 4 - 2　Chloasma

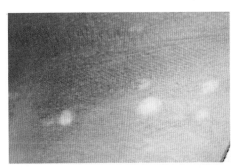

Color Figure 4 - 3　Vitiligo—depigmentation
macules

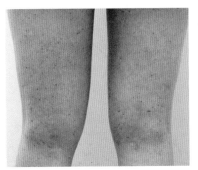

Color Figure 4 - 4　Thrombocytolytic
purpura—blood spots

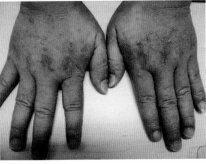

Color Figure 4 - 5　Flat wart—planate
papules

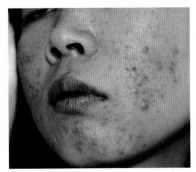

Color Figure 4 - 6　Acne—inflammation
papules

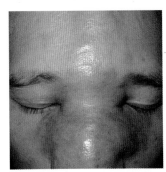

Color Figure 4 - 7　Conidiobolomycosis

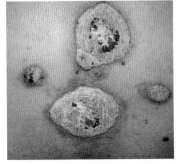

Color Figure 4 - 8　Psoriasis

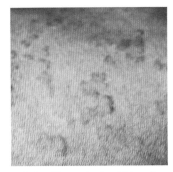

Color Figure 4 - 9　Urticaria

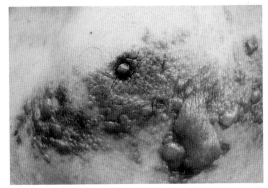

Color Figure 4 - 10　Herpes zoster

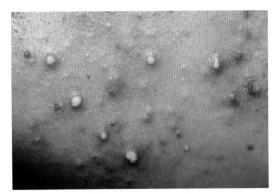

Color Figure 4 - 11　Acne

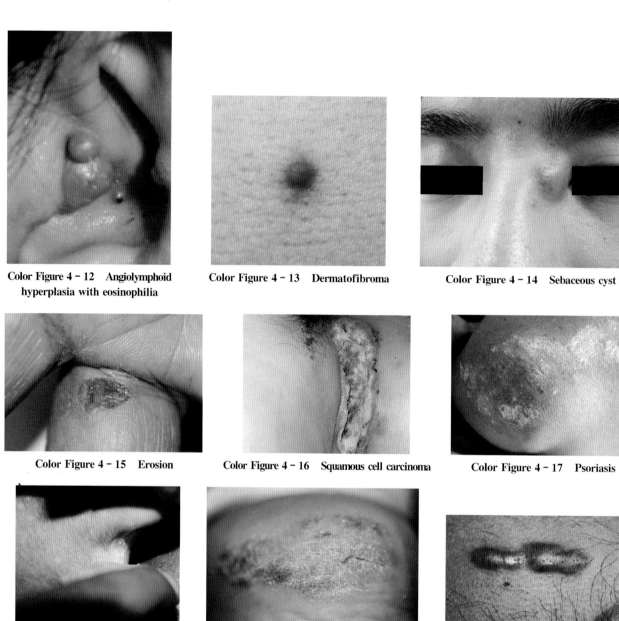

Color Figure 4 - 12   Angiolymphoid
hyperplasia with eosinophilia

Color Figure 4 - 13   Dermatofibroma

Color Figure 4 - 14   Sebaceous cyst

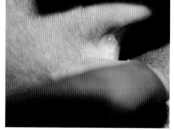

Color Figure 4 - 15   Erosion

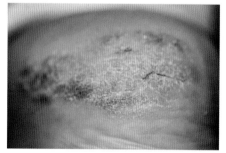

Color Figure 4 - 16   Squamous cell carcinoma

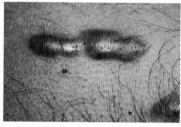

Color Figure 4 - 17   Psoriasis

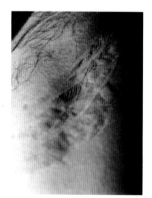

Color Figure 4 - 18   Tinea pedis

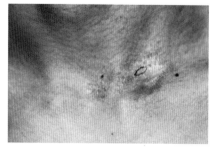

Color Figure 4 - 19   Fissure

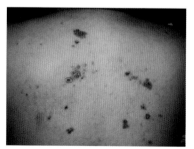

Color Figure 4 - 20   After acne scar

Color Figure 4 - 21   Striae
atrophicae

Color Figure 4 - 22   Striae atrophicae

Color Figure 4 - 23   Bullous pemphigoid

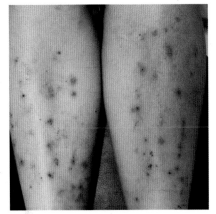

Color Figure 4 – 24　Excoriation

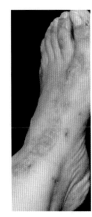

Color Figure 4 – 25　Neurodermatitis

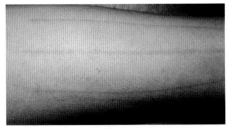

Color Figure 4 – 26　Dermatograph test

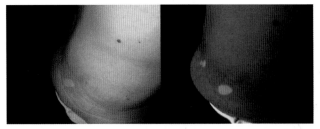

Color Figure 4 – 27　Filtered ultraviolet light examination

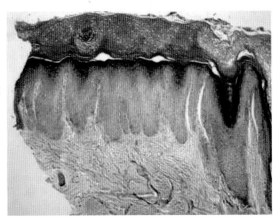

Color Figure 5 – 1　Hyperkeratosis

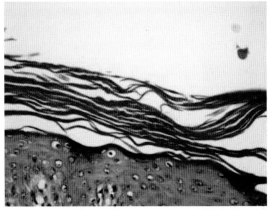

Color Figure 5 – 2　Parakeratosis

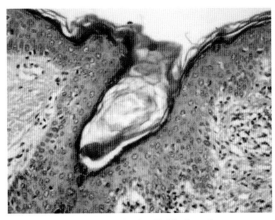

Color Figure 5 – 3　Follicular plug

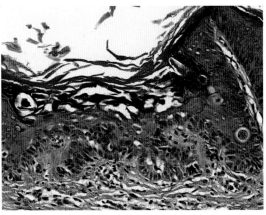

Color Figure 5 – 4　Dyskeratosis

（By Professor Tianwen Gao）

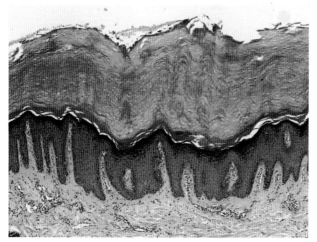

Color Figure 5－5　Hypergranulosis
（By Professor Tianwen Gao）

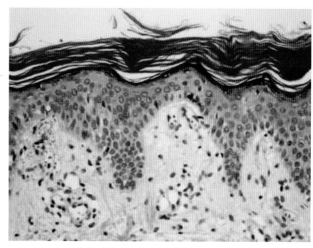

Color Figure 5－6　Hypogranulosis

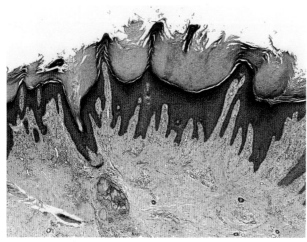

Color Figure 5－7　Acanthosis
（By Professor Tianwen Gao）

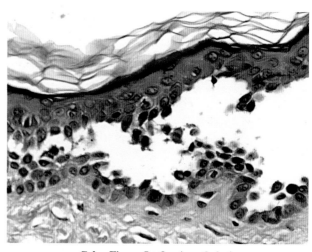

Color Figure 5－8　Acantholysis
（By Professor Tianwen Gao）

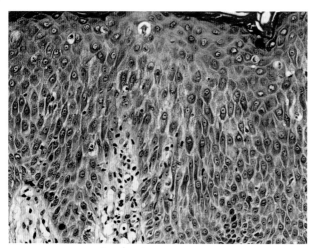

Color Figure 5－9　Spongiosis
（By Professor Tianwen Gao）

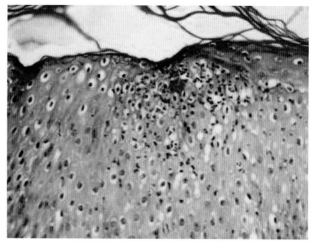

Color Figure 5－10　Kogoj spongiform pustule

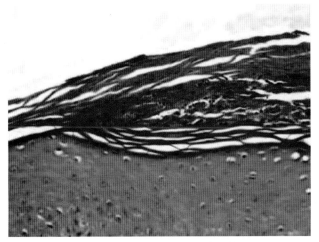

Color Figure 5 - 11　Munro microabscess

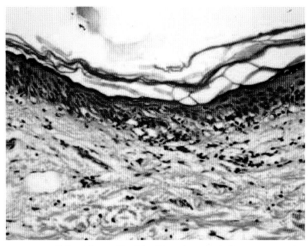

Color Figure 5 - 12　Pautrier microabscess

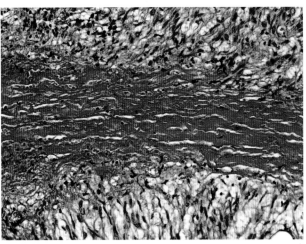

Color Figure 5 - 13　Collagen degeneration
（By Professor Tianwen Gao）

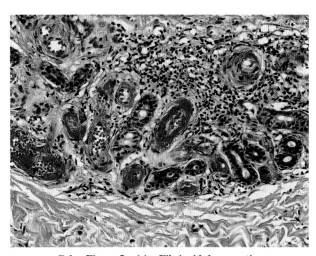

Color Figure 5 - 14　Fibrinoid degeneration
（By Professor Tianwen Gao）

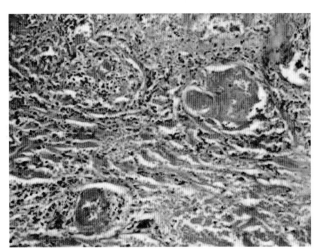

Color Figure 5 - 15　Necrosis

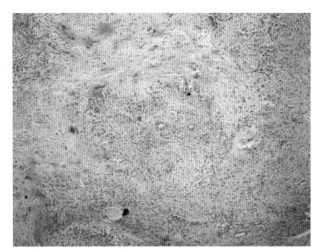

Color Figure 5 - 16　Granuloma

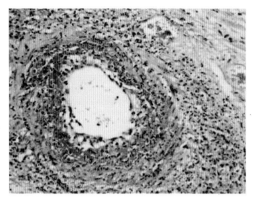

Color Figure 5 - 17　Vasculitis

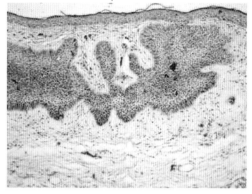

Color Figure 5 - 18　Neoplasm

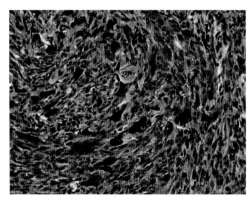

Color Figure 5 - 19　Atypia

（By Professor Tianwen Gao）

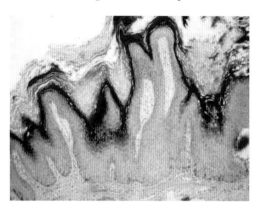

Color Figure 5 - 20　Papilloma

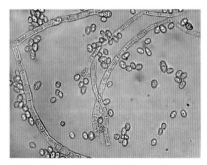

Color Figure 6 - 1　Hyphae and spores

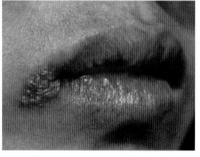

Color Figure 9 - 1　Herpetic
gingivostomatitis

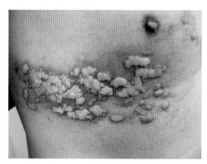

Color Figure 9 - 2　Herpes zoster

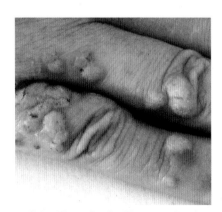

Color Figure 9 - 3　Verruca vulgaris

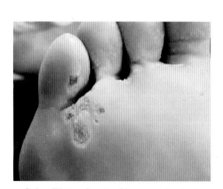

Color Figure 9 - 4　Verruca plantaris

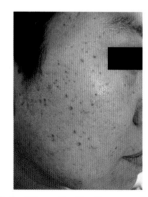

Color Figure 9 - 5　Verruca plana

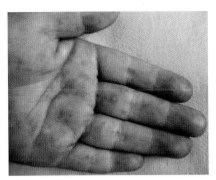

Color Figure 9 - 6   The hand, foot and mouth disease

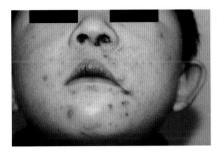

Color Figure 10 - 1   Impetigo contagiosa

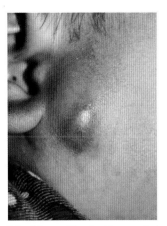

Color Figure 10 - 2   Furunculosis

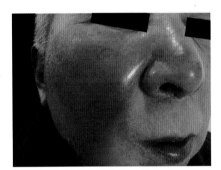

Color Figure 10 - 3   Erysipelas

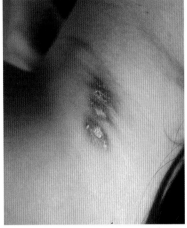

Color Figure 10 - 4   Lupus vulgaris
（By Professor Zhihua Wu）

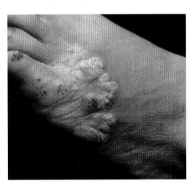

Color Figure 10 - 5   Tuberculosis verrucosa cutis
（By Professor Zhihua Wu）

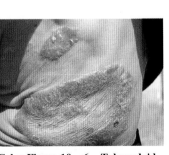

Color Figure 10 - 6   Tuberculoid leprosy
（By Professor Zhihua Wu）

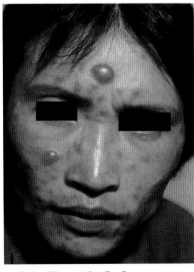

Color Figure 10 - 7   Lepromatous leprosy
（By Professor Zhihua Wu）

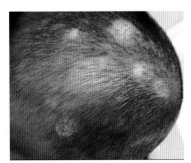

Color Figure 11 - 1   White tinea capitis

8

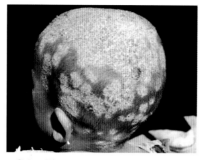

Color Figure 11 - 2   Black-dot tinea capitis
（By Professor Zhihua Wu）

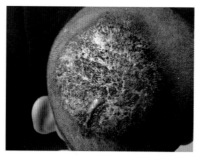

Color Figure 11 - 3   Pustular tinea capitis
（By Professor Zhihua Wu）

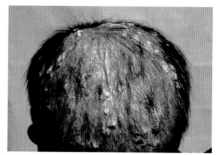

Color Figure 11 - 4   Crusted tinea capitis
（By Professor Zhihua Wu）

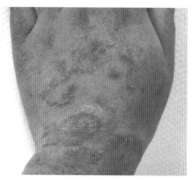

Color Figure 11 - 5   Tinea corporis

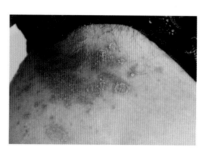

Color Figure 11 - 6   Tinea cruris

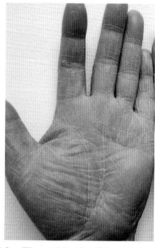

Color Figure 11 - 7   Tinea manuum

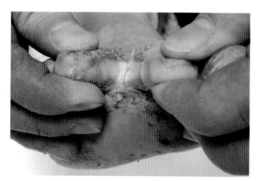

Color Figure 11 - 8   Tinea pedis

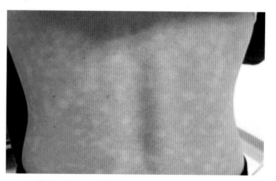

Color Figure 11 - 9   Pityriasis versicolor

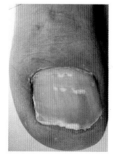

Color Figure 11 - 10   SWO

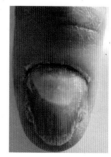

Color Figure 11 - 11   DLSO

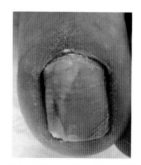

Color Figure 11 - 12   PSO

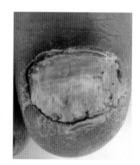

Color Figure 11 - 13   TDO

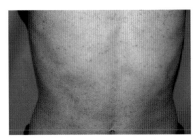

Color Figure 12 - 1　Scabies on the prothorax and the abdomen

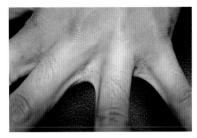

Color Figure 12 - 2　Scabies on the finger webs

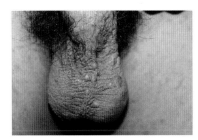

Color Figure 12 - 3　Scabies
Note lesion on scrotum

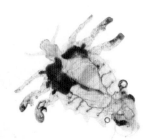

Color Figure 12 - 4　The crab louse

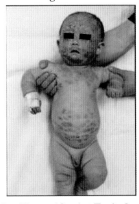

Color Figure 13 - 1　Typical well-defined erythema and edema in acute contact dermatitis

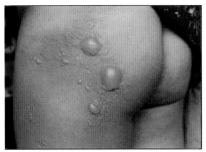

Color Figure 13 - 2　Bullae in severe acute contact dermatitis

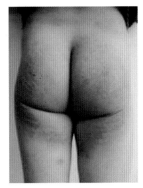

Color Figure 13 - 3　Scaly, erythematous patch in chronic contact dermatitis

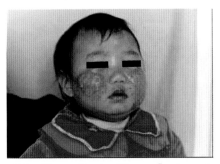

Color Figure 13 - 4　Edema, weeping and oozing in acute phase of eczema

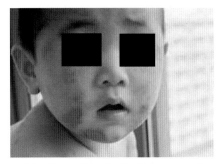

Color Figure 13 - 5　Erythema, papule and dry scales in subacute phase of eczema

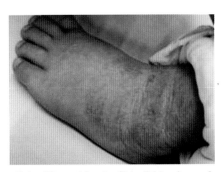

Color Figure 13 - 6　Skin thickening and lichenification in chronic phase of eczema

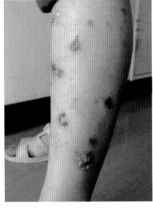

Color Figure 13 - 7　Typical nummular plaques with crusting, oozing and pustules in discoid eczema

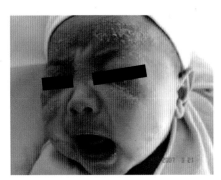

Color Figure 13 - 8　Facial involvement in a baby with atopic dermatitis

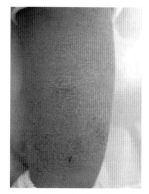

Color Figure 13 - 9　Xerosis in an AD child

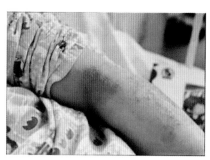

Color Figure 13 - 10　Typical lesion in flexural fold

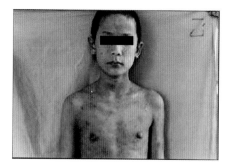

Color Figure 13 - 11　Generalized eczematous lesions in childhood atopic dermatitis

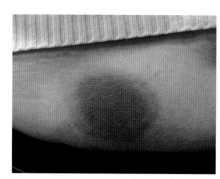

Color Figure 14 - 1　Fixed drug eruption

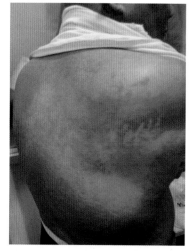

Color Figure 14 - 2　Urticarial drug eruption

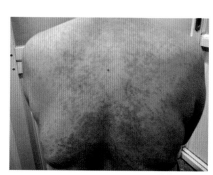

Color Figure 14 - 3　Morbilliform drug eruption

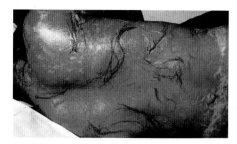

Color Figure 14 - 4　Drug-induced bullae epidermolysis
(By Professor Zhihua Wu)

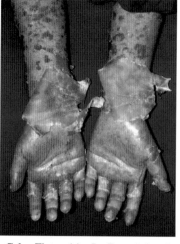

Color Figure 14 - 5　Drug-induced exfoliative dermatitis
(By Professor Zhihua Wu)

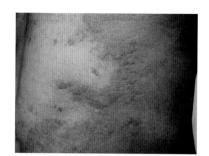

Color Figure 15 - 1　Acute urticaria

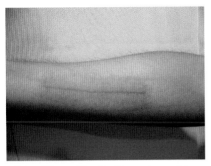

Color Figure 15 - 2　Dermatographism

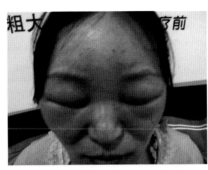

Color Figure 15 - 3　Acquired
angioedema

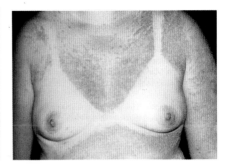

Color Figure 16 - 1　Sunburn
(By Professor Zhihua Wu)

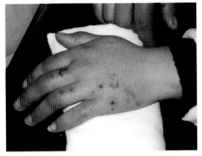

Color Figure 16 - 2　Pernio
(By Professor Zhihua Wu)

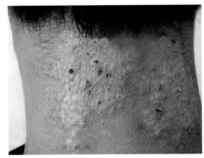

Color Figure 17 - 1　Lichen simplex
chronicus

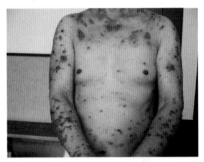

Color Figure 17 - 2　Acute prurigo

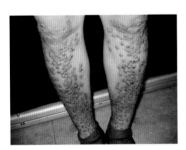

Color Figure 17 - 3　Prurigo
nodularis

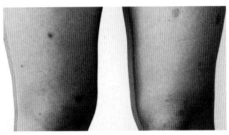

Color Figure 18 - 1　The typical "target lesion"
or "iris lesion"

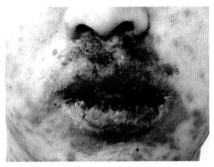

Color Figure 18 - 2　Involvement
of the lips

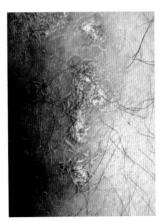

Color Figure 18 - 3　The typical lesion
of psoriasis vulgaris

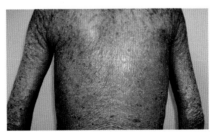

Color Figure 18 - 4　Erythrodermic
psoriasis

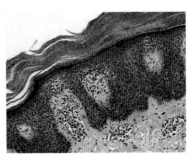

Color Figure 18 - 5　Pathologic
appearances

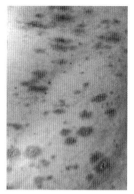

Color Figure 18 - 6　Oval patches of pityriasis rosea

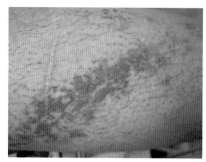

Color Figure 18 - 7　The typical lesion of LP

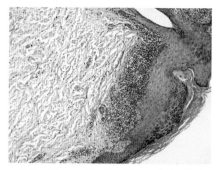

Color Figure 18 - 8　The pathological appearance of LP

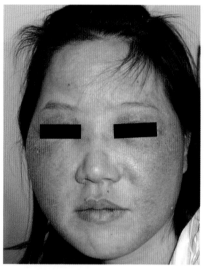

Color Figure 19 - 1　The butterfly rash

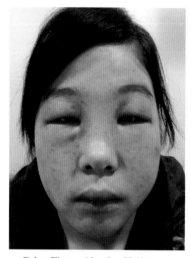

Color Figure 19 - 2　Heliotrope erythema of eyelids

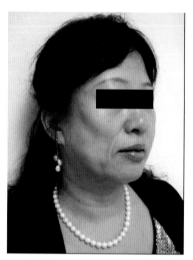

Color Figure 19 - 3　Morphea

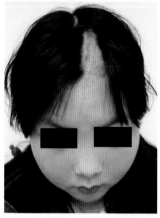

Color Figure 19 - 4　Linear scleroderma return to limited scleroderma
(CREST syndrome)

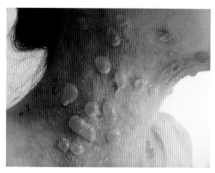

Color Figure 20 - 1　Pemphigus vulgaris

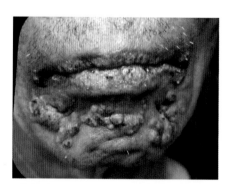

Color Figure 20 - 2　Pemphigus vegetans
(By Professor Zhihua Wu)

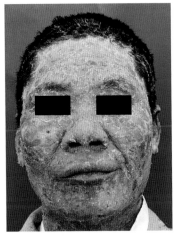

Color Figure 20 - 3　Pemphigus foliaceus
(By Professor Zhihua Wu)

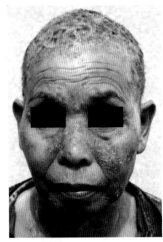

Color Figure 20 - 4　Pemphigus erythematosus
(By Professor Zhihua Wu)

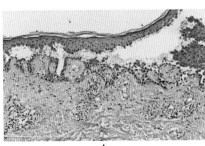

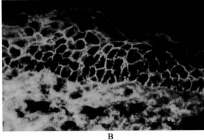

Color Figure 20 - 5　Histopathology and immunopathology of pemphigus
（A：histopathology，B：immunopathology）　(By Professor Zhihua Wu)

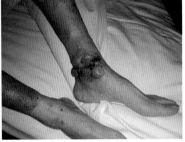

**Color Figure 20 - 6　Bullous
pemphigoid**

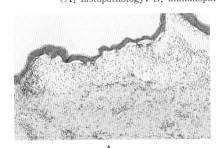

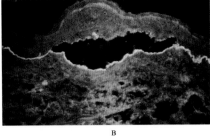

Color Figure 20 - 7　Histopathology and immunopathology of bullous pemphigoid
（A：Histopathology，B：immunopathology）
(By Professor Zhihua Wu)

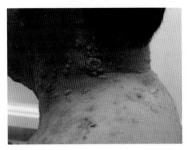

**Color Figure 20 - 8　Dermatitis
herpetiformis**

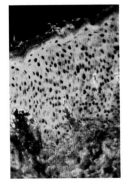

**Color Figure 20 - 9　Immunopathology
of dermatitis herpetiformis**
(By Professor Zhihua Wu)

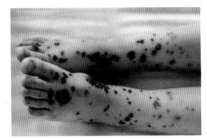

Color Figure 21 - 1　Anaphylactoid purpura

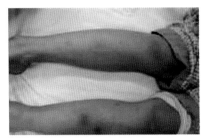

Color Figure 21 - 2　Erythema nodosum

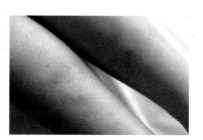

Color Figure 21 - 3   Allergic cutaneous vasculitis

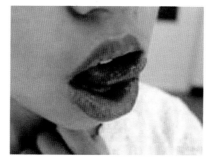

Color Figure 21 - 4   Aphthous stomatitis in Behçet's disease

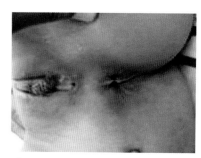

Color Figure 21 - 5   Genital aphthae in Behçet's disease

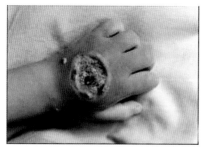

Color Figure 21 - 6   Cutaneous lesion in Behçet's disease

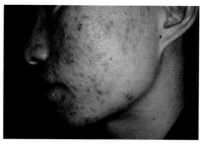

Color Figure 22 - 1   Acne vulgaris
Note comedones, inflammation, papules, pustules and pitted scars

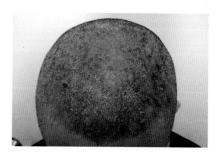

Color Figure 22 - 2   Seborrheic dermatitis
Note yellow-red, white, dry, scaling macules on scalp

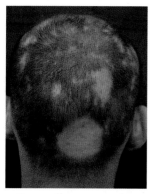

Color Figure 22 - 3   Multiple sharply outlined patches of alopecia without abnormal scaling

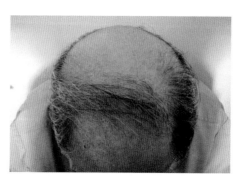

Color Figure 22 - 4   Androgenetic alopecia
Note loss of hair in the frontotemporal and vertex areas

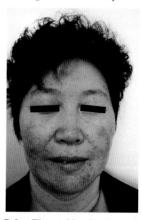

Color Figure 22 - 5   Rosacea
Note clusters of papulopustules on the cheek, forehead and chin

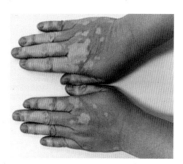

Color Figure 23 - 1   Vitiligo

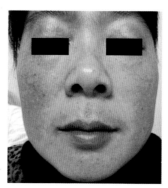

Color Figure 23 - 2   Chloasma

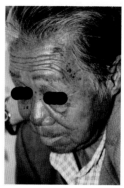

Color Figure 23 - 3   Melanosis

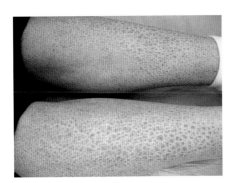

Color Figure 24 - 1   Ichthyosis vulgaris, dry

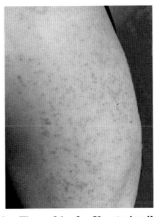

Color Figure 24 - 2   Keratosis pilaris

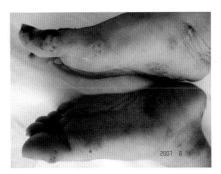

Color Figure 24 - 3   Punctate keratoderma
Multiple small hyperkeratotic papules on the soles

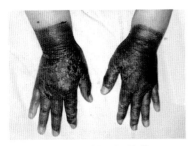

Color Figure 25 - 1   Pellagra
(niacin deficiency)
(By Professor Zhihua Wu)

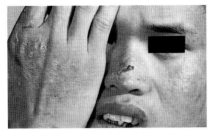

Color Figure 25 - 2   Porphyria cutanea tarda
(By Professor Zhihua Wu)

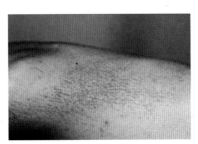

Color Figure 25 - 3   Macular amyloidosis, upper arm extensor aspect

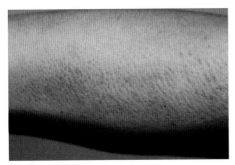

Color Figure 25 - 4   Macular amyloidosis, forearm extensor aspect

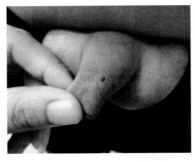

Color Figure 26 - 1   Junctional nevus

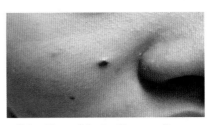

Color Figure 26 - 2   Compound nevus

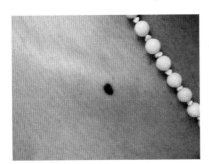

Color Figure 26 - 3   Intradermal nevus

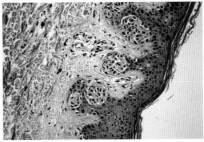

Color Figure 26 - 4   Junctional nevus(×400)

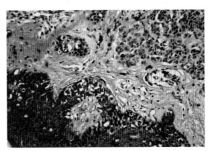

Color Figure 26 - 5   Compound nevus(×400)

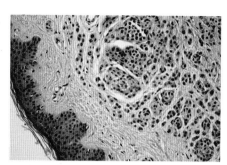

Color Figure 26 – 6　Intradermal nevus(×400)

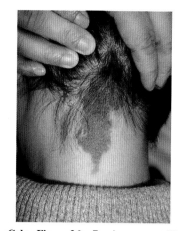

Color Figure 26 – 7　A woman with port-wine stain on the back of neck

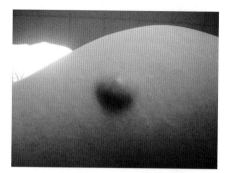

Color Figure 26 – 8　VM of haunch
(Presented by Fang Liu)

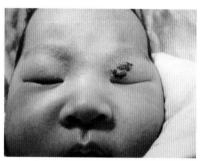

Color Figure 26 – 9　IH located on the left upper eyelid

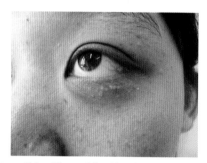

Color Figure 26 – 10　Syringomas on the eyelid

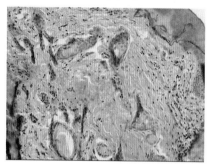

Color Figure 26 – 11　The strands of epithelial cells and the dilated cystic sweat ducts in the dermis

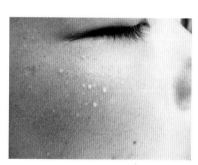

Color Figure 26 – 12　Milium

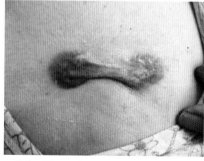

Color Figure 26 – 13　Keloid with no history of preceding trauma on the chest

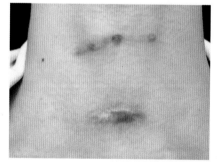

Color Figure 26 – 14　Hypertrophic scar with the history of preceding trauma on the neck

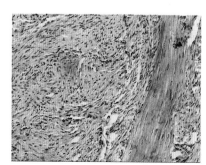

Color Figure 26 – 15　The new growth of fibroblasts and collagen in the dermis

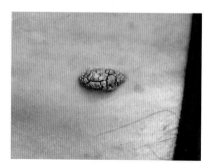

Color Figure 26 – 16　Seborrheic keratosis on the abdomen

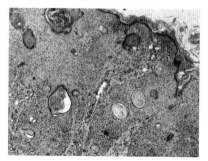

Color Figure 26 – 17　Hyperkeratotic surface, hypertrophic stratum spinosum and numerous horn pseudocysts

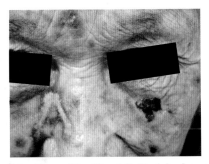

Color Figure 26－18 A light-pink plaque with crust on the left cheek
（Presented by Mei Cao）

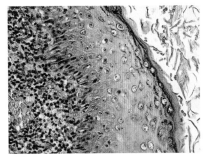

Color Figure 26－19 Marked atypism is observed，especially in the lower epidermal layer

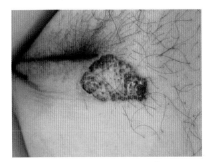

Color Figure 26－20 Bowen's disease on the vulva skin

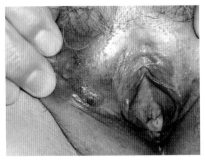

Color Figure 26－21 Extramammary Paget's disease of vulva skin

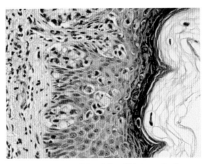

Color Figure 26－22 Histopathology of Paget's disease

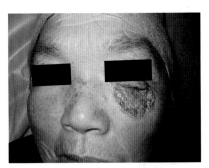

Color Figure 26－23 Noduloulcerative basal cell carcinoma（BCC）of left face

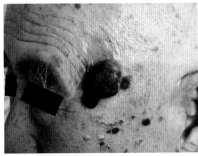

Color Figure 26－24 Noduloulcerative basal cell carcinoma （BCC）of left tempus

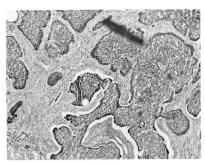

Color Figure 26－25 Histopathology of basal cell carcinoma（BCC）

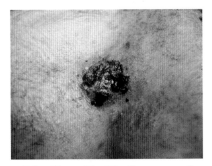

Color Figure 26－26 Squamous cell carcinoma（SCC）of right face

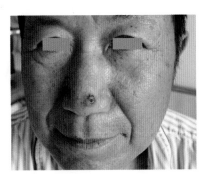

Color Figure 26－27 Squamous cell carcinoma（SCC）on the nose

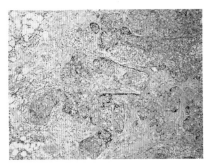

Color Figure 26－28 Histopathology of squamous cell carcinoma （SCC）

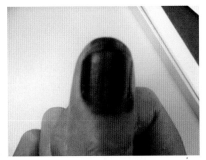

Color Figure 26－29 Subungual acral lentiginous melanoma （ALM）of right thumb

18

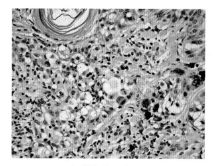
A. H－E staining

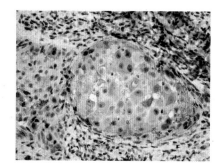
B. S－100 staining

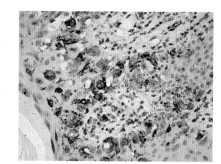
C. HMB－45 staining

Color Figure 26－30　The expression of melanoma by H－E(A),S－100(B) and HMB－45 (C) immunohistochemical staining

Atypical melanocytes proliferate in the epidermis and dermis. Classical melanoma tumor cells contain large quantities of melanin pigment

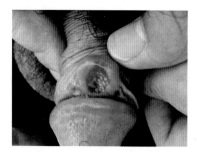
Color Figure 27－1　Chancre

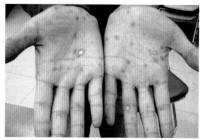
Color Figure 27－2　Secondary syphilis on the palms

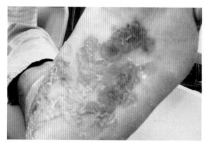
Color Figure 27－3　Secondary syphilis on the left sole

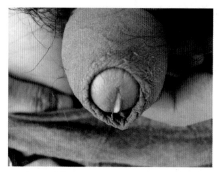
Color Figure 27－4　Male gonorrhea

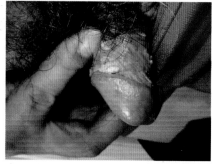
Color Figure 27－5　Condyloma acuminatum

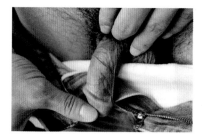
Color Fig 27－6　Genital herpes

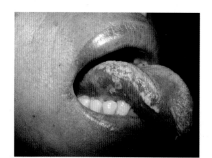
Color Figure 27－7　Mucocutaneous candidiasis

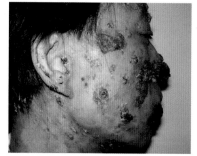
Color Figure 27－8　Fungal infections

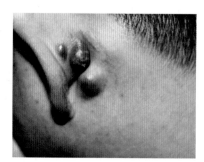
Color Figure 27－9　Kaposi sarcoma